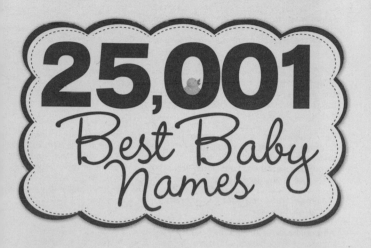

25,001 Best Baby Names

Lesley Bolton

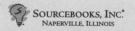

SOURCEBOOKS, INC.
NAPERVILLE, ILLINOIS

Published by Sourcebooks, Inc.
P.O. Box 4410, Naperville, Illinois 60567-4410
(630) 961-3900
Fax: (630) 961-2168
www.sourcebooks.com

Library of Congress Cataloging-in-Publication Data

Bolton, Lesley.
    25,001 best baby names / Lesley Bolton.
        p. cm.
    1. Names, Personal—Dictionaries. 2. Names, Personal—United States—Dictionaries I. Title.

CS2377.B65 2006
929.4′4—dc22

2006011688

Printed and bound in the United States of America.
QW 10 9 8 7 6 5 4 3 2 1

Contents

Introduction...v

13 Easy Essentials to Help You Choose the Perfect Name.......vi

Part 1: 57 Fun Lists 1

  1. Classic Names
  2. Influential Names
  3. Biblical Names
  4. Hip Names that Sound Classic
  5. Presidential Names
  6. Patriotic Names
  7. Gender-Neutral Names
  8. Super Surnames
  9. Big-City Names
  10. Under the Radar Names
  11. Familiar yet Unique Names
  12. Names that Make an Impression
  13. Names that Mean *Wise*
  14. Names that Mean *Strong*
  15. Names that Mean *Gift*
  16. Names that Command Respect
  17. British Names
  18. Irish Names
  19. Hispanic Names
  20. African American Names
  21. Saint Names
  22. Celebrity Baby Names
  23. Most Popular Names of the 1950s
  24. Most Popular Names of the 1960s
  25. Most Popular Names of the 1970s
  26. Most Popular Names of the 1980s
  27. Most Popular Names of the 1990s
  28. Most Popular Names of the 2000s
  29. Most Popular Names of 2008
  30. Most Popular Twin Names of 2008
  31. Hot Names on the Rise

Part 2: Boys 15

Part 3: Girls 177

Introduction

Let's face it: you have enough to worry about in anticipation of your new arrival. So why make the baby-naming process any more stressful than it has to be? Sure, you know how important it is to give your child a name he or she will be proud of for the rest of his or her life. In fact, a name is one of the greatest gifts you'll ever give your child. But choosing it can be an enjoyable experience.

If you are looking for a quick, convenient, fun, and—most important—painless approach to baby-naming, *25,001 Best Baby Names* will be invaluable. This book has been designed to give you the best of the best, from the most popular new names to the treasured classics. Plus, there are plenty of names from countries around the world.

Whether you are looking for a specific meaning, origin, or a variation of a popular name, this guide makes it easier than ever to make an informed decision. *25,001 Best Baby Names* has the most up-to-date information on trends and variety, all in one handy, parent-friendly book. So if you're an expectant parent who wants an easy guide to the best baby names out there, welcome. Happy baby naming!

13 Easy Essentials to Help You Choose the Perfect Name

1. **Say the Names out Loud:** Think about how the name sounds in a variety of situations; listen for rhythm and harmony; try out the first name with the middle name and last name.

2. **Make it Meaningful:** Think carefully about the feelings, thoughts, and associations the name evokes. What do you want people to think of when they hear the name? What does it mean to you?

3. **Avoid Negative Connotations:** Watch out for general stereotypes as well as names from your past.

4. **Test Nicknames:** Will the name hold up on the playground?

5. **Be Creative:** Playing thoughtfully with spellings, variations, and nicknames can yield fresh results, but...

6. **Keep in Mind Spelling and Pronunciation:** Will the name often be mispronounced or misspelled?

7. **Consider Gender Sensitivity:** Think carefully about using feminine names for boys and masculine ones for girls

8. **Origin/Ancestry:** Honor your heritage by combing the family tree for names, both first and last; connect your child with the richness of his or her past.

9. **The Most Popular Problem:** The most-used names are popular for a reason—they're likable and pleasing. Just be aware that there might be five other little Avas in kindergarten.

10. **Ask for Suggestions:** You don't have to use them! People who have recently had children can be very helpful.

11. **Scour the Media:** Think about names from books, TV shows, movies, and celebrities.

12. **Consider the Classics:** They've stood the test of time for a reason.

13. **Play it Safe:** Pick at least one name for each gender—ultrasounds can be wrong!

Part 1

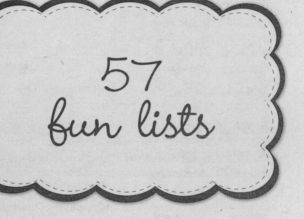

57
fun lists

Boys	Girls
Classic Names	
John	Emily
Charles	Ann
George	Elizabeth
Alexander	Mary
Michael	Sarah
Richard	Jane
William	Katherine
Thomas	Margaret
David	Helen
Edward	Christine

Boys	Girls
Biblical Names	
Aaron	Eve
Darius	Sarah
Ezekiel	Deborah
Caleb	Anne
John	Mary
Elijah	Rachel
Zion	Naomi
Samuel	Rebecca
Levi	Dinah
Isaiah	Delilah

Influential Names

Boys	Girls
Winston	Amelia
Albert	Madonna
Franklin	Betty
William	Margaret
Bill	Isabella
Warren	Josephine
Elvis	Helen
Jonas	Angela
Nelson	Ruth
Wyatt	Diana

Hip Names that Sound Classic

Albert	Hannah
Benjamin	Leonie
Christian	Lauren
Nathan	Lillian
Noah	Matilda
Oscar	Natalie
Oliver	Sadie
Samuel	Sarah
Saul	Sophia
Josiah	Violet

Presidential Names

Lincoln	Washington
Jefferson	Madison
Reagan	Jackson
Clinton	Hayes
Harrison	Pierce
McKinley	Roosevelt
Grant	Cleveland
Monroe	Wilson
Truman	Ford
Kennedy	Carter

Gender-Neutral Names

Avery	London
Cameron	Parker
Charlie	Lyric
Dylan	Payton
Finley	Quinn
Harley	Riley
Jayden	Rease
Jordan	Rowan
Kendall	Skyler
Logan	Teagan

Patriotic Names

Lincoln	Liberty
Free	Washington
Norman	Justice
Columbus	Spirit
Knox	Starr
Crane	America
William	Peace
Almo	Independence
Bragg	Eagle
Librada	Leavenworth

Super Surnames

Sawyer	Tanner
Hunter	Keaton
Archer	Cortland
Dexter	Everett
Hadley	McKenzie
Bailey	Wade
Fletcher	Taylor
Grant	Tanner
Lynden	Blane
Otis	Dalton

Boys	Girls
Big-City Names	
Paris	Orly
Troy	Ankara
Dallas	Sydney
Kobe	Lourdes
Berlin	Adelaide
Boston	Charlotte
Kingston	Florence
Dublin	Cairo
London	Andorra
Athens	Geneva

Boys	Girls
Familiar yet Unique Names	
Brody	Zoey
Devin	Amy
Jesse	Sadie
Kaleb	Lola
Marcus	Eva
Patrick	Katryn
Seth	Bellamy
Colton	Mya
Riley	Rebecca
Bryce	Ruby

Under the Radar Names

Gage	Bianca
Malachi	Piper
Asher	Bethany
Cash	Iris
Declan	Sylvie
Judah	Bel
Simeon	Penelope
Rhys	Tessa
Sullivan	Lydia
Trace	Tuesday

Names that Make an Impression

Jagger	Lulu
Jovan	Roxana
Ace	Fiona
Ryder	Vivica
Rodeo	Harley
Happy	Pixie
Jazz	Bliss
Tru	Charlie
Preston	Blakesley
Chaz	Veronica

Boys	Girls
Names that Mean *Wise*	
Akili	Athena
Bathasar	Avery
Conaire	Dara
Conroy	Keyla
Drew	Landra
Eldrick	Medora
Hakim	Monique
Raymond	Rayna
Sarat	Sage
Shanahan	Sennet

Boys	Girls
Names that Mean *Gift*	
Cathan	Amaariah
Jesse	Chip
Mathias	Adia
Nathaniel	Dori
Niaz	Daryn
Seanan	Emsley
Shai	Grace
Ted	Makalo
Tesher	Theodora
Zani	Matea

Names that Mean *Strong*

Arthur	Andrea
Cale	Bridget
Everett	Charla
Magglio	Jerica
Nardo	Karla
Pierce	Mirit
Quinlan	Petronelle
Steele	Sela
Terrian	Sloane
Valerian	Trudy

Names that Command Respect

William	Elizabeth
Edward	Alexandra
Graham	Jacqueline
Henry	Magdalena
Richard	Katherine
Jefferson	Isabella
Augustus	Mary
John	Anne
Caesar	Cleopatra
Phillip	Clara

Boys	Girls
British Names	
Ian	Sienna
Nigel	Nicola
Clive	Poppy
Winston	Maisie
Percy	Pippa
Trevor	Tamsin
Alastair	Gemma
Hewitt	Portia
Leland	Saffron
Cedric	Bridget

Boys	Girls
Hispanic Names	
José	Graciela
Miguel	Gabriella
Juan	María
Pablo	Juliana
Alfonso	Liliana
Joel	Estrella
Jesús	Alejandra
Luis	Camila
Carlos	Marisol
Diego	Eliana

Irish Names	
Aidan	Briana
Colin	Ciara
Connor	Fiona
Kyan	Moira
Neal	Naimh
Quinn	Maura
Declan	Saoirse
Killian	Siobhan
Eamon	Aoife
Devin	Roina

African American Names	
Antwon	Cherise
Denzel	Imani
Gervaise	Jada
Imari	Jayla
Jamar	Kalinda
Juwan	Keisha
Malik	Leteisha
Nile	Nakari
Rashaun	Raisha
Tariq	Zeleka

Boys	Girls
Saint Names	
George	Catherine
Francis	Anne
Patrick	Mary
David	Theresa
Stephen	Bridget
Peter	Cecilia
Thomas	Elizabeth
Paul	Agnes
John	Joan
Anthony	Agatha

Boys	Girls
Celebrity Baby Names	
Max	Kai
Jagger	Seraphina
Liam	Emme
Romeo	Shiloh
Maddox	Vivienne
Knox	Matilda
Moses	Harlow
Bronx	Grier
Stellan	Finley
Rafferty	Carys

Boys	Girls
Most Popular Names of the 1950s	
James	Mary
Michael	Linda
Robert	Patricia
John	Susan
David	Deborah
William	Barbara
Richard	Debra
Thomas	Karen
Mark	Nancy
Charles	Donna

Boys	Girls
Most Popular Names of the 1960s	
Michael	Lisa
David	Mary
John	Susan
James	Karen
Robert	Kimberly
Mark	Patricia
William	Linda
Richard	Donna
Thomas	Michelle
Jeffrey	Cynthia

Most Popular Names of the 1970s

Boys	Girls
Michael	Jennifer
Christopher	Amy
➤ Jason	Melissa
David	Michelle
James	Kimberly
John	Lisa
Robert	Angela
Brian	Heather
William	Stephanie
Matthew	Nicole

Most Popular Names of the 1990s

Boys	Girls
Michael	Jessica
Christopher	Ashley
Matthew	Emily
Joshua	Samantha
Jacob	Sarah
Nicholas	Amanda
Andrew	Brittany
Daniel	Elizabeth
Tyler	Taylor
Joseph	Megan

Most Popular Names of the 1980s

Boys	Girls
Michael	Jessica
Christopher	Jennifer
Matthew	Amanda
Joshua	Ashley
David	Sarah
James	Stephanie
Daniel	Melissa
Robert	Nicole
John	Elizabeth
Joseph	Heather

Most Popular Names of the 2000s

Boys	Girls
Jacob	Emily
Michael	Madison
Joshua	Emma
Matthew	Hannah
Christopher	Olivia
Andrew	Abigail
Daniel	Isabella
Ethan	Ashley
Joseph	Samantha
William	Elizabeth

★ Most Popular Names of 2008
★ — All names with a ★ in the text denote
Top 100 Names of 2008.

Most Popular Boys' Names

1. Jacob
2. Michael
3. Ethan
4. Joshua
5. Daniel
6. Alexander
7. Anthony
8. William
9. Christopher
10. Matthew
11. Jayden
12. Andrew
13. Joseph
14. David
15. Noah
16. Aiden
17. James
18. Ryan
19. Logan
20. John
21. Nathan
22. Elijah
23. Christian
24. Gabriel
25. Benjamin
26. Jonathan
27. Tyler
28. Samuel
29. Nicholas
30. Gaven
31. Dylan
32. Jackson
33. Brandon
34. Caleb
35. Mason
36. Angel
37. Isaac
38. Evan
39. Jack
40. Kevin
41. José
42. Isaiah
43. Luke
44. Landon
45. Justin
46. Lucas
47. Zachary
48. Jordan
49. Robert
50. Aaron
51. Brayden
52. Thomas
53. Cameron
54. Hunter
55. Austin
56. Adrian
57. Connor
58. Owen
59. Aidan
60. Jason
61. Julian
62. Wyatt
63. Charles
64. Luis
65. Carter
66. Juan

67. Chase	79. Jesús	91. Ayden
68. Diego	80. Ian	92. Cooper
69. Jeremiah	81. Tristan	93. Dominic
70. Brody	82. Bryan	94. Brady
71. Xavier	83. Sean	95. Caden
72. Adam	84. Cole	96. Josiah
73. Carlos	85. Alex	97. Kyle
74. Sebastian	86. Eric	98. Colton
75. Liam	87. Brian	99. Kaden
76. Hayden	88. Jaden	100. Eli
77. Nathaniel	89. Carson	
78. Henry	90. Blake	

★ Most Popular Names of 2008

Most Popular Girls' Names

1. Emma	11. Samantha	21. Grace
2. Isabella	12. Addison	22. Taylor
3. Emily	13. Natalie	23. Brianna
4. Madison	14. Mia	24. Lily
5. Ava	15. Alexis	25. Hailey
6. Olivia	16. Alyssa	26. Anna
7. Sophia	17. Hannah	27. Victoria
8. Abigail	18. Ashley	28. Kayla
9. Elizabeth	19. Ella	29. Lillian
10. Chloe	20. Sarah	30. Lauren

31. Kaylee
32. Allison
33. Savannah
34. Nevaeh
35. Gabriella
36. Sofia
37. Makayla
38. Avery
39. Riley
40. Julia
41. Leah
42. Aubrey
43. Jasmine
44. Audrey
45. Katherine
46. Morgan
47. Brooklyn
48. Destiny
49. Sydney
50. Alexa
51. Kylie
52. Brooke
53. Kaitlyn
54. Evelyn
55. Layla

56. Madeline
57. Kimberly
58. Zoe
59. Jessica
60. Peyton
61. Alexandra
62. Claire
63. Madelyn
64. Maria
65. Mackenzie
66. Arianna
67. Jocelyn
68. Amelia
69. Angelina
70. Trinity
71. Andrea
72. Maya
73. Valeria
74. Sophie
75. Rachel
76. Vanessa
77. Aaliyah
78. Mariah
79. Gabrielle
80. Katelyn

81. Ariana
82. Bailey
83. Camila
84. Jennifer
85. Melanie
86. Gianna
87. Charlotte
88. Paige
89. Autumn
90. Payton
91. Faith
92. Sara
93. Isabelle
94. Caroline
95. Genesis
96. Isabel
97. Mary
98. Zoey
99. Gracie
100. Megan

T Most Popular Twin Names of 2008

T — All names with a **T** in the text denote
Top Twin Names of 2008.

1. Jacob, Joshua
2. Daniel, David
3. Jayden, Jordan
4. Ethan, Evan
5. Taylor, Tyler
6. Gabriella, Isabella
7. Isaac, Isaiah
8. Madison, Morgan
9. Elijah, Isaiah
10. Ella, Emma
11. Landon, Logan
12. Logan, Lucas
13. Matthew, Michael
14. Faith, Hope
15. Isabella, Sophia
16. Olivia, Sophia
17. James, John
18. Madison, Mason
19. Brandon, Bryan
20. Hailey, Hannah
21. Mackenzie, Madison
22. Nathan, Nicholas
23. Addison, Aiden
24. Caleb, Joshua
25. Christian, Christopher
26. Emma, Ethan
27. Jayden, Jaylen
28. Ava, Emma
29. Ava, Olivia
30. Joseph, Joshua
31. Andrew, Matthew
32. Makayla, Makenzie
33. Benjamin, Samuel
34. Brandon, Brian
35. Abigail, Emma
36. Jacob, Matthew
37. Jordan, Justin
38. Nathan, Noah
39. Alexander, Andrew
40. Emily, Ethan
41. Ethan, Nathan
42. Gabriel, Michael
43. Hayden, Hunter
44. Jacob, Joseph

45. Addison, Avery

46. Faith, Grace

47. Jayda, Jayden

48. Joshua, Justin

49. Joshua, Matthew

50. Alexander, Nicholas

51. Emma, Sophie

52. Jada, Jaden

53. Logan, Luke

54. Aaron, Andrew

55. Andrew, Anthony

56. Anna, Emma

57. Autumn, Summer

58. Isabella, Olivia

59. Jacob, Jordan

60. Jacob, Lucas

61. Kyle, Ryan

62. Nicholas, Noah

63. Valeria, Vanessa

64. Abigail, Benjamin

65. Aiden, Ava

66. Alexander, Benjamin

67. Alexander, Christopher

68. Ashley, Emily

69. Benjamin, William

70. Christopher, Matthew

71. Daniel, Michael

72. Dylan, Tyler

73. Emma, Sophia

74. Hannah, Sarah

75. Heaven, Neveah

76. Jake, Luke

77. Jennifer, Jessica

78. Mackenzie, Makayla

79. Matthew, William

80. Natalie, Nathan

81. Ryan, Tyler

82. Samuel, Sophia

83. Samuel, William

84. Addison, Emma

85. Adrian, Adriana

86. Aiden, Austin

87. Alexander, Alexis

88. Ava, Mia

89. Benjamin, Jacob

90. Benjamin, Matthew

91. Caleb, Christian

92. Caleb, Jacob

93. Elijah, Ethan

94. Jada, Jayden

95. James, William

96. John, William

97. Lily, Logan

98. Mark, Matthew

99. Matthew, Nicholas

100. Maxwell, Samuel

^Hot Names on the Rise

^ — All names with a ^ in the text denote hot names
rising in popularity in 2008.

Boys		
Jacoby	Kellen	Paisley
Kane	Maximus	Miley
Beckett	Cruz	Lyla
Paxton	Graham	Harper
Kale	Colten	Dayana
August	Grady	Valentina
Braylon	Jonas	London
Ryker	Titus	Jimena
Kingston	Karson	Mylee
Kolton	Easton	Lyric
Zayden	Johan	Kayden
Brycen		Emery
River	**Girls**	Lia
Milo	Amari	Rihanna
Landyn	Amira	Delilah
Alijah	Khloe	Madilyn
Cash	Marlee	Teagan
Alvin	Marely	Madelynn
Jude	Audrina	Lila
Byron	Marley	Madalyn
Kobe	Danna	Janiyah
Reid	Jaslene	Cara
	Lilah	Brielle

Part 2

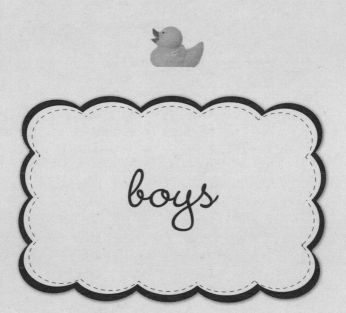

boys

a

Aabha (Indian) One who shines
Abha, Abbha

Aabharan (Hindu) One who is treasured; jewel
Abharan, Abharen, Aabharen, Aabharon

Aaden (Irish) Form of Aidan, meaning "a fiery young man"
Adan, Aden

Aage (Norse) Representative of ancestors
Age, Ake, Aake

Aarif (Arabic) A learned man
Arif, Aareef, Areef, Aareaf, Areaf, Aareif, Areif, Aarief

Aaron (Hebrew) One who is exalted; from the mountain of strength
Aaran, Aaren, Aarin, Aaro, Aaronas, Aaronn, Aarron, Aaryn, Eron, Aron, Eran

Abdi (Hebrew) My servant
Abdie, Abdy, Abdey, Abdee

Abdul (Arabic) A servant of God
Abdal, Abdall, Abdalla, Abdallah, Abdel, Abdell, Abdella, Abdellah

Abedi (African) One who worships God
Abedie, Abedy, Abedey, Abedee, Abedea

Abednago (Aramaic) Servant of the god of wisdom, Nabu
Abednego

Abejundio (Spanish) Resembling a bee
Abejundo, Abejundeo, Abedjundiyo, Abedjundeyo

Abel (Hebrew) The life force, breath
Abele, Abell, Abelson, Able, Avel, Avele

Abraham (Hebrew) Father of a multitude; father of nations
Abarran, Avraham, Aberham, Abrahamo, Abrahan, Abrahim, Abram, Abrami, Ibrahim

Absalom (Hebrew) The father of peace
Absalon, Abshalom, Absolem, Absolom, Absolon, Avshalom, Avsholom

Abu (African) A father
Abue, Aboo, Abou

Abundio (Spanish) A man of plenty
Abbondio, Abondio, Aboundio, Abundo, Abundeo, Aboundeo

Adael (Hebrew) God witnesses
Adaele, Adayel, Adayele

•Adam (Hebrew) Of the earth
Ad, Adamo, Adams, Adan, Adao, Addam, Addams, Addem

Adamson (English) The son of Adam
Adamsson, Addamson, Adamsun, Adamssun

Addy (Teutonic) One who is awe-inspiring
Addey, Addi, Addie, Addee, Addea, Adi, Ady, Adie

Adelpho (Greek) A brotherly man
Aldelfo, Adelfus, Adelfio, Adelphe

Adil (Arabic) A righteous man; one who is fair and just
Adyl, Adiel, Adeil, Adeel, Adeal, Adyeel

Aditya (Hindi) Of the sun
Adithya, Adithyan, Adityah, Aditeya, Aditeyah

Adonis (Greek) In mythology, a handsome young man loved by Aphrodite
Addonia, Adohnes, Adonys

•ᴛAdrian (Latin) A man from Hadria
Adrien, Adrain, Adrean, Adreean, Adreyan, Adreeyan, Adriaan

Adriel (Hebrew) From God's flock
Adriell, Adriele, Adryel, Adryell, Adryele

Afif (Arabic) One who is chaste; pure
Afeef, Afief, Afeif, Affeef, Affif, Afyf, Afeaf

Agamemnon (Greek) One who works slowly; in mythology, the leader of the Greeks at Troy
Agamemno, Agamenon

Ahmed (Arabic) One who always thanks God; a name of Muhammed
Ahmad

•ᴛAidan (Irish) A fiery young man
Aiden, Aedan, Aeden, Aidano, Aidyn, Ayden, Aydin, Aydan

Aiken (English) Constructed of oak; sturdy
Aikin, Aicken, Aickin, Ayken, Aykin, Aycken, Ayckin

Ainsworth (English) From Ann's estate
Answorth, Annsworth, Ainsworthe, Answorthe, Annsworthe

Ajax (Greek) In mythology, a hero of the Trojan war
Aias, Aiastes, Ajaxx, Ajaxe

Ajit (Indian) One who is invincible
Ajeet, Ajeat, Ajeit, Ajiet, Ajyt

Akiko (Japanese) Surrounded by bright light
Akyko

Akin (African) A brave man; a hero
Akeen, Akean, Akein, Akien, Akyn

Akiva (Hebrew) One who protects or provides shelter
Akyva, Akeeva, Akeava, Akieva, Akeiva, Akeyva

Akmal (Arabic) A perfect man
Aqmal, Akmall, Aqmall, Acmal, Acmall, Ackmal, Ackmall

Alaire (French) Filled with joy
Alair, Alaer, Alaere, Alare, Alayr, Alayre

Alamar (Arabic) Covered with gold
Alamarr, Alemar, Alemarr, Alomar, Alomarr

Alard (German) Of noble strength
Aliard, Allard, Alliard

Albert (German) One who is noble and bright
Alberto, Albertus, Alburt, Albirt, Aubert, Albyrt, Albertos, Albertino

Alan (German / Gaelic) One who is precious / resembling a little rock
Alain, Alann, Allan, Alson, Allin, Allen, Allyn

Alden (English) An old friend
Aldan, Aldin, Aldyn, Aldon, Aldun

Aldo (German) Old or wise one; elder
Aldous, Aldis, Aldus, Alldo, Aldys

Aldred (English) An old advisor
Alldred, Aldraed, Alldraed, Aldread, Alldread

Alejandro (Spanish) Form of Alexander, meaning "a helper and defender of mankind"
Alejandrino, Alejo

Alex (English) Form of Alexander, meaning "a helper and defender of mankind"
Aleks, Alecks, Alecs, Allex, Alleks, Allecks, Alexis

∗τAlexander (Greek) A helper and defender of mankind
Alex, Alec, Alejandro, Alaxander, Aleksandar, Aleksander, Aleksandr, Alessandro, Alexzander, Zander

Alfonso (Italian) Prepared for battle; eager and ready
Alphonso, Alphonse, Affonso, Alfons, Alfonse, Alfonsin, Alfonsino, Alfonz, Alfonzo

Ali (Arabic) The great one; one who is exalted
Alie, Aly, Aley, Alee

∧Alijah (American) Form of Elijah, meaning Jehovah is my god

Alon (Hebrew) Of the oak tree
Allona, Allon, Alonn

Alonzo (Spanish) Form of Alfonso, meaning "prepared for battle; eager and ready"
Alonso, Alanso, Alanzo, Allonso, Allonzo, Allohnso, Allohnzo, Alohnso

Aloysius (German) A famous warrior
Ahlois, Aloess, Alois, Aloisio, Aloisius, Aloisio, Aloj, Alojzy

Alpha (Greek) The first-born child; the first letter of the Greek alphabet
Alphah, Alfa, Alfah

Alter (Hebrew) One who is old
Allter, Altar, Alltar

Alton (English) From the old town
Aldon, Aldun, Altun, Alten, Allton, Alltun, Allten

∧Alvin (English) Friend of the elves
Alven, Alvan, Alvyn

Amani (African / Arabic) One who is peaceful / one with wishes and dreams
Amanie, Amany, Amaney, Amanee, Amanye, Amanea, Amaneah

Amari (African) Having great strength; a builder
Amarie, Amaree, Amarea, Amary, Amarey

Amil (Hindi) One who is invaluable
Ameel, Ameal, Ameil, Amiel, Amyl

Amit (Hindi) Without limit; endless
Ameet, Ameat, Ameit, Amiet, Amyt

Amory (German) Ruler and lover of one's home
Aimory, Amery, Amorey, Amry, Amori, Amorie, Amoree, Amorea

Amos (Hebrew) To carry; hardworking
Amoss, Aymoss, Aymos

Andre (French) Form of Andrew, meaning "manly, a warrior" *Andreas, Andrei, Andrej, Andres, Andrey*

Andino (Italian) Form of Andrew, meaning "one who is manly; a warrior" *Andyno, Andeeno, Andeano, Andieno, Andeino*

*ᵀ**Andrew** (Greek) One who is manly; a warrior *Andy, Aindrea, Andreas, Andie, Andonia, Andor, Andresj, Anderson*

Andrik (Slavic) Form of Andrew, meaning "one who is manly; a warrior" *Andric, Andrick, Andryk, Andryck, Andryc*

***Angel** (Greek) A messenger of God *Andjelko, Ange, Angelino, Angell, Angelmo, Angelo, Angie, Angy*

Angus (Scottish) One force; one strength; one choice *Aengus, Anngus, Aonghus*

Anicho (German) An ancestor *Anico, Anecho, Aneco, Anycho, Anyco*

Ankur (Indian) One who is blossoming; a sapling

Annan (Celtic) From the brook *Anan*

Ansley (English) From the noble's pastureland *Ansly, Anslie, Ansli, Anslee, Ansleigh, Anslea, Ansleah, Anslye*

Antenor (Spanish) One who antagonizes *Antener, Antenar, Antenir, Antenyr, Antenur*

Antonio (Italian) Form of Anthony, meaning "a flourishing man, from an ancient Roman family" *Antonin, Antonino, Antonius, Antonyo*

*ᵀ**Anthony** (Latin) A flourishing man; of an ancient Roman family *Antal, Antony, Anthoney, Anntoin, Antin, Anton, Antone, Antonello, **Antonio***

Antoine (French) Form of Anthony, meaning "a flourishing man; of an ancient Roman family" *Antione, Antjuan, Antuan, Antuwain, Antuwaine, Antuwayne, Antuwon, Antwahn*

Ara (Armenian / Latin) A legendary king / of the altar; the name of a constellation *Araa, Aira, Arah, Arae, Ahraya*

Aram (Assyrian) One who is exalted *Arram*

Arcadio (Greek) From an ideal country paradise
Alcadio, Alcado, Alcedio, Arcadios, Arcadius, Arkadi, Arkadios, Arkadius

Arcelio (Spanish) From the altar of heaven
Arcelios, Arcelius, Aricelio, Aricelios, Aricelius

Archard (German) A powerful holy man
Archerd, Archird, Archyrd

Archelaus (Greek) The ruler of the people
Archelaios, Arkelaos, Arkelaus, Arkelaios, Archelaos

Ardal (Gaelic) Having the valor of a bear
Ardghal

Ardell (Latin) One who is eager
Ardel, Ardelle, Ardele

Arden (Latin / English) One who is passionate and enthusiastic / from the valley of the eagles
Ardan, Arrden, Arrdan, Ardin, Arrdin, Ard, Ardyn, Arrdyn

Arduino (German) A valued friend
Ardwino, Arrduino, Ardueno

Ari (Hebrew) Resembling a lion or an eagle
Aree, Arie, Aristide, Aristides, Arri, Ary, Arye, Arrie

Ariel (Hebrew) A lion of God
Arielle, Ariele, Ariell, Arriel, Ahriel, Airial, Arieal, Arial

Aries (Latin) Resembling a ram; the first sign of the zodiac; a constellation
Arese, Ariese

Arion (Greek) A poet or musician
Arian, Arien, Aryon

Aristotle (Greek) Of high quality
Aristotelis, Aristotellis

Arius (Greek) Enduring life; everlasting; immortal
Areos, Areus, Arios

Arley (English) From the hare's meadow
Arlea, Arleigh, Arlie, Arly, Arleah, Arli, Arlee

Arliss (Hebrew) Of the pledge
Arlyss, Aryls, Arlis, Arlisse, Arlysse

Arnold (German) The eagle ruler
Arnaldo, Arnaud, Arnauld, Arnault, Arnd, Arndt, Arnel, Arnell

Arthur (Celtic) As strong
as a bear; a hero
*Aart, Arrt, Art, Artair, Arte,
Arther, Arthor, Arthuro*

Arvad (Hebrew) A wan-
derer; voyager
Arpad

Arvin (English) A friend to
everyone
*Arvinn, Arvinne, Arven,
Arvenn, Arvenne, Arvyn,
Arvynn, Arvynne*

Asa (Hebrew) One who
heals others
Asah

Asaph (Hebrew) One who
gathers or collects
*Asaf, Asaphe, Asafe, Asiph,
Asiphe, Asif, Asife*

Ash (English) From the
ash tree
Ashe

Asher (Hebrew) Filled with
happiness Ashar, *Ashor,
Ashir, Ashyr, Ashur*

Ashley (English) From the
meadow of ash trees
*Ashely, Asheley, Ashelie,
Ashlan, Ashleigh, Ashlen,
Ashli, Ashlie*

Ashton (English) From the
ash-tree town
*Asheton, Ashtun, Ashetun,
Ashtin, Ashetin, Ashtyn,
Ashetyn, Aston*

Aslan (Turkish)
Resembling a lion
Aslen, Azlan, Azlen

Athens (Greek) From the
capital of Greece
*Athenios, Athenius,
Atheneos, Atheneus*

Atticus (Latin) A man
from Athens
*Attikus, Attickus, Aticus,
Atickus, Atikus*

Atwell (English) One who
lives at the spring
Attwell, Atwel, Attwel

Aubrey (English) One who
rules with elf-wisdom
*Aubary, Aube, Aubery,
Aubry, Aubury, Aubrian,
Aubrien, Aubrion*

Auburn (Latin) Having a
reddish-brown color
*Aubirn, Auburne, Aubyrn,
Abern, Abirn, Aburn,
Abyrn, Aubern*

Audley (English) From the
old meadow
*Audly, Audleigh, Audlee,
Audlea, Audleah, Audli,
Audlie*

^**August** (Irish) One who is
venerable; majestic
*Austin, Augustine,
Agoston, Aguistin, Agustin,
Augustin, Augustyn,
Avgustin, Augusteen,
Agosteen*

*†**Austin** (English) Form of August, meaning "one who is venerable; majestic"
Austen, Austyn, Austan, Auston, Austun

†**Avery** (English) One who is a wise ruler; of the nobility
Avrie, Averey, Averie, Averi, Averee

Aviram (Hebrew) My Father is mighty
Avyram, Avirem, Avyrem

Axel (German / Latin / Hebrew) Source of life; small oak / axe / peace
Aksel, Ax, Axe, Axell, Axil, Axill, Axl

Aya (Hebrew) Resembling a bird
Ayah

•**Ayden** (Irish) form of Aiden, meaning "a fiery young man"

Ayo (African) Filled with happiness
Ayoe, Ayow, Ayowe

Azamat (Arabic) A proud man; one who is majestic

Azi (African) One who is youthful
Azie, Azy, Azey, Azee, Azea

Azmer (Islamic) Resembling a lion
Azmar, Azmir, Azmyr, Azmor, Azmur

b

Baakir (African) The eldest child
Baakeer, Baakyr, Baakear, Baakier, Baakeir

Bachir (Hebrew) The oldest son
Bacheer, Bachear, Bachier, Bacheir, Bachyr

Baha (Arabic) A glorious and splendid man
Bahah

Bailintin (Irish) A valiant man
Bailinten, Bailentin, Bailenten, Bailintyn, Bailentyn

Bain (Irish) A fair-haired man
Baine, Bayn, Bayne, Baen, Baene, Bane, Baines, Baynes

Bajnok (Hungarian) A victorious man
Bajnock, Bajnoc

Bakari (Swahili) One who is promised
Bakarie, Bakary, Bakarey, Bakaree, Bakarea

Bakhit (Arabic) A lucky man
Bakheet, Bakheat, Bakheit, Bakhiet, Bakhyt, Bukht

Bala (Hindi) One who is youthful
Balu, Balue, Balou

Balark (Hindi) Born with the rising sun

Balasi (Basque) One who is flat-footed
Balasie, Balasy, Balasey, Balasee, Balasea

Balbo (Latin) One who mutters
Balboe, Balbow, Balbowe, Ballbo, Balbino, Balbi, Balbie, Balby

Baldwin (German) A brave friend
Baldwine, Baldwinn, Baldwinne, Baldwen, Baldwenn, Baldwenne, Baldwyn, Baldwynn

Balint (Latin) A healthy and strong man
Balent, Balin, Balen, Balynt, Balyn

Balloch (Scottish) From the grazing land

Bancroft (English) From the bean field
Bancrofte, Banfield, Banfeld, Bankroft, Bankrofte

Bandana (Spanish) A brightly colored headwrap
Bandanah, Bandanna, Bandannah

Bandy (American) A fiesty man
Bandey, Bandi, Bandie, Bandee, Bandea

Bansi (Indian) One who plays the flute
Bansie, Bansy, Bansey, Bansee, Bansea

Bao (Vietnamese / Chinese) To order / one who is prized

Baqir (Arabic) A learned man
Baqeer, Baqear, Baqier, Baqeir, Baqyr, Baqer

Barak (Hebrew) Of the lightning flash
Barrak, Barac, Barrac, Barack, Barrack

Baram (Hebrew) The son of the nation
Barem, Barum, Barom, Barim, Barym

Bard (English) A minstrel; a poet
Barde, Bardo

Barden (English) From the barley valley; from the boar's valley
Bardon, Bardun, Bardin, Bardyn, Bardan, Bardene

Bardol (Basque) A farmer
Bardo, Bartol

Bardrick (Teutonic) An axe ruler
Bardric, Bardrik, Bardryck, Bardryk, Bardryc, Bardarick, Bardaric, Bardarik

Barek (Arabic) One who is noble
Barec, Bareck

Barend (German) The hard bear
Barende, Barind, Barinde, Barynd, Barynde

Barnett (English) Of honorable birth
Barnet, Baronet, Baronett

Baron (English) A title of nobility
Barron

Barr (English) A lawyer
Barre, Bar

Barra (Gaelic) A fair-haired man

Barrett (German / English) Having the strength of a bear / one who argues
Baret, Barrat, Barratt, Barret, Barrette

Barry (Gaelic) A fair-haired man
Barrey, Barri, Barrie, Barree, Barrea, Barrington, Barryngton, Barringtun

Bartholomew (Aramaic) The son of the farmer
Bart, Bartel, Barth, Barthelemy, Bartho, Barthold, Bartholoma, Bartholomaus, Bartlett, Bartol

Bartlett (French) Form of Bartholomew, meaning "the son of the farmer"
Bartlet, Bartlitt, Bartlit, Bartlytt, Bartlyt

Bartley (English) From the meadow of birch trees
Bartly, Bartli, Bartlie, Bartlee, Bartlea, Bartleah, Bartleigh

Bartoli (Spanish) Form of Bartholomew, meaning "the son of the farmer"
Bartolie, Bartoly, Bartoley, Bartolee, Bartoleigh, Bartolea, Bartolo, Bartolio

Barton (English) From the barley town
Bartun, Barten, Bartan, Bartin, Bartyn

Barwolf (English) The ax-wolf
Barrwolf, Barwulf, Barrwulf

Basant (Arabic) One who smiles often
Basante

Bassett (English) A little person
Baset, Basset, Basett

Basy (American) A home-body
Basey, Basi, Basie, Basee, Basea, Basye

Baurice (American) Form of Maurice, meaning "a dark-skinned man; Moorish"
Baurell, Baureo, Bauricio, Baurids, Baurie, Baurin

Bay (Vietnamese / English) The seventh-born child; born during the month of July / from the bay
Baye, Bae, Bai

Beal (French) A handsome man
Beals, Beale, Beall, Bealle

Beamer (English) One who plays the trumpet
Beamor, Beamir, Beamyr, Beamur, Beamar, Beemer, Beemar, Beemir

Beau (French) A handsome man, an admirer
Bo

Becher (Hebrew) The first-born son

^**Beckett** (English) From the small stream; from the brook
Becket

Bedar (Arabic) One who is attentive
Beder, Bedor, Bedur, Bedyr, Bedir

Beircheart (Anglo-Saxon) Of the intelligent army

Bela (Slavic) A white-skinned man
Belah, Bella, Bellah

Belden (English) From the beautiful valley
Beldan, Beldon, Beldun, Beldin, Beldyn, Bellden, Belldan, Belldon, Belldun, Belldin, Belldyn

Belen (Greek) Of an arrow
Belin, Belyn, Belan, Belon, Belun

Belindo (English) A handsome and tender man
Belyndo, Belindio, Belyndio, Belindeo, Belyndeo, Belindiyo, Belyndiyo, Belindeyo

Bellarmine (Italian) One who is handsomely armed
Bellarmin, Bellarmeen, Bellarmeene, Bellarmean, Bellarmeane, Bellarmyn, Bellarmyne

Belton (English) From the beautiful town
Bellton, Beltun, Belltun, Belten, Bellten

Belvin (American) Form of Melvin, meaning "a friend who offers counsel"
Belven, Belvyn, Belvon, Belvun, Belvan

Bem (African) A peaceful man

Ben (English) Form of Benjamin, meaning "son of the south; son of the right hand"
Benn, Benni, Bennie, Bennee, Benney, Benny, Bennea, Benno

*∗†**Benjamin** (Hebrew) Son of the south; son of the right hand
Ben, Benejamen, Beniamino, Benjaman, Benjamen, Benjamino, Benjamon, Benjiman, Benjimen

Bennett (English) Form of Benedict, meaning one who is blessed
Benett, Bennet, Benet

Berdy (German) Having a brilliant mind
Berdey, Berdee, Berdea, Berdi, Berdie

Bentley (English) From the meadow of bent grass
Bently, Bentleigh, Bentlee, Bentlie

Beresford (English) From the barley ford
Beresforde, Beresfurd, Beresfurde, Beresferd, Beresferde, Berford, Berforde, Berfurd

Berkeley (English) From the meadow of birch trees
Berkely, Berkeli, Berkelie, Berkelea, Berkeleah, Berkelee, Berkeleigh, Berkley

Bernard (German) As strong and brave as a bear
Barnard, Barnardo, Barnhard, Barnhardo, Bearnard, Bernardo, Bernarr, Bernd

Berry (English) Resembling a berry fruit
Berrey, Berri, Berrie, Berree, Berrea

Bert (English) One who is illustrious
Berte, Berti, Bertie, Bertee, Bertea, Berty, Bertey

Bethel (Hebrew) The house of God
Bethell, Bethele, Bethelle, Betuel, Betuell, Betuele, Betuelle

Bevis (Teutonic) An archer
Beviss, Bevys, Bevyss, Beavis, Beaviss, Beavys, Beavyss

Biagio (Italian) One who has a stutter
Biaggio

Birney (English) From the island with the brook
Birny, Birnee, Birnea, Birni, Birnie

Black (English) A dark-skinned man
Blak, Blac, Blacke

Blackwell (English) From the dark spring
Blackwel, Blackwelle, Blackwele

Blade (English) One who wields a sword or knife
Blayd, Blayde, Blaid, Blaide, Blaed, Blaede

Blagden (English) From the dark valley
Blagdon, Blagdan, Blagdun, Blagdin, Blagdyn

Blaine (Scottish / Irish) A saint's servant / a thin man
Blayne, Blane, Blain, Blayn, Blaen, Blaene, Blainy, Blainey

Blaise (Latin / American) One with a lisp or a stutter / a fiery man
Blaze, Blaize, Blaiz, Blayze, Blayz, Blaez, Blaeze

Blake (English) A dark, handsome man
Blayk, Blayke, Blaik, Blaike, Blaek, Blaeke

Bliss (English) Filled with happiness
Blis, Blyss, Blys

Blondell (English) A fair-haired boy
Blondel, Blondele, Blondelle

Boaz (Hebrew) One who is swift
Boaze, Boas, Boase

Bob (English) Form of Robert, meaning "one who is bright with fame"
Bobbi, Bobbie, Bobby, Bobbey, Bobbee, Bobbea

Bogart (French) One who is strong with the bow
Bogaard, Bogaart, Bogaerd, Bogey, Bogie, Bogi, Bogy, Bogee

Bolivar (Spanish) A mighty warrior
Bolevar, Bolivarr, Bolevarr, Bollivar, Bollivarr, Bollevar, Bollevarr

Bonaventure (Latin) One who undertakes a blessed venture
Bonaventura, Buenaventure, Buenaventura, Bueaventure, Bueaventura

Booker (English) One who binds books; a scribe
Bookar, Bookir, Bookyr, Bookur, Bookor

Bosley (English) From the meadow near the forest
Bosly, Boslee, Boslea, Bosleah, Bosleigh, Bosli, Boslie, Bozley

Boston (English) From the town near the forest; from the city of Boston
Bostun, Bostin, Bostyn, Bosten, Bostan

Boyce (French) One who lives near the forest
Boice, Boyse, Boise

Boyd (Celtic) A blond-haired man
Boyde, Boid, Boide, Boyden, Boydan, Boydin, Boydyn, Boydon

Boynton (Irish) From the town near the river Boyne
Boyntun, Boynten, Boyntin, Boyntan, Boyntyn

Bracken (English) Resembling the large fern
Braken, Brackan, Brakan, Brackin, Brakin, Brackyn

Braddock (English) From the broadly spread oak
Bradock, Braddoc, Bradoc, Braddok, Bradok

***Braden** (Gaelic / English) Resembling salmon / from the wide valley
Bradan, Bradon, Bradin, Bradyn, Braeden, Braddan, Braddin, Brayden

Bradford (English) From the wide ford
Bradforde, Bradferd, Bradferde, Bradfurd

Bradley (English) From the wide meadow
Bradly, Bradlea, Bradleah, Bradlee, Bradleigh, Bradli

***Brady** (Irish) The son of a large-chested man
Bradey, Bradee, Bradea, Bradi, Bradie, Braidy, Braidey, Braidee

Bramley (English) From the wild gorse meadow; from the raven's meadow
Bramly, Bramlee, Bramlea, Bramleah, Bramleigh, Bramli, Bramlie

Branch (Latin) An extension
Branche

*ᵀ**Brandon** (English) From the broom or gorse hill
Brandun, Brandin, Brandyn, Brandan, Branden, Brannon, Brannun, Brannen

Branson (English) The son of Brand or Brandon
Bransun, Bransen, Bransan, Bransin, Bransyn

Braxton (English) From Brock's town
Braxtun, Braxten, Braxtan, Braxtyn

***Brayden** (Gaelic / English) Form of Braden, meaning "resembling salmon / from the wide valley"
Braydon, Braydan, Braydin, Braydyn

^**Braylon** (American) Combination of Brayden and Lynn
Braylen

Brendan (Irish) Born to royalty; a prince
Brendano, Brenden, Brendin, Brendon, Brendyn, Brendun

Brennan (Gaelic) A sorrowful man; a teardrop
Brenan, Brenn, Brennen, Brennin, Brennon, Brenin, Brennun, Brennyn

Brent (English) From the hill
Brendt, Brennt, Brentan, Brenten, Brentin, Brenton, Brentun, Brentyn

Brett (Latin) A man from Britain or Brittany
Bret, Breton, Brette, Bretton, Brit, Briton, Britt, Brittain

Brewster (English) One who brews
Brewer, Brewstere

*ᵀ**Brian** (Gaelic / Celtic) Of noble birth / having great strength
*Briano, Briant, Brien, Brion, **Bryan**, Bryant, Bryen, Bryent*

Briar (English) Resembling a thorny plant
Brier, Bryar, Bryer

Brock (English) Resembling a badger
Broc

Broderick (English) From the wide ridge
Broderik, Broderic, Brodrick, Brodryk, Brodyrc, Brodrik, Broderyc, Brodrig

•**Brody** (Gaelic / Irish) From the ditch
Brodie, Brodey, Brodi, Brodee

Brogan (Gaelic) One who is sturdy
Broggan, Brogen, Broggen, Brogon, Broggon, Brogun, Broggun, Brogin, Broggin, Brogyn

Brooks (English) From the running stream
Brookes

Bruce (Scottish) A man from Brieuse; one who is well-born; from an influential family
Brouce, Brooce, Bruci, Brucie, Brucey, Brucy

Bruno (German) A brown-haired man
Brunoh, Brunoe, Brunow, Brunowe, Bruin, Bruine, Brunon, Brunun

Bryce (Scottish / Anglo-Saxon) One who is speckled / the son of a nobleman
Brice, Bricio, Brizio, Brycio

^**Bryson** (Welsh) The son of Brice
*Brisen, Brysin, Brysun, Brysyn, **Brycen***

Bud (English) One who is brotherly
Budd, Buddi, Buddie, Buddee, Buddey, Buddy

Budha (Hindi) Another name for the planet Mercury
Budhan, Budhwar

Bulat (Russian) Having great strength
Bulatt

Burbank (English) From the riverbank of burrs
Burrbank, Burhbank

Burgess (German) A free citizen of the town
Burges, Burgiss, Burgis, Burgyss, Burgys, Burgeis

Burne (English) Resembling a bear; from the brook; the brown-haired one
Burn, Beirne, Burnis, Byrn, Byrne, Burns, Byrnes

Burnet (French) Having brown hair
Burnett, Burnete, Burnette, Bernet, Bernett, Bernete, Bernette

Burton (English) From the fortified town
Burtun, Burten, Burtin, Burtyn, Burtan

Butler (English) The keeper of the bottles (wine, liquor)
Buttler, Butlar, Butlor, Butlir, Buttlir, Butlyr

^**Byron** (English) One who lives near the cow sheds
Byrom, Beyren, Beyron, Biren, Biron, Buiron, Byram, Byran

C

Cable (French) One who makes rope
Cabel, Caibel, Caible, Caybel, Cayble, Caebel, Caeble, Cabe

Caddis (English) Resembling a worsted fabric
Caddys, Caddiss, Caddice

•**Cade** (English / French) One who is round / of the cask
Caid, Caide, Cayd, Cayde, Caed, Caede

Cadell (Welsh) Having the spirit of battle
Cadel, Caddell, Caddel

•**Caden** (Welsh) Spirit of Battle
Caiden, Cayden

Cadmus (Greek) A man from the east; in mythology, the man who founded Thebes
Cadmar, Cadmo, Cadmos, Cadmuss

Cadogan (Welsh) Having glory and honor during battle
Cadogawn, Cadwgan, Cadwgawn, Cadogaun

Caesar (Latin) An emperor
Caezar, Casar, Cezar, Chezare, Caesarius, Ceasar, Ceazer

Cain (Hebrew) One who wields a spear; something acquired; in the Bible, Adam and Eve's first son who killed his brother Abel
Cayn, Caen, Cane, Caine, Cayne, Caene

Caird (Scottish) A traveling metal worker
Cairde, Cayrd, Cayrde, Caerd, Caerde

Cairn (Gaelic) From the mound of rocks
Cairne, Cairns, Caern, Caerne, Caernes

Caith (Irish) Of the battle-field
Caithe, Cayth, Caythe, Cathe, Caeth, Caethe

Calbert (English) A cowboy
Calberte, Calburt, Calburte, Calbirt, Calbirte, Calbyrt, Calbyrte

Cale (English) Form of Charles, meaning "one who is manly and strong / a free man"
Cail, Caile, Cayl, Cayle, Cael, Caele

*ᵀ**Caleb** (Hebrew) Resembling a dog
Cayleb, Caileb, Caeleb, Calob, Cailob, Caylob, Caelob, Kaleb

Calian (Native American) A warrior of life
Calien, Calyan, Calyen

Callum (Gaelic) Resembling a dove
Calum

Calvin (French) The little bald one
Cal, Calvyn, Calvon, Calven, Calvan, Calvun, Calvino

Camara (African) One who teaches others

Camden (Gaelic) From the winding valley
Camdene, Camdin, Camdyn, Camdan, Camdon, Camdun

Cameo (English) A small, perfect child
Cammeo

•**Cameron** (Scottish)
Having a crooked nose
*Cameren, Cameran,
Camerin, Cameryn,
Camerun, Camron,
Camren, Camran, Tameron*

Campbell (Scottish)
Having a crooked mouth
*Campbel, Cambell, Cambel,
Camp, Campe, Cambeul,
Cambeull, Campbeul*

Candan (Turkish) A sincere man
*Canden, Candin, Candyn,
Candon, Candun*

Cannon (French) An official of the church
*Canon, Cannun, Canun,
Cannin, Canin*

Canyon (Spanish / English)
From the footpath / from
the deep ravine
Caniyon, Canyun, Caniyun

Capricorn (Latin) The tenth
sign of the zodiac; the goat

Cargan (Gaelic) From the
small rock
*Cargen, Cargon, Cargun,
Cargin, Cargyn*

•**Carl** (German) Form of
Karl, meaning "a free man"
*Carel, Carlan, Carle,
Carlens, Carlitis, Carlin,
Carlo, **Carlos***

•**Carlos** (Spanish) Form
of Karl, meaning "a free
man"
Carolos, Carolo, Carlito

Carlsen (Scandinavian)
The son of Carl
*Carlssen, Carlson, Carlsson,
Carlsun, Carllsun, Carlsin,
Carllsin, Carlsyn*

Carlton (English) From
the free man's town
*Carltun, Carltown, Carston,
Carstun, Carstown,
Carleton, Carletun, Carlten*

Carmichael (Scottish) A
follower of Michael

Carmine (Latin / Aramaic)
A beautiful song / the color
crimson
*Carman, Carmen, Carmin,
Carmino, Carmyne,
Carmon, Carmun, Carmyn*

•ᴛ**Carson** (Scottish) The
son of a marsh dweller
*Carsen, Carsun, Carsan,
Carsin, Carsyn*

•**Carter** (English) One who
transports goods; one who
drives a cart
*Cartar, Cartir, Cartyr,
Cartor, Cartur, Cartere,
Cartier, Cartrell*

Cartland (English) From
Carter's land
*Carteland, Cartlan,
Cartlend, Cartelend,
Cartlen*

Cary (Celtic / Welsh / Gaelic) From the river / from the fort on the hill / having dark features
Carey, Cari, Carie, Caree, Carea, Carry, Carrey, Carri

Case (French) Refers to a chest or box
Cace

^**Cash** (Latin) money

Cassander (Spanish) A brother of heroes
Casander, Casandro, Cassandro, Casandero

Cassius (Latin) One who is empty; hollow; vain
Cassios, Cassio, Cach, Cache, Cashus, Cashos, Cassian, Cassien

Castel (Spanish) From the castle
Castell, Castal, Castall, Castol, Castoll, Castul, Castull, Castil

Castor (Greek) Resembling a beaver; in mythology, one of the Dioscuri
Castur, Caster, Castar, Castir, Castyr, Castorio, Castoreo, Castoro

Cat (American) Resembling the animal
Catt, Chait, Chaite

Cathmore (Irish) A renowned fighter
Cathmor, Cathemore

Cato (Latin) One who is all-knowing
Cayto, Caito, Caeto

Caton (Spanish) One who is knowledgable
Caten, Catun, Catan, Catin, Catyn

Cavell (Teutonic) One who is bold
Cavel, Cavele, Cavelle

Caxton (English) From the lump settlement
Caxtun, Caxten

Celesto (Latin) From heaven
Célestine, Celestino, Celindo, Celestyne, Celestyno

Cephas (Hebrew) As solid as a rock

Cesar (Spanish) form of Caesar, meaning "an emperor"
Cesare, Cesaro, Cesario

Chad (English) One who is warlike
Chaddie, Chadd, Chadric, Chadrick, Chadrik, Chadryck, Chadryc, Chadryk

Chadwick (English) From Chad's dairy farm
Chadwik, Chadwic, Chadwyck, Chadwyk, Chadwyc

Chai (Hebrew) A giver of life
Chaika, Chaim, Cahyim, Cahyyam

Chalkley (English) From the chalk meadow
Chalkly, Chalkleigh, Chalklee, Chalkleah, Chalkli, Chalklie, Chalklea

Champion (English) A warrior; the victor
Champeon, Champiun, Champeun, Champ

Chan (Spanish / Sanskrit) Form of John, meaning "God is gracious" / a shining man
Chayo, Chano, Chawn, Chaun

Chanan (Hebrew) God is compassionate
Chanen, Chanin, Chanyn, Chanun, Chanon

Chance (English) Having good fortune

Chandler (English) One who makes candles
Chandlar, Chandlor

Chaniel (Hebrew) The grace of God
Chanyel, Chaniell, Chanyell

Channing (French / English) An official of the church / resembling a young wolf
Channyng, Canning, Cannyng

Chao (Chinese) The great one

Chappel (English) One who works in the chapel
Capel, Capell, Capello, Cappel, Chappell

*•***Charles** (English / German) One who is manly and strong / a free man
Charls, Chas, Charli, Charlie, Charley, Charly, Charlee, Charleigh, Cale, Chuck, Chick

Charleson (English) The son of Charles
Charlesen, Charlesin, Charlesyn, Charlesan, Charlesun

Charlton (English) From the free man's town
Charleton, Charltun, Charletun, Charleston, Charlestun

Charro (Spanish) A cowboy
Charo

*•***Chase** (English) A huntsman
Chace, Chasen, Chayce, Chayse, Chaise, Chaice, Chaece, Chaese

Chatwin (English) A warring friend
Chatwine, Chatwinn, Chatwinne, Chatwen, Chatwenn, Chatwenne, Chatwyn, Chatwynn

Chaviv (Hebrew) One who is dearly loved
Chaveev, Chaveav, Chaviev, Chaveiv, Chavyv, Chavivi, Chavivie, Chavivy

Chay (Gaelic) From the fairy place
Chaye, Chae

Chelsey (English) From the landing place for chalk
Chelsee, Chelseigh, Chelsea, Chelsi, Chelsie, Chelsy, Chelcey, Chelcy

Cheslav (Russian) From the fortified camp
Cheslaw

Chester (Latin) From the camp of the soldiers
Chet, Chess, Cheston, Chestar, Chestor, Chestur, Chestir, Chestyr

Chico (Spanish) A boy; a lad

Chien (Vietnamese) A combative man

Chiron (Greek) A wise tutor
Chyron, Chirun, Chyrun

Chogan (Native American) Resembling a blackbird
Chogen, Chogon, Chogun, Chogin, Chogyn

Choni (Hebrew) A gracious man
Chonie, Chony, Choney, Chonee, Chonea

✝**Christian** (Greek) A follower of Christ
Chrestien, Chretien, Chris, Christan, Christer, Christiano, Cristian

✝**Christopher** (Greek) One who bears Christ inside
Chris, Kit, Christof, Christofer, Christoffer, Christoforo, Christoforus, Christoph, Christophe, Cristopher, Cristofer

Chuchip (Native American) A deer spirit

Chuck (English) Form of Charles, meaning "one who is manly and strong / a free man"
Chucke, Chucki, Chuckie, Chucky, Chuckey, Chuckee, Chuckea

Chul (Korean) One who stands firm

Chun (Chinese) Born during the spring

Cid (Spanish) A lord
Cyd

Cillian (Gaelic) One who suffers strife

Ciqala (Native American) The little one

Cirrus (Latin) A lock of hair; resembling the cloud
Cyrrus

Clair (Latin) One who is bright
Clare, Clayr, Claer, Clairo, Claro, Claero

Clancy (Celtic) Son of the red-haired warrior
Clancey, Clanci, Clancie, Clancee, Clancea, Clansey, Clansy, Clansi

Clark (English) A cleric; a clerk
Clarke, Clerk, Clerke, Clerc

Claude (English) One who is lame
Claud, Claudan, Claudell, Claidianus, Claudicio, Claudien, Claudino, Claudio

Clay (English) Of the earth's clay

Clayton (English) From the town settled on clay
Claytun, Clayten, Claytin, Claytyn, Claytan, Cleyton, Cleytun, Cleytan

Cleon (Greek) A well-known man
Cleone, Clion, Clione, Clyon, Clyone

Clifford (English) From the ford near the cliff
Cliff, Clyfford, Cliford, Clyford

Cliffton (English) From the town near the cliff
Cliff, Cliffe, Clyff, Clyffe, Clifft, Clift, Clyfft, Clyft

Clinton (English) From the town on the hill
Clynton, Clintun, Clyntun, Clint, Clynt, Clinte, Clynte

Clive (English) One who lives near the cliff
Clyve, Cleve

Cluny (Irish) From the meadow
Cluney, Cluni, Clunie, Clunee, Clunea, Cluneah

Cobden (English) From the cottage in the valley
Cobdenn, Cobdale, Cobdail, Cobdaile, Cobdell, Cobdel, Cobdayl, Cobdayle

Coby (English) Form of Jacob, meaning he who supplants
Cobey

Cody (Irish / English) One who is helpful; a wealthy man / acting as a cushion
Codi, Codie, Codey, Codee, Codeah, Codea, Codier, Codyr

Colbert (French) A famous and bright man
Colvert, Culbert, Colburt, Colbirt, Colbyrt, Colbart, Culburt, Culbirt

Colby (English) From the coal town
Colbey, Colbi, Colbie, Colbee, Collby, Coalby, Colbea, Colbeah

•Cole (English) Having dark features; having coal-black hair
Coley, Coli, Coly, Colie, Colee, Coleigh, Colea, Colson

Coleridge (English) From the dark ridge
Colerige, Colridge, Colrige

Colgate (English) From the dark gate
Colegate, Colgait, Colegait, Colgayt, Colegayt, Colgaet

•Colin (Scottish) A young man; a form of Nicholas, meaning "of the victorious people"
Cailean, Colan, Colyn, Colon, Colen, Collin, Collan

Colt (English) A young horse; from the coal town
Colte

^Colton (English) From the coal town
Colten, Coltun, Coltan, Coltin, Coltyn, Coltrain

Colter (English) A horse herdsman
Coltere, Coltar, Coltor, Coltir, Coltyr, Coulter, Coultar, Coultir

Comanche (Native American) A tribal name
Comanchi, Comanchie, Comanchee, Comanchea, Comanchy, Comanchey

Comus (Latin) In mythology, the god of mirth and revelry
Comas, Comis, Comys

Conan (English / Gaelic) Resembling a wolf / one who is high and mighty
Conant

Condon (Celtic) A dark, wise man
Condun, Condan, Conden, Condin, Condyn

Cong (Chinese) A clever man

Conn (Irish) The chief
Con

Connecticut (Native American) From the place beside the long river / from the state of Connecticut

Connery (Scottish) A daring man
Connary, Connerie, Conneri, Connerey, Connarie, Connari, Connarey, Conary

•Connor (Gaelic) A wolf lover
Conor, Conner, Coner, Connar, Conar, Connur, Conur, Connir, Conir

Conroy (Irish) A wise advisor
Conroye, Conroi

Constantine (Latin) One who is steadfast; firm
Dinos

Consuelo (Spanish) One who offers consolation
Consuel, Consuelio, Consueleo, Consueliyo, Consueleyo

Conway (Gaelic) The hound of the plain; from the sacred river
Conwaye, Conwai, Conwae, Conwy

Cook (English) One who prepares meals for others
Cooke

Cooney (Irish) A handsome man
Coony, Cooni, Coonie, Coonee, Coonea

·Cooper (English) One who makes barrels
Coop, Coopar, Coopir, Coopyr, Coopor, Coopur, Coopersmith, Cupere

Corbett (French) Resembling a young raven
Corbet, Corbete, Corbette, Corbit, Corbitt, Corbite, Corbitte

Corcoran (Gaelic) Having a ruddy complexion
Cochran

Cordero (Spanish) Resembling a lamb
Corderio, Corderiyo, Cordereo, Cordereyo

Corey (Irish) From the hollow; of the churning waters
Cory, Cori, Corie, Coree, Corea, Correy, Corry, Corri

Coriander (Greek) A romantic man; resembling the spice
Coryander, Coriender, Coryender

Corlan (Irish) One who wields a spear
Corlen, Corlin, Corlyn, Corlon, Corlun

Corrado (German) A bold counselor
Corrade, Corradeo, Corradio

Corridon (Irish) One who wields a spear
Corridan, Corridun, Corriden, Corridin, Corridyn

Cortez (Spanish) A courteous man
Cortes

Cosmo (Greek) The order of the universe
Cosimo, Cosmé, Cosmos, Cosmas, Cozmo, Cozmos, Cozmas

Cotton (American)
Resembling or farmer of
the plant
Cottin, Cotten, Cottyn,
Cottun, Cottan

Courtney (English) A
courteous man; courtly
Cordney, Cordni, Cortenuy,
Corteney, Cortni, Cortnee,
Cortneigh, Cortney

Covert (English) One who
provides shelter
Couvert

Covey (English) A brood
of birds
Covy, Covi, Covie, Covee,
Covea, Covvey, Covvy, Covvi

Covington (English) From
the town near the cave
Covyngton, Covingtun,
Covyngtun

Cox (English) A coxswain
Coxe, Coxi, Coxie, Coxey,
Coxy, Coxee, Coxea

Coyle (Irish) A leader during battle
Coyl, Coil, Coile

Craig (Gaelic) From the
rocks; from the crag
Crayg, Craeg, Craige,
Crayge, Craege, Crage, Crag

Crandell (English) From
the valley of cranes
Crandel, Crandale, Crandail,
Crandaile, Crandayl, Crandayle,
Crandael, Crandaele

Crawford (English) From
the crow's ford
Crawforde, Crawferd,
Crawferde, Crawfurd,
Crawfurde

Creed (Latin) A guiding
principle; a belief
Creede, Cread, Creade,
Creedon, Creadon, Creedun,
Creadun, Creedin

Creek (English) From the
small stream
Creeke, Creak, Creake,
Creik, Creike

Creighton (Scottish) From
the border town
Creightun, Crayton,
Craytun, Craiton, Craitun,
Craeton, Craetun, Crichton

Crescent (French) One who
creates; increasing; growing
Creissant, Crescence,
Cressant, Cressent, Crescant

^**Cruz** (Spanish) Of the Cross

Cuarto (Spanish) The
fourth-born child
Cuartio, Cuartiyo, Cuarteo

Cullen (Gaelic) A good-
looking young man
Cullin, Cullyn, Cullan,
Cullon, Cullun

Cunningham (Gaelic)
From the village of milk
*Conyngham, Cuningham,
Cunnyngham, Cunyngham*

Curcio (French) One who
is courteous
Curceo

Cuthbert (English) One
who is bright and famous
*Cuthbeorht, Cuthburt,
Cuthbirt, Cuthbyrt*

Cyneley (English) From
the royal meadow
*Cynely, Cyneli, Cynelie,
Cynelee, Cynelea, Cyneleah,
Cyneleigh*

Czar (Russian) An emperor

d

Dacey (Gaelic / Latin) A
man from the south / a
man from Dacia
*Dacy, Dacee, Dacea, Daci,
Dacie, Daicey, Daicy*

Dack (English) From the
French town of Dax
Dacks, Dax

Daedalus (Greek) A crafts-
man
Daldalos, Dedalus

Dag (Scandinavian) Born
during the daylight
*Dagney, Dagny, Dagnee,
Dagnea, Dagni, Dagnie,
Daeg, Dagget*

Daijon (American) A gift
of hope
Dayjon, Daejon, Dajon

Dainan (Australian) A
kind-hearted man
*Dainen, Dainon, Dainun,
Dainyn, Dainin, Daynan,
Daynen, Daynon*

Daire (Irish) A wealthy man
*Dair, Daere, Daer, Dayr,
Dayre, Dare, Dari, Darie*

Daivat (Hindi) A powerful
man

Dakarai (African) Filled
with happiness

Dakota (Native American)
A friend to all
*Daccota, Dakoda, Dakodah,
Dakotah, Dakoeta, Dekota,
Dekohta, Dekowta*

Dallan (Irish) One who is
blind
*Dalan, Dallen, Dalen,
Dalin, Dallin, Dallyn,
Dalyn, Dallon, Dalon,
Dallun, Dalun*

Dallas (Scottish) From the
dales
*Dalles, Dallis, Dallys,
Dallos*

Dalton (English) from the town in the valley
Daltun, Dalten, Daltan, Daltin, Daltyn, Daleten, Dalte, Daulten

Damario (Greek / Spanish) Resembling a calf / one who is gentle
Damarios, Damarius, Damaro, Damero, Damerio, Damereo, Damareo, Damerios

Damian (Greek) One who tames or subdues others
Daemon, Daimen, Daimon, Daman, Damen, Dameon, Damiano, Damianos

Dane (English) A man from Denmark
Dain, Daine, Dayn, Dayne

Danely (Scandinavian) A man from Denmark
Daneley, Daneli, Danelie, Danelee, Daneleigh, Danelea, Daineley, Dainely

Daniachew (African) A mediator

Daniel (Hebrew) God is my judge
Dan, Danal, Daneal, Danek, Danell, Danial, Daniele, Danil, Danilo

Danso (African) A reliable man
Dansoe, Dansow, Dansowe

Dante (Latin) An enduring man; everlasting
Dantae, Dantay, Dantel, Daunte, Dontae, Dontay, Donte, Dontae

Daoud (Arabian) Form of David, meaning "the beloved one"
Daoude, Dawud, Doud, Daud, Da'ud

Daphnis (Greek) In mythology, the son of Hermes
Daphnys

Dar (Hebrew) Resembling a pearl
Darr

Darcel (French) Having dark features
Darcell, Darcele, Darcelle, Darcio, Darceo

Dardanus (Greek) In mythology, the founder of Troy
Dardanio, Dardanios, Dardanos, Dard, Darde

Darek (English) Form of Derek, meaning "the ruler of the tribe"
Darrek, Darec, Darrec, Darreck, Dareck

Darion (Greek) A gift
Darian, Darien, Dariun, Darrion, Darrian, Darrien, Daryon, Daryan

Darius (Greek) A kingly
man; one who is wealthy
*Darias, Dariess, Dario,
Darious, Darrius, Derrius,
Derrious, Derrias*

Darlen (American) A
sweet man; a darling
*Darlon, Darlun, Darlan,
Darlin, Darlyn*

Darnell (English) From the
hidden place
*Darnall, Darneil, Darnel,
Darnele, Darnelle*

Darold (English) Form
of Harold, meaning "the
ruler of an army"
*Darrold, Derald, Derrald,
Derold, Derrold*

Darren (Gaelic / English) A
great man / a gift from God
*Darran, Darrin, Darryn,
Darron, Darrun, Daren,
Darin, Daran*

Dart (English / American)
From the river / one who
is fast
*Darte, Darrt, Darrte, Darti,
Dartie, Dartee, Dartea, Darty*

Darvell (French) From the
eagle town
Darvel, Darvele, Darvelle

Dasras (Indian) A handsome man

Dasya (Indian) A servant

David (Hebrew) The
beloved one
*Dave, Davey, Davi,
Davidde, Davide, Davie,
Daviel, Davin, Daoud*

Davis (English) The son
of David
*Davies, Daviss, Davys,
Davyss*

Davu (African) Of the
beginning
*Davue, Davoo, Davou,
Davugh*

Dawson (English) The son
of David
*Dawsan, Dawsen, Dawsin,
Dawsun*

Dayton (English) From the
sunny town

Dax (French) From the
French town Dax
Daxton

Deacon (Greek) The dusty
one; a servant
*Deecon, Deakon, Deekon,
Deacun, Deecun, Deakun,
Deekun, Deacan*

Dean (English) From the
valley; a church official
*Deane, Deen, Deene, Dene,
Deans, Deens, Deani, Deanie*

DeAndre (American) A
manly man
*D'André, DeAndrae,
DeAndray, Diandray,
Diondrae, Diondray*

Dearon (American) One who is much loved
Dearan, Dearen, Dearin, Dearyn, Dearun

Decker (German / Hebrew) One who prays / a piercing man
Deker, Decer, Dekker, Deccer, Deck, Decke

Declan (Irish) The name of a saint

Dedrick (English) Form of Dietrich, meaning "the ruler of the tribe"
Dedryck, Dedrik, Dedryk, Dedric, Dedryc

Deegan (Irish) A black-haired man
Deagan, Degan, Deegen, Deagen, Degen, Deegon, Deagon, Degon

Deinorus (American) A lively man
Denorius, Denorus, Denorios, Deinorius, Deinorios

Dejuan (American) A talkative man
Dejuane, Dewon, Dewonn, Dewan, Dewann, Dwon, Dwonn, Dajuan

Delaney (Irish / French) The dark challenger / from the elder-tree grove
Delany, Delanee, Delanea, Delani, Delanie, Delainey, Delainy, Delaini

Delaware (English) From the state of Delaware
Delawair, Delaweir, Delwayr, Delawayre, Delawaire, Delawaer, Delawaere

Delius (Greek) A man from Delos
Delios, Delos, Delus, Delo

Dell (English) From the small valley
Delle, Del

Delmon (English) A man of the mountain
Delmun, Delmen, Delmin, Delmyn, Delmont, Delmonte, Delmond, Delmonde

Delsi (American) An easy-going guy
Delsie, Delsy, Delsey, Delsee, Delsea, Delci, Delcie, Delcee

Delvin (English) A godly friend
Delvinn, Delvinne, Delvyn, Delvynn, Delvynne, Delven, Delvenn, Delvenne

Demarcus (American) The son of Marcus
DeMarcus, DaMarkiss, DeMarco, Demarkess, DeMarko, Demarkus, DeMarques, DeMarquez

Dembe (African) A peaceful man
Dembi, Dembie, Dembee, Dembea, Dembey, Demby

Denali (American) From the national park
Denalie, Denaly, Denaley, Denalee, Denalea, Denaleigh

Denley (English) From the meadow near the valley
Denly, Denlea, Denleah, Denlee, Denleigh, Denli, Denlie

Denman (English) One who lives in the valley
Denmann, Denmin, Denmyn, Denmen, Denmon, Denmun

Dennis (French) A follower of Dionysus
Den, Denies, Denis, Dennes, Dennet, Denney, Dennie, Denys, Dennys

Dennison (English) The son of Dennis
Denison, Dennisun, Denisun, Dennisen, Denisen, Dennisan, Denisan

Deo (Greek) A godly man

Deonte (French) An outgoing man
Deontay, Deontaye, Deontae, Dionte, Diontay, Diontaye, Diontae

Deotis (American) A learned man; a scholar
Deotiss, Deotys, Deotyss, Deotus, Deotuss

Derek (English) The ruler of the tribe
Dereck, Deric, Derick, Derik, Deriq, Derk, Derreck, Derrek, Derrick

Dervin (English) A gifted friend
Dervinn, Dervinne, Dervyn, Dervynn, Dervynne, Dervon, Dervan, Dervun

Deshan (Hindi) Of the nation
Deshal, Deshad

Desiderio (Latin) One who is desired; hoped for
Derito, Desi, Desideratus, Desiderios, Desiderius, Desiderus, Dezi, Diderot

Desmond (Gaelic) A man from South Munster
Desmonde, Desmund, Desmunde, Dezmond, Dezmonde, Dezmund, Dezmunde, Desmee

Desperado (Spanish) A renegade

Destin (French) Recognizing one's certain fortune; fate
Destyn, Deston, Destun, Desten, Destan

Destrey (American) A cowboy
Destry, Destree, Destrea, Destri, Destrie

Deutsch (German) A
German

Devanshi (Hindi) A divine
messenger
*Devanshie, Devanshy,
Devanshey, Devanshee*

Devante (Spanish) One
who fights wrongdoing

Deverell (French) From
the riverbank
*Deverel, Deveral, Deverall,
Devereau, Devereaux,
Devere, Deverill, Deveril*

Devlin (Gaelic) Having
fierce bravery; a misfortu-
nate man
*Devlyn, Devlon, Devlen,
Devlan, Devlun*

Devon (English) From the
beautiful farmland; of the
divine
*Devan, Deven, Devenn,
Devin, Devonn, Devone,
Deveon, Devonne*

Dewitt (Flemish) A blond-
haired man
*DeWitt, Dewytt, DeWytt,
Dewit, DeWit, Dewyt, DeWyt*

Dexter (Latin) A right-
handed man; one who is
skillful
*Dextor, Dextar, Dextur,
Dextir, Dextyr, Dexton,
Dextun, Dexten*

Dhyanesh (Indian) One
who meditates
*Dhianesh, Dhyaneshe,
Dhianeshe*

Dice (American) A gam-
bling man
Dyce

Dichali (Native American)
One who talks a lot
*Dichalie, Dichaly, Dichaley,
Dichalee, Dichalea, Dichaleigh*

·Diego (Spanish) Form of
James, meaning "he who
supplants"
Dyego, Dago

Diesel (American) Having
great strength
Deisel, Diezel, Deizel, Dezsel

Dietrich (German) The
ruler of the tribe
Dedrick

Digby (Norse) From the
town near the ditch
*Digbey, Digbee, Digbea,
Digbi, Digbie*

Diji (African) A farmer
*Dijie, Dijee, Dijea, Dijy,
Dijey*

Dillon (Gaelic) Resembling
a lion; a faithful man
*Dillun, Dillen, Dillan, Dillin,
Dillyn, Dilon, Dilan, Dilin*

Dino (Italian) One who
wields a little sword
*Dyno, Dinoh, Dynoh,
Deano, Deanoh, Deeno,
Deenoh, Deino*

Dinos (Greek) Form of
Constantine, meaning "one
who is steadfast; firm"
*Dynos, Deanos, Deenos,
Deinos, Dinose, Dinoz*

Dins (American) One who
climbs to the top
Dinz, Dyns, Dynz

Dionysus (Greek) The god
of wine and revelry
*Dion, Deion, Deon, Deonn,
Deonys, Deyon, Diandre*

Dior (French) The golden one
*D'Or, Diorr, Diorre, Dyor,
Deor, Dyorre, Deorre*

Diron (American) Form of
Darren, meaning "a great
man / a gift from God"
*Dirun, Diren, Diran, Dirin,
Diryn, Dyron, Dyren*

Dixon (English) The son
of Dick
*Dixen, Dixin, Dixyn,
Dixan, Dixun*

Doane (English) From the
rolling hills
Doan

Dobber (American) An
independent man
*Dobbar, Dobbor, Dobbur,
Dobbir, Dobbyr*

Dobbs (English) A fiery
man
Dobbes, Dobes, Dobs

Domevlo (African) One
who doesn't judge others
Domivlo, Domyvlo

Domingo (Spanish) Born
on a Sunday
*Domyngo, Demingo,
Demyngo*

·Dominic (Latin) A lord
*Demenico, Dom, Domenic,
Domenico, Domenique,
Domini, Dominick,
Dominico*

Domnall (Gaelic) A world
ruler
*Domhnall, Domnull,
Domhnull*

Don (Scottish) From of
Donald, meaning "ruler of
the world"
*Donn, Donny, Donney,
Donnie, Donni, Donnee,
Donnea, Donne*

Donald (Scottish) Ruler of
the world
*Don, Donold, Donuld,
Doneld, Donild, Donyld*

Donovan (Irish) A brown-
haired chief
*Donavan, Donavon,
Donevon, Donovyn*

Donato (Italian) A gift
from God

Dor (Hebrew) Of this generation
Doram, Doriel, Dorli, Dorlie, Dorlee, Dorlea, Dorleigh, Dorly

Doran (Irish) A stranger; one who has been exiled
Doren, Dorin, Doryn

Dorsey (Gaelic) From the fortress near the sea
Dorsy, Dorsee, Dorsea, Dorsi, Dorsie

Dost (Arabic) A beloved friend
Doste, Daust, Dauste, Dawst, Dawste

Dotson (English) The son of Dot
Dotsen, Dotsan, Dotsin, Dotsyn, Dotsun, Dottson, Dottsun, Dottsin

Dove (American) A peaceful man
Dovi, Dovie, Dovy, Dovey, Dovee, Dovea

Drade (American) A serious-minded man
Draid, Draide, Drayd, Drayde, Draed, Draede, Dradell, Dradel

Drake (English) Resembling a dragon
Drayce, Drago, Drakie

Drew (Welsh) One who is wise
Drue, Dru

Driscoll (Celtic) A mediator; one who is sorrowful; a messenger
Dryscoll, Driscol, Dryscol, Driskoll, Dryskoll, Driskol, Dryskol, Driskell

Druce (Gaelic / English) A wise man; a druid / the son of Drew
Drews, Drewce, Druece, Druse, Druson, Drusen

Drummond (Scottish) One who lives on the ridge
Drummon, Drumond, Drumon, Drummund, Drumund, Drummun

Duane (Gaelic) A dark or swarthy man
Dewain, Dewayne, Duante, Duayne, Duwain, Duwaine, Duwayne, Dwain

Dublin (Irish) From the capital of Ireland
Dublyn, Dublen, Dublan, Dublon, Dublun

Duc (Vietnamese) One who has upstanding morals

Due (Vietnamese) A virtuous man

Duke (English) A title of nobility; a leader
Dooke, Dook, Duki, Dukie, Dukey, Duky, Dukee, Dukea

Dumi (African) One who inspires others
Dumie, Dumy, Dumey, Dumee, Dumea

Dumont (French) Man of the mountain
Dumonte, Dumount, Dumounte

Duncan (Scottish) A dark warrior
Dunkan, Dunckan, Dunc, Dunk, Dunck

Dundee (Scottish) From the town on the Firth of Tay
Dundea, Dundi, Dundie, Dundy, Dundey

Dung (Vietnamese) A brave man; a heroic man

Dunton (English) From the town on the hill
Duntun, Dunten, Duntan, Duntin, Duntyn

Durin (Norse) In mythology, one of the fathers of the dwarves
Duryn, Duren, Duran, Duron, Durun

Durjaya (Hindi) One who is difficult to defeat

Durrell (English) One who is strong and protective
Durrel, Durell, Durel

Dustin (English / German) From the dusty area / a courageous warrior
Dustyn, Dusten, Dustan, Duston, Dustun, Dusty, Dustey, Dusti

Duvall (French) From the valley
Duval, Duvale

Dwade (English) A dark traveler
Dwaid, Dwaide, Dwayd, Dwayde, Dwaed, Dwaede

Dwight (Flemish) A white- or blond-haired man
Dwite, Dwhite, Dwyght, Dwighte

Dyami (Native American) Resembling an eagle
Dyamie, Dyamy, Dyamey, Dyamee, Dyamea, Dyame

Dyer (English) A creative man
Dier, Dyar, Diar, Dy, Dye, Di, Die

Dylan (Welsh) Son of the sea
Dyllan, Dylon, Dyllon, Dylen, Dyllen, Dylun, Dyllun, Dylin

Dzigbode (African) One who is patient

e

Eagan (Irish) A fiery man
*Eegan, Eagen, Eegen,
Eagon, Eegon, Eagun,
Eegun*

Eagle (Native American)
Resembling the bird
Eegle, Eagel, Eegel

Eamon (Irish) Form of
Edmund, meaning "a
wealthy protector"
*Eaman, Eamen, Eamin,
Eamyn, Eamun, Eamonn,
Eames, Eemon*

Ean (Gaelic) Form of John,
meaning "God is gracious"
Eion, Eyan, Eyon, Eian

Earl (English) A nobleman
Earle, Erle, Erl, Eorl

Easey (American) An easy-
going man
*Easy, Easi, Easie, Easee,
Easea, Eazey, Eazy, Eazi*

Eastman (English) A man
from the east
East, Easte, Eeste

^**Easton** (English) Eastern
place.
Eastan, Easten, Eastyn

Eckhard (German) Of the
brave sword point
*Eckard, Eckardt, Eckhardt,
Ekkehard, Ekkehardt,
Ekhard, Ekhardt*

Ed (English) Form of
Edward, meaning "a
wealthy protector"
*Edd, Eddi, Eddie, Eddy,
Eddey, Eddee, Eddea, Edi*

Edan (Celtic) One who is
full of fire
Edon, Edun

Edbert (English) One who
is prosperous and bright
*Edberte, Edburt, Edburte,
Edbirt, Edbirte, Edbyrt,
Edbyrte*

Edenson (English) Son of
Eden
*Eadenson, Edensun,
Eadensun, Edinson*

Edgar (English) A power-
ful and wealthy spearman
*Eadger, Edgardo, Edghur,
Edger*

Edison (English) Son of
Edward
*Eddison, Edisun, Eddisun,
Edisen, Eddisen, Edisyn,
Eddisyn, Edyson*

Edlin (Anglo-Saxon) A
wealthy friend
*Edlinn, Edlinne, Edlyn,
Edlynn, Edlynne, Eadlyn,
Eadlin, Edlen*

Edmund (English) A
wealthy protector
Ed, Eddie, Edmond, Eamon

Edom (Hebrew) A red-
haired man
*Edum, Edam, Edem, Edim,
Edym*

Edred (Anglo-Saxon) A
king
Edread, Edrid, Edryd

Edward (English) A
wealthy protector
*Ed, Eadward, Edik,
Edouard, Eduard, Eduardo,
Edvard, Edvardas, Edwardo*

Edwardson (English) The
son of Edward
*Edwardsun, Eadwardsone,
Eadwardsun*

Edwin (English) A wealthy
friend
*Edwinn, Edwinne, Edwine,
Edwyn, Edwynn, Edwynne,
Edwen, Edwenn*

Effiom (African)
Resembling a crocodile
*Efiom, Effyom, Efyom,
Effeom, Efeom*

Efigenio (Greek) Form of
Eugene, meaning "a well-
born man"
*Ephigenio, Ephigenios,
Ephigenius, Efigenios*

Efrain (Spanish) Form of
Ephraim, meaning "one
who is fertile; productive"
*Efraine, Efrayn, Efrayne,
Efraen, Efraene, Efrane*

Efrat (Hebrew) One who is
honored
Efratt, Ephrat, Ephratt

Egesa (Anglo-Saxon) One
who creates terror
*Egessa, Egeslic, Egeslick,
Egeslik*

Eghert (German) An intel-
ligent man
*Egherte, Eghurt, Eghurte,
Eghirt, Eghirte, Eghyrt*

Egidio (Italian) Resembling
a young goat
*Egydio, Egideo, Egydeo,
Egidiyo, Egydiyo, Egidius*

Eilert (Scandinavian) Of
the hard point
*Elert, Eilart, Elart, Eilort,
Elort, Eilurt, Elurt, Eilirt*

Eilon (Hebrew) From the
oak tree
Eilan, Eilin, Eilyn, Eilen, Eilun

Einar (Scandinavian) A
leading warrior
*Einer, Ejnar, Einir, Einyr,
Einor, Einur, Ejnir, Ejnyr*

Einri (Teutonic) An intel-
ligent man
*Einrie, Einry, Einrey,
Einree, Einrea*

Eisig (Hebrew) One who laughs often
Eisyg

Eladio (Spanish) A man from Greece
Eladeo, Eladiyo, Eladeyo

Elbert (English / German) A well-born man / a bright man
Elberte, Elburt, Elburte, Elbirt, Elbirte, Ethelbert, Ethelburt, Ethelbirt

Eldan (English) From the valley of the elves

Eldon (English) From the sacred hill
Eldun

Eldorado (Spanish) The golden man

Eldred (English) An old, wise advisor
Eldrid, Eldryd, Eldrad, Eldrod, Edlrud, Ethelred

Eldrick (English) An old, wise ruler
Eldrik, Eldric, Eldryck, Eldryk, Eldryc, Eldrich

Eleazar (Hebrew) God will help
Elazar, Eleasar, Eliezer, Elazaro, Eleazaro, Elazer

Elias (Hebrew) Form of Elijah, meaning "Jehovah is my god"
Eliyas

Eliachim (Hebrew) God will establish
Eliakim, Elyachim, Elyakim, Eliakym

*⁎**Eli** (Hebrew) One who has ascended; my God on High
Ely

Elian (Spanish) A spirited man
Elyan, Elien, Elyen, Elion, Elyon, Eliun, Elyun

Elihu (Hebrew) My God is He
Elyhu, Elihue, Elyhue

*⁎⁎**Elijah** (Hebrew) Jehovah is my God
Elija, Eliyahu, Eljah, Elja, Elyjah, Elyja, Elijuah, Elyjuah

Elimu (African) Having knowledge of science
Elymu, Elimue, Elymue, Elimoo, Elymoo

Elisha (Hebrew) God is my salvation
Elisee, Eliseo, Elisher, Eliso, Elisio, Elysha, Elysee, Elyseo

Elliott (English) Form of Elijah, meaning "Jehovah is my God"
Eliot, Eliott, Elliot, Elyot

Ellory (Cornish) Resembling a swan
Ellorey, Elloree, Ellorea, Ellori, Ellorie, Elory, Elorey

Ellsworth (English) From
the nobleman's estate
*Elsworth, Ellswerth, Elswerth,
Ellswirth, Elswirth, Elzie*

Elman (English) A nobleman
Elmann, Ellman, Ellmann

Elmo (English / Latin) A
protector / an amiable man
Elmoe, Elmow, Elmowe

Elmot (American) A lovable man
Elmott, Ellmot, Ellmott

Elof (Swedish) The only heir
*Eluf, Eloff, Eluff, Elov, Ellov,
Eluv, Elluv*

Elois (German) A famous
warrior
Eloys, Eloyis, Elouis

Elpidio (Spanish) A fear-
less man; having heart
*Elpydio, Elpideo, Elpydeo,
Elpidios, Elpydios, Elpidius*

Elroy (Irish / English) A red-
haired young man / a king
*Elroi, Elroye, Elric, Elryc,
Elrik, Elryk, Elrick, Elryck*

Elston (English) From the
nobleman's town
*Ellston, Elstun, Ellstun,
Elson, Ellson, Elsun, Ellsun*

Elton (English) From the
old town
*Ellton, Eltun, Elltun, Elten,
Ellten, Eltin, Elltin, Eltyn*

Eluwilussit (Native
American) A holy man

Elvey (English) An elf
warrior
*Elvy, Elvee, Elvea, Elvi,
Elvie*

Elvis (Scandinavian) One
who is wise
Elviss, Elvys, Elvyss

Elzie (English) Form of
Ellsworth, meaning "from
the nobleman's estate"
*Elzi, Elzy, Elzey, Elzee,
Elzea, Ellzi, Ellzie, Ellzee*

Emest (German) One who
is serious
*Emeste, Emesto, Emestio,
Emestiyo, Emesteo,
Emesteyo, Emo, Emst*

Emil (Latin) One who is
eager; an industrious man
*Emelen, Emelio, Emile,
Emilian, Emiliano,
Emilianus, Emilio, Emilion*

Emmanuel (Hebrew) God
is with us
*Manuel, Manny, Em,
Eman, Emmannuel*

Emmett (German) A uni-
versal man
*Emmet, Emmit, Emmitt,
Emmot*

Emrys (Welsh) An immortal man

Enapay (Native American) A brave man
Enapaye, Enapai, Enapae

Enar (Swedish) A great warrior
Ener, Enir, Enyr, Enor, Enur

Engelbert (German) As bright as an angel
Englebert, Englbert, Engelburt, Engleburt, Englburt, Englebirt, Engelbirt, Englbirt

Enoch (Hebrew) One who is dedicated to God
Enoc, Enok, Enock

Enrique (Spanish) The ruler of the estate
Enrico, Enriko, Enricko, Enriquez, Enrikay, Enreekay, Enrik, Enric

Enyeto (Native American) One who walks like a bear

Enzo (Italian) The ruler of the estate
Enzio, Enzeo, Enziyo, Enzeyo

Eoin Baiste (Irish) Refers to John the Baptist

Ephraim (Hebrew) One who is fertile; productive
Eff, Efraim, Efram, Efrem, Efrain

•Eric (Scandinavian) Ever the ruler
Erek, Erich, Erick, Erik, Eriq, Erix, Errick, Eryk

Ernest (English) One who is sincere and determined; serious
Earnest, Ernesto, Ernestus, Ernst, Erno, Ernie, Erni, Erney

Eron (Spanish) Form of Aaron, meaning "one who is exalted"
Erun, Erin, Eran, Eren, Eryn

Errigal (Gaelic) From the small church
Errigel, Errigol, Errigul, Errigil, Errigyl, Erigal, Erigel, Erigol

Erskine (Gaelic) From the high cliff
Erskin, Erskyne, Erskyn, Erskein, Erskeine, Erskien, Erskiene

Esam (Arabic) A safeguard
Essam

Esben (Scandinavian) Of God
Esbin, Esbyn, Esban, Esbon, Esbun

Esmé (French) One who is esteemed
Esmay, Esmaye, Esmai, Esmae, Esmeling, Esmelyng

Esmun (American) A kind man
Esmon, Esman, Esmen, Esmin, Esmyn

Esperanze (Spanish) Filled with hope
Esperance, Esperence, Esperenze, Esperanzo, Esperenzo

Estcott (English) From the eastern cottage
Estcot

Esteban (Spanish) One who is crowned in victory
Estebon, Estevan, Estevon, Estefan, Estefon, Estebe, Estyban, Estyvan

*ᴛ**Ethan** (Hebrew) One who is firm and steadfast
Ethen, Ethin, Ethyn, Ethon, Ethun, Eitan, Etan, Eithan

Ethanael (American) God has given me strength
Ethaniel, Ethaneal, Ethanail, Ethanale

Ethel (Hebrew) One who is noble
Ethal, Etheal

Etlelooaat (Native American) One who shouts

Eudocio (Greek) One who is respected
Eudoceo, Eudociyo, Eudoceyo, Eudoco

***Eugene** (Greek) A wellborn man
*Eugean, Eugenie, Ugene, Efigenio, Gene, **Owen***

Eulogio (Greek) A reasonable man
Eulogiyo, Eulogo, Eulogeo, Eulogeyo

Euodias (Greek) Having good fortune
Euodeas, Euodyas

Euphemios (Greek) One who is well-spoken
Eufemio, Eufemius, Euphemio, Eufemios, Euphemius, Eufemius

Euphrates (Turkish) From the great river
Eufrates, Euphraites, Eufraites, Euphraytes, Eufraytes

Eusebius (Greek) One who is devout
Esabio, Esavio, Esavius, Esebio, Eusabio, Eusaio, Eusebio, Eusebios

Eustace (Greek) Having an abundance of grapes
Eustache, Eustachios, Eustachius, Eustachy, Eustaquio, Eustashe, Eustasius, Eustatius

***Evan** (Welsh) Form of John, meaning "God is gracious"
Evann, Evans, Even, Evin, Evon, Evyn, Evian, Evien

Evander (Greek) A benevolent man
Evandor, Evandar, Evandir, Evandur, Evandyr

Evers (English) Resembling a wild boar
Ever, Evert, Everte

Evett (American) A bright
man
*Evet, Evatt, Evat, Evitt,
Evit, Evytt, Evyt*

Eyal (Hebrew) Having
great strength

Eze (African) A king

Ezeji (African) The king of
yams
*Ezejie, Ezejy, Ezejey, Ezejee,
Ezejea*

Ezekiel (Hebrew)
Strengthened by God
*Esequiel, Ezechiel,
Eziechiele, Eziequel,
Ezequiel, Ezekial, Ezekyel,
Esquevelle, Zeke*

f

Factor (English) A busi-
nessman
*Facter, Factur, Factir,
Factyr, Factar*

Fairbairn (Scottish) A fair-
haired boy
*Fayrbairn, Faerbairn,
Fairbaern, Fayrbaern,
Faerbaern, Fairbayrn,
Fayrbayrn, Faerbayrn*

Fairbanks (English) From
the bank along the path
*Fayrbanks, Faerbanks,
Farebanks*

Faisal (Arabic) One who is
decisive; resolute
*Faysal, Faesal, Fasal,
Feisal, Faizal, Fusel,
Fayzal, Faezal*

Fakhir (Arabic) A proud
man
*Fakheer, Fakhear, Fakheir,
Fakhier, Fakhyr, Faakhir,
Faakhyr, Fakhr*

Fakih (Arabic) A legal
expert
*Fakeeh, Fakeah, Fakieh,
Fakeih, Fakyh*

Falco (Latin) Resembling
a falcon; one who works
with falcons
*Falcon, Falconer,
Falconner, Falk, Falke,
Falken, Falkner, Faulconer*

Fam (American) A family-
oriented man

Fang (Scottish) From the
sheep pen
Faing, Fayng, Faeng

Faraji (African) One who
provides consolation
*Farajie, Farajy, Farajey,
Farajee, Farajea*

Fardoragh (Irish) Having
dark features

Fargo (American) One who is jaunty
Fargoh, Fargoe, Fargouh

Farha (Arabic) Filled with happiness
Farhah, Farhad, Farhan, Farhat, Farhani, Farhanie, Farhany, Farhaney

Fariq (Arabic) One who holds rank as lieutenant general
Fareeq, Fareaq, Fareiq, Farieq, Faryq, Farik, Fareek, Fareak

Farnell (English) From the fern hill
Farnel, Farnall, Farnal, Fernauld, Farnauld, Fernald, Farnald

Farold (English) A mighty traveler
Farould, Farald, Farauld, Fareld

Farran (Irish / Arabic / English) Of the land / a baker / one who is adventurous
Fairran, Fayrran, Faerran, Farren, Farrin, Farron, Ferrin, Ferron

Farrar (English) A blacksmith
Farar, Farrer, Farrier, Ferrar, Ferrars, Ferrer, Ferrier, Farer

Farro (Italian) Of the grain
Farroe, Faro, Faroe, Farrow, Farow

Fatik (Indian) Resembling a crystal
Fateek, Fateak, Fatyk, Fatiek, Fateik

Faust (Latin) Having good luck
Fauste, Faustino, Fausto, Faustos, Faustus, Fauston, Faustin, Fausten

Fawcett (American) An audacious man
Fawcet, Fawcette, Fawcete, Fawce, Fawci, Fawcie, Fawcy, Fawcey

Fawwaz (Arabic) A successful man
Fawaz, Fawwad, Fawad

Fay (Irish) Resembling a raven
Faye, Fai, Fae, Feich

Februus (Latin) A pagan god

Fedor (Russian) A gift from God
Faydor, Feodor, Fyodor, Fedyenka, Fyodr, Fydor, Fjodor

Feechi (African) One who worships God
Feechie, Feechy, Feechey, Feechee, Feachi, Feachie

Feivel (Hebrew) The brilliant one
Feival, Feivol, Feivil, Feivyl, Feivul, Feiwel, Feiwal, Feiwol

Felim (Gaelic) One who is always good
Felym, Feidhlim, Felimy, Felimey, Felimee, Felimea, Felimi, Felimie

Felipe (Spanish) Form of Phillip, meaning "one who loves horses"
Felippe, Filip, Filippo, Fillip, Flip, Fulop, Fullop, Fulip

Felix (Latin) One who is happy and prosperous

Felton (English) From the town near the field
Feltun, Felten, Feltan, Feltyn, Feltin

Fenn (English) From the marsh
Fen

Ferdinand (German) A courageous voyager
Ferdie, Ferdinando, Fernando

Fergus (Gaelic) The first and supreme choice
Fearghas, Fearghus, Feargus, Fergie, Ferguson, Fergusson, Furgus, Fergy

Ferrell (Irish) A brave man; a hero
Ferell, Ferel, Ferrel

Fiacre (Celtic) Resembling a raven
Fyacre, Fiacra, Fyacra, Fiachra, Fyachra, Fiachre, Fyachre

Fielding (English) From the field
Fieldyng, Fielder, Field, Fielde, Felding, Feldyng, Fields

Fiero (Spanish) A fiery man
Fyero

Finbar (Irish) A fair-haired man
Finnbar, Finnbarr, Fionn, Fionnbharr, Fionnbar, Fionnbarr, Fynbar, Fynnbar

Finch (English) Resembling the small bird
Fynch, Finche, Fynche, Finchi, Finchie, Finchy, Finchey, Finchee

Fineas (Egyptian) A dark-skinned man
Fyneas, Finius, Fynius

Finian (Irish) A handsome man; fair
Finan, Finnian, Fionan, Finien, Finnien, Finghin, Finneen, Fineen

Finnley (Gaelic) A fair-haired hero
Findlay, Findley, Finly, Finlay, Finlee, Finnly, Finnley

Finn (Gaelic) A fair-haired man
Fin, Fynn, Fyn, Fingal, Fingall

Finnegan (Irish) A fair-haired man
Finegan, Finnegen, Finegen, Finnigan, Finigan

Fiorello (Italian) Resembling a little flower
Fiorelo, Fiorelio, Fioreleo, Fiorellio, Fiorelleo

Fisher (English) a fisherman
Fischer, Fysher

Fitch (English) Resembling an ermine
Fytch, Fich, Fych, Fitche, Fytche

Fitzgerald (English) The son of Gerald
Fytzgerald

Flann (Irish) One who has a ruddy complexion
Flan, Flainn, Flannan, Flannery, Flanneri, Flannerie, Flannerey

Fletcher (English) One who makes arrows
Fletch, Fletche, Flecher

Flynn (Irish) One who has a ruddy complexion
Flyn, Flinn, Flin, Flen, Flenn, Floinn

Fogarty (Irish) One who has been exiled
Fogartey, Fogartee, Fogartea, Fogarti, Fogartie, Fogerty, Fogertey, Fogerti

Foley (English) A creative man
Foly, Folee, Foli, Folie

Folker (German) A guardian of the people
Folkar, Folkor, Folkur, Folkir, Folkyr, Folke, Folko, Folkus

Fonso (German) Form of Alfonso, meaning "prepared for battle; eager and ready"
Fonzo, Fonsie, Fonzell, Fonzie, Fonsi, Fonsy, Fonsey, Fonsee

Fontaine (French) From the water source
Fontayne, Fontaene, Fontane, Fonteyne, Fontana, Fountain

Ford (English) From the river crossing
Forde, Forden, Fordan, Fordon, Fordun, Fordin, Fordyn, Forday

Fouad (Arabic) One who has heart
Fuad

Francisco (Spanish) A man from France
Francesco, Franchesco, Fransisco

Frank (Latin) Form of Francis, meaning "a man from France; one who is free."
Franco, Frankie

Fred (German) Form of Frederick, meaning "a peaceful ruler"
Freddi, Freddie, Freddy, Freddey, Freddee, Freddea, Freddis, Fredis

Frederick (German) A peaceful ruler
Fred, Fredrick, Federico, Federigo, Fredek, Frederic, Frederich, Frederico, Frederik, Fredric

Freeborn (English) One who was born a free man
Freeborne, Freebourn, Freebourne, Freeburn, Freeburne, Free

Fremont (French) The protector of freedom
Freemont, Fremonte

Frigyes (Hungarian) A mighty and peaceful ruler

Frode (Norse) A wise man
Froad, Froade

Froyim (Hebrew) A kind man
Froiim

Fructuoso (Spanish) One who is fruitful
Fructo, Fructoso, Fructuso

Fu (Chinese) A wealthy man

Fudail (Arabic) Of high moral character
Fudaile, Fudayl, Fudayle, Fudale, Fudael, Fudaele

Fulbright (English) A brilliant man
Fullbright, Fulbrite, Fullbrite, Fulbryte, Fullbryte, Fulbert, Fullbert

Fulki (Indian) A spark
Fulkie, Fulkey, Fulky, Fulkee, Fulkea

Fullerton (English) From Fuller's town
Fullertun, Fullertin, Fullertyn, Fullertan, Fullerten

Fursey (Gaelic) The name of a missionary saint
Fursy, Fursi, Fursie, Fursee, Fursea

Fyfe (Scottish) A man from Fifeshire
Fife, Fyffe, Fiffe, Fibh

Fyren (Anglo-Saxon) A wicked man
Fyrin, Fyryn, Fyran, Fyron, Fyrun

g

Gabai (Hebrew) A delightful man

Gabbana (Italian) A creative man
Gabbanah, Gabana, Gabanah, Gabbanna, Gabanna

Gabbo (English) To joke or scoff
Gabboe, Gabbow, Gabbowe

Gabor (Hebrew) God is my strength
Gabur, Gabar, Gaber, Gabir, Gabyr

Gabra (African) An offering
Gabre

*ᵀ**Gabriel** (Hebrew) A hero of God
Gabrian, Gabriele, Gabrielli, Gabriello, Gaby, Gab, Gabbi, Gabbie

Gad (Hebrew / Native American) Having good fortune / from the juniper tree
Gadi, Gadie, Gady, Gadey, Gadee, Gadea

Gadiel (Arabic) God is my fortune
Gadiell, Gadiele, Gadielle, Gaddiel, Gaddiell, Gadil, Gadeel, Gadeal

Gaffney (Irish) Resembling a calf
Gaffny, Gaffni, Gaffnie, Gaffnee, Gaffnea

Gage (French) Of the pledge
Gaige, Gaege, Gauge

Gahuj (African) A hunter

Gair (Gaelic) A man of short stature
Gayr, Gaer, Gaire, Gayre, Gaere, Gare

Gaius (Latin) One who rejoices
Gaeus

Galal (Arabic) A majestic man
Galall, Gallal, Gallall

Galbraith (Irish) A foreigner; a Scot
Galbrait, Galbreath, Gallbrait, Gallbreath, Galbraithe, Gallbraithe, Galbreathe, Gallbreathe

Gale (Irish / English) A foreigner / one who is cheerful
Gail, Gaill, Gaille, Gaile, Gayl, Gayle, Gaylle, Gayll

Galen (Greek) A healer; one who is calm
Gaelan, Gaillen, Galan, Galin, Galyn, Gaylen, Gaylin, Gaylinn

Gali (Hebrew) From the
fountain
*Galie, Galy, Galey, Galee,
Galea, Galeigh*

Galip (Turkish) A victori-
ous man
*Galyp, Galup, Galep,
Galap, Galop*

Gallagher (Gaelic) An
eager helper
*Gallaghor, Gallaghar,
Gallaghur, Gallaghir,
Gallaghyr, Gallager,
Gallagar, Gallagor*

Galt (English) From the
high, wooded land
Galte, Gallt, Gallte

Galtero (Spanish) Form
of Walter, meaning "the
commander of the army"
*Galterio, Galteriyo,
Galtereo, Galtereyo,
Galter, Galteros, Galterus,
Gualterio*

Gamaliel (Hebrew) God's
reward
*Gamliel, Gamalyel,
Gamlyel, Gamli, Gamlie,
Gamly, Gamley, Gamlee*

Gameel (Arabic) A hand-
some man
*Gameal, Gamil, Gamiel,
Gameil, Gamyl*

Gamon (American) One
who enjoys playing games
*Gamun, Gamen, Gaman,
Gamin, Gamyn, Gammon,
Gammun, Gamman*

Gan (Chinese) A wanderer

Gandy (American) An
adventurer
*Gandey, Gandi, Gandie,
Gandee, Gandea*

Gann (English) One who
defends with a spear
Gan

Gannon (Gaelic) A fair-
skinned man
*Gannun, Gannen,
Gannan, Gannin, Gannyn,
Ganon, Ganun, Ganin*

Garcia (Spanish) One who
is brave in battle
*Garce, Garcy, Garcey, Garci,
Garcie, Garcee, Garcea*

Gared (English) Form of
Gerard, meaning "one
who is mighty with a
spear"
*Garad, Garid, Garyd,
Garod, Garud*

Garman (English) A spear-
man
*Garmann, Garmen,
Garmin, Garmon,
Garmun, Garmyn, Gar,
Garr*

Garrison (French) Prepared
Garris, Garrish, Garry, Gary

Garrett (English) Form of Gerard, meaning "one who is mighty with a spear"
Garett, Garret, Garretson, Garritt, Garrot, Garrott, Gerrit, Gerritt

Garson (English) The son of Gar (Garrett, Garrison, etc.)
Garrson, Garsen, Garrsen, Garsun, Garrsun, Garsone, Garrsone

Garth (Scandinavian) The keeper of the garden
Garthe, Gart, Garte

Garvey (Gaelic) A rough but peaceful man
Garvy, Garvee, Garvea, Garvi, Garvie, Garrvey, Garrvy, Garrvee

Garvin (English) A friend with a spear
Garvyn, Garven, Garvan, Garvon, Garvun

Gary (English) One who wields a spear
Garey, Gari, Garie, Garea, Garee, Garry, Garrey, Garree

Gassur (Arabic) A courageous man
Gassor, Gassir, Gassyr, Gassar, Gasser

Gaston (French) A man from Gascony
Gastun, Gastan, Gasten, Gascon, Gascone, Gasconey, Gasconi, Gasconie

Gate (American) One who is close-minded
Gates, Gait, Gaite, Gaits

⋅**Gavin** (Welsh) A little white falcon
Gavan, Gaven, Gavino, Gavyn, Gavynn, Gavon, Gavun, Gavyno

Gazali (African) A mystic
Gazalie, Gazaly, Gazaley, Gazalee, Gazalea, Gazaleigh

Geirleif (Norse) A descendant of the spear
Geirleaf, Geerleif, Geerleaf

Geirstein (Norse) One who wields a rock-hard spear
Geerstein, Gerstein

Gellert (Hungarian) A mighty soldier
Gellart, Gellirt, Gellyrt, Gellort, Gellurt

Genaro (Latin) A dedicated man
Genaroh, Genaroe, Genarow, Genarowe

Gene (English) Form of Eugene, meaning "a well-born man"
Genio, Geno, Geneo, Gino, Ginio, Gineo

Genet (African) From Eden
Genat, Genit, Genyt, Genot, Genut

Genoah (Italian) From the
city of Genoa
Genoa, Genovise, Genovize

Geoffrey (English) Form
of Jeffrey, meaning "a
man of peace"
*Geffrey, Geoff, Geoffery,
Geoffroy, Geoffry, Geofrey,
Geofferi, Geofferie*

George (Greek) One who
works the earth; a farmer
*Georas, Geordi, Geordie,
Georg, Georges, Georgi,
Georgie, Georgio, Yegor,
Jurgen, Joren*

Gerald (German) One who
rules with the spear
*Jerald, Garald, Garold,
Gearalt, Geralde, Geraldo,
Geraud, Gere, Gerek*

Gerard (French) One who
is mighty with a spear
*Gerord, Gerrard, Gared,
Garrett*

Geremia (Italian) Form of
Jeremiah, meaning "one
who is exalted by the Lord"
*Geremiah, Geremias,
Geremija, Geremiya,
Geremyah, Geramiah,
Geramia*

Germain (French / Latin)
A man from Germany /
one who is brotherly
*Germaine, German,
Germane, Germanicus,
Germano, Germanus,
Germayn, Germayne*

Gerry (German) Short
form of names beginning
with Ger-, such as Gerald
or Gerard
*Gerrey, Gerri, Gerrie,
Gerrea, Gerree*

Gershom (Hebrew) One
who has been exiled
*Gersham, Gershon,
Gershoom, Gershem,
Gershim, Gershym,
Gershum, Gersh*

Getachew (African) Their
master

Ghazi (Arabic) An invader;
a conqueror
*Ghazie, Ghazy, Ghazey,
Ghazee, Ghazea*

Ghoukas (Armenian)
Form of Lucas, meaning
"a man from Lucania"
Ghukas

Giancarlo (Italian) One
who is gracious and mighty
Gyancarlo

Gideon (Hebrew) A mighty
warrior; one who fells trees
*Gideone, Gidi, Gidon,
Gidion, Gid, Gidie, Gidy,
Gidey*

Gilam (Hebrew) The joy of
the people
*Gylam, Gilem, Gylem,
Gilim, Gylim, Gilym,
Gylym, Gilom*

Gilbert (French / English)
Of the bright promise /
one who is trustworthy
*Gib, Gibb, Gil, Gilberto,
Gilburt, Giselbert,
Giselberto, Giselbertus*

Gildas (Irish / English)
One who serves God / the
golden one
*Gyldas, Gilda, Gylda, Gilde,
Gylde, Gildea, Gyldea,
Gildes*

Giles (Greek) Resembling
a young goat
*Gyles, Gile, Gil, Gilles,
Gillis, Gilliss, Gyle, Gyl*

Gill (Gaelic) A servant
*Gyll, Gilly, Gilley, Gillee,
Gillea, Gilli, Gillie, Ghill*

Gillivray (Scottish) A servant of God
Gillivraye, Gillivrae, Gillivrai

Gilmat (Scottish) One who
wields a sword
Gylmat, Gilmet, Gylmet

Gilmer (English) A famous
hostage
*Gilmar, Gilmor, Gilmur,
Gilmir, Gilmyr, Gillmer,
Gillmar, Gillmor*

Gilon (Hebrew) Filled with
joy
*Gilun, Gilen, Gilan, Gilin,
Gilyn, Gilo*

Ginton (Arabic) From the
garden
*Gintun, Gintan, Ginten,
Gintin, Gintyn*

Giovanni (Italian) Form
of John, meaning "God is
gracious"
*Geovani, Geovanney,
Geovanni, Geovanny,
Geovany, Giannino,
Giovan, Giovani, Yovanny*

Giri (Indian) From the
mountain
*Girie, Giry, Girey, Giree,
Girea*

Girvan (Gaelic) The small
rough one
*Gyrvan, Girven, Gyrven,
Girvin, Gyrvin, Girvyn,
Gyrvyn, Girvon*

Giulio (Italian) One who is
youthful
Giuliano, Giuleo

Giuseppe (Italian) Form
of Joseph, meaning "God
will add"
*Giuseppi, Giuseppie,
Giuseppy, Giuseppee,
Giuseppea, Giuseppey,
Guiseppe, Guiseppi*

Gizmo (American) One
who is playful
*Gismo, Gyzmo, Gysmo,
Gizmoe, Gismoe, Gyzmoe,
Gysmoe*

Glade (English) From the clearing in the woods
Glayd, Glayde, Glaid, Glaide, Glaed, Glaede

Glaisne (Irish) One who is calm; serene
Glaisny, Glaisney, Glaisni, Glaisnie, Glaisnee, Glasny, Glasney, Glasni

Glasgow (Scottish) From the city in Scotland
Glasgo

Glen (Gaelic) From the secluded narrow valley
Glenn, Glennard, Glennie, Glennon, Glenny, Glin, Glinn, Glyn

Glover (English) One who makes gloves
Glovar, Glovir, Glovyr, Glovur, Glovor

Gobind (Sanskrit) The cow finder
Gobinde, Gobinda, Govind, Govinda, Govinde

Goby (American) An audacious man
Gobi, Gobie, Gobey, Gobee, Gobea

Godfrey (German) God is peace
Giotto, Godefroi, Godfry, Godofredo, Goffredo, Gottfrid, Gottfried, Godfried

Godfried (German) God is peace
Godfreed, Gjord

Gogo (African) A grandfatherly man

Goldwin (English) A golden friend
Goldwine, Goldwinn, Goldwinne, Goldwen, Goldwenn, Goldwenne, Goldwyn, Goldwynn

Goode (English) An upstanding man
Good, Goodi, Goodie, Goody, Goodey, Goodee, Goodea

Gordon (Gaelic) From the great hill; a hero
Gorden, Gordin, Gordyn, Gordun, Gordan, Gordi, Gordie, Gordee

Gormley (Irish) The blue spearman
Gormly, Gormlee, Gormlea, Gormleah, Gormleigh, Gormli, Gormlie, Gormaly

Goro (Japanese) The fifth-born child

Gotzon (Basque) A heavenly messenger; an angel

Gower (Welsh) One who is pure; chaste
Gwyr, Gowyr, Gowir, Gowar, Gowor, Gowur

Gozal (Hebrew)
Resembling a baby bird
*Gozall, Gozel, Gozell,
Gozale, Gozele*

^**Grady** (Gaelic) One who
is famous; noble
*Gradey, Gradee, Gradea,
Gradi, Gradie, Graidy,
Graidey, Graidee*

^**Graham** (English) From
the gravelled area; from
the gray home
Graem

Grand (English) A supe-
rior man
*Grande, Grandy, Grandey,
Grandi, Grandie, Grandee,
Grandea, Grander*

Granger (English) A farmer
*Grainger, Graynger,
Graenger, Grange, Graynge,
Graenge, Grainge, Grangere*

Grant (English) A tall
man; a great man
Grante, Graent

Granville (French) From
the large village
*Granvylle, Granvil,
Granvyl, Granvill,
Granvyll, Granvile,
Granvyle, Grenvill*

Gray (English) A gray-
haired man
*Graye, Grai, Grae, Greye,
Grey, Graylon, Graylen,
Graylin*

Grayson (English) The son
of a gray-haired man
*Graysen, Graysun, Graysin,
Greyson, Graysan, Graison,
Graisun, Graisen*

Greenwood (English)
From the green forest
Greenwode

Gregory (Greek) One who
is vigilant; watchful
*Greg, Greggory, Greggy,
Gregori, Gregorie, Gregry,
Grigori*

Gremian (Anglo-Saxon)
One who enrages others
*Gremien, Gremean,
Gremyan*

Gridley (English) From the
flat meadow
*Gridly, Gridlee, Gridlea,
Gridleah, Gridleigh, Gridli,
Gridlie*

Griffin (Latin) Having a
hooked nose
*Griff, Griffen, Griffon,
Gryffen, Gryffin, Gryphen*

Griffith (Welsh) A mighty
chief
Griffyth, Gryffith, Gryffyth

Grimsley (English) From
the dark meadow
*Grimsly, Grimslee, Grimslea,
Grimsleah, Grimsleigh,
Grimsli, Grimslie*

Griswold (German) From the gray forest
Griswald, Gryswold, Gryswald, Greswold, Greswald

Guban (African) One who has been burnt
Guhen, Gubin, Gubyn, Gubon, Gubun

Guedado (African) One who is unwanted

Guerdon (English) A warring man
Guerdun, Guerdan, Guerden, Guerdin, Guerdyn

Guido (Italian) One who acts as a guide
Guidoh, Gwedo, Gwido, Gwydo, Gweedo

Guillaume (French) Form of William, meaning "the determined protector"
Gillermo, Guglielmo, Guilherme, Guillermo, Gwillyn, Gwilym, Guglilmo

Gulshan (Hindi) From the gardens

Gunnar (Scandinavian) A bold warrior
Gunner, Gunnor, Gunnur, Gunnir, Gunnyr

Gunnolf (Norse) A warrior wolf
Gunolf, Gunnulf, Gunulf

Gur (Hebrew) Resembling a lion cub
Guryon, Gurion, Guriel, Guriell, Guryel, Guryell, Guri, Gurie

Gurpreet (Indian) A devoted follower
Gurpreat, Gurpriet, Gurpreit, Gurprit, Gurpryt

Guru (Indian) A teacher; a religious head

Gurutz (Basque) Of the holy cross
Guruts

Gus (German) A respected man; one who is exalted
Guss

Gustav (Scandinavian) Of the staff of the gods
Gus, Gustave, Gussie, Gustaf, Gustof, Tavin

Gusty (American) Of the wind; a revered man
Gustey, Gustee, Gustea, Gusti, Gustie, Gusto

Guwayne (American) Form of Wayne, meaning "one who builds wagons"
Guwayn, Guwain, Guwaine, Guwaen, Guwaene, Guwane

Gwalchmai (Welsh) A battle hawk

Gwandoya (African) Suffering a miserable fate

Gwydion (Welsh) In mythology, a magician
Gwydeon, Gwydionne, Gwydeonne

Gylfi (Scandinavian) A king
Gylfie, Gylfee, Gylfea, Gylfi, Gylfie, Gylphi, Gylphie, Gylphey

Gypsy (English) A wanderer; a nomad
Gipsee, Gipsey, Gipsy, Gypsi, Gypsie, Gypsey, Gypsee, Gipsi

h

Habimama (African) One who believes in God
Habymama

Hadden (English) From the heather-covered hill
Haddan, Haddon, Haddin, Haddyn, Haddun

Hadriel (Hebrew) The splendor of God
Hadryel, Hadriell, Hadryell

Hadwin (English) A friend in war
Hadwinn, Hadwinne, Hadwen, Hadwenn, Hadwenne, Hadwyn, Hadwynn, Hadwynne

Hafiz (Arabic) A protector
Haafiz, Hafeez, Hafeaz, Hafiez, Hafeiz, Hafyz, Haphiz, Haaphiz

Hagar (Hebrew) A wanderer

Hagen (Gaelic) One who is youthful
Haggen, Hagan, Haggan, Hagin, Haggin, Hagyn, Haggyn, Hagon

Hagop (Armenian) Form of James, meaning "he who supplants"
Hagup, Hagap, Hagep, Hagip, Hagyp

Hagos (African) Filled with happiness

Hahnee (Native American) A beggar
Hahnea, Hahni, Hahnie, Hahny, Hahney

Haim (Hebrew) A giver of live
Hayim, Hayyim

Haines (English) From the vined cottage; from the hedged enclosure
Haynes, Haenes, Hanes, Haine, Hayne, Haene, Hane

Hajari (African) One who takes flight
Hajarie, Hajary, Hajarey, Hajaree, Hajarea

Haji (African) Born during the hajj
Hajie, Hajy, Hajey, Hajee, Hajea

Hakan (Norse / Native American) One who is noble / a fiery man

Hakim (Arabic) One who is wise; intelligent
Hakeem, Hakeam, Hakeim, Hakiem, Hakym

Hal (English) A form of Henry, meaning "the ruler of the house"; a form of Harold, meaning "the ruler of an army"

Halford (English) From the hall by the ford
Hallford, Halfurd, Hallfurd, Halferd, Hallferd

Halil (Turkish) A beloved friend
Haleel, Haleal, Haleil, Haliel, Halyl

Halla (African) An unexpected gift
Hallah, Hala, Halah

Hallberg (Norse) From the rocky mountain
Halberg, Hallburg, Halburg

Halle (Norse) As solid as a rock

Halley (English) From the hall near the meadow
Hally, Halli, Hallie, Halleigh, Hallee, Halleah, Hallea

Halliwell (English) From the holy spring
Haligwell

Hallward (English) The guardian of the hall
Halward, Hallwerd, Halwerd, Hallwarden, Halwarden, Hawarden, Haward, Hawerd

Hamid (Arabic / Indian) A praiseworthy man / a beloved friend
Hameed, Hamead, Hameid, Hamied, Hamyd, Haamid

Hamidi (Swahili) One who is commendable
Hamidie, Hamidy, Hamidey, Hamidee, Hamidea, Hamydi, Hamydie, Hamydee

Hamilton (English) From the flat-topped hill
Hamylton, Hamiltun, Hamyltun, Hamilten, Hamylten, Hamelton, Hameltun, Hamelten

Hamlet (German) From the little home
Hamlett, Hammet, Hammett, Hamnet, Hamnett, Hamlit, Hamlitt, Hamoelet

Hammer (German) One who makes hammers; a carpenter
Hammar, Hammor, Hammur, Hammir, Hammyr

Hampden (English) From the home in the valley
Hampdon, Hampdan, Hampdun, Hampdyn, Hampdin

Hancock (English) One who owns a farm
Hancok, Hancoc

Hanford (English) From the high ford
Hanferd, Hanfurd, Hanforde, Hanferde, Hanfurde

Hanisi (Swahili) Born on a Thursday
Hanisie, Hanisy, Hanisey, Hanisee, Hanisea, Hanysi, Hanysie, Hanysy

Hank (English) Form of Henry, meaning "the ruler of the house"
Hanke, Hanks, Hanki, Hankie, Hankee, Hankea, Hanky, Hankey

Hanley (English) From the high meadow
Hanly, Hanleigh, Hanleah, Hanlea, Hanlie, Hanli

Hanoch (Hebrew) One who is dedicated
Hanock, Hanok, Hanoc

Hanraoi (Irish) Form of Henry, meaning "the ruler of the house"

Hansraj (Hindi) The swan king

Hardik (Indian) One who has heart
Hardyk, Hardick, Hardyck, Hardic, Hardyc

Hare (English) Resembling a rabbit

Harence (English) One who is swift
Harince, Harense, Harinse

Hari (Indian) Resembling a lion
Harie, Hary, Harey, Haree, Harea

Harim (Arabic) A superior man
Hareem, Haream, Hariem, Hareim, Harym

Harkin (Irish) Having dark red hair
Harkyn, Harken, Harkan, Harkon, Harkun

Harlemm (American) A soulful man
Harlam, Harlom, Harlim, Harlym, Harlem

Harlow (English) From the army on the hill
Harlowe, Harlo, Harloe

Harold (Scandinavian) The ruler of an army
Hal, Harald, Hareld, Harry, Darold

Harper (English) One who plays or makes harps
Harpur, Harpar, Harpir, Harpyr, Harpor, Hearpere

Harrington (English) From of Harry's town; from the herring town
Harringtun, Harryngton, Harryngtun, Harington, Haringtun, Haryngton, Haryntun

Harrison (English) The son of Harry
Harrisson, Harris, Harriss, Harryson

Harshad (Indian) A bringer of joy
Harsh, Harshe, Harsho, Harshil, Harshyl, Harshit, Harshyt

Hartford (English) From the stag's ford
Harteford, Hartferd, Harteferd, Hartfurd, Hartefurd, Hartforde, Harteforde, Hartferde

Haru (Japanese) Born during the spring

Harvey (English / French) One who is ready for battle / a strong man
Harvy, Harvi, Harvie, Harvee, Harvea, Harv, Harve, Hervey

Hasim (Arabic) One who is decisive
Haseem, Haseam, Hasiem, Haseim, Hasym

Haskel (Hebrew) An intelligent man
Haskle, Haskell, Haskil, Haskill, Haske, Hask

Hasso (German) Of the sun
Hassoe, Hassow, Hassowe

Hassun (Native American) As solid as a stone

Hastiin (Native American) A man

Hastin (Hindi) Resembling an elephant
Hasteen, Hastean, Hastien, Hastein, Hastyn

Hawes (English) From the hedged place
Haws, Hayes, Hays, Hazin, Hazen, Hazyn, Hazon, Hazan

Hawiovi (Native American) One who descends on a ladder
Hawiovie, Hawiovy, Hawiovey, Hawiovee, Hawiovea

Hawkins (English) Resembling a small hawk
Haukins, Hawkyns, Haukyn

Hawthorne (English) From the hawthorn tree
Hawthorn

*ᴛ**Hayden** (English) From the hedged valley
Haydan, Haydon, Haydun, Haydin, Haydyn, Haden, Hadan, Hadon

Haye (Scottish) From the stockade
Hay, Hae, Hai

Hazaiah (Hebrew) God will decide
Hazaia, Haziah, Hazia

Hazleton (English) From the hazel tree town
Hazelton, Hazletun, Hazelton, Hazleten, Hazelten

Heath (English) From the untended land of flowering shrubs
Heathe, Heeth, Heethe

Heaton (English) From the town on high ground
Heatun, Heeton, Heetun, Heaten, Heeten

Heber (Hebrew) A partner or companion
Heeber, Hebar, Heebar, Hebor, Heebor, Hebur, Heebur, Hebir

Hector (Greek) One who is steadfast; in mythology, the prince of Troy
Hecter, Hekter, Heckter

Helio (Greek) Son of the sun
Heleo, Helios, Heleos

Hem (Indian) The golden son

Hemendu (Indian) Born beneath the golden moon
Hemendue, Hemendoo

Hemi (Maori) Form of James, meaning "he who supplants"
Hemie, Hemy, Hemee, Hemea, Hemey

Henderson (Scottish) The son of Henry
Hendrie, Hendries, Hendron, Hendri, Hendry, Hendrey, Hendree, Hendrea

Hendrick (English) Form of Henry, meaning "the ruler of the house"
Hendryck, Hendrik, Hendryk, Hendric, Hendryc

Henley (English) From the high meadow
Henly, Henleigh, Henlea, Henleah, Henlee, Henli, Henlie

*Henry (German) The ruler of the house
Hal, Hank, Harry, Henny, Henree, Henri, Hanraoi, Hendrick

Heraldo (Spanish) Of the divine

Hercules (Greek) In mythology, a son of Zeus who possessed superhuman strength
Herakles, Hercule, Herculi, Herculie, Herculy, Herculey, Herculee

Herman (German) A soldier
Hermon, Hermen, Hermun, Hermin, Hermyn, Hermann, Hermie

Herne (English) Resembling a heron
Hern, Hearn, Hearne

Hero (Greek) The brave defender
Heroe, Herow, Herowe

Hershel (Hebrew) Resembling a deer
Hersch, Herschel, Herschell, Hersh, Hertzel, Herzel, Herzl, Heschel

Herwin (Teutonic) A friend of war
Herwinn, Herwinne, Herwen, Herwenn, Herwenne, Herwyn, Herwynn, Herwynne

Hesed (Hebrew) A kind man

Hesutu (Native American) A rising yellow-jacket nest
Hesutou, Hesoutou

Hewson (English) The son of Hugh
Hewsun

Hiawatha (Native American) He who makes rivers
Hiawathah, Hyawatha, Hiwatha, Hywatha

Hickok (American) A famous frontier marshal
Hickock, Hickoc, Hikock, Hikoc, Hikok, Hyckok, Hyckock, Hyckoc

Hidalgo (Spanish) The noble one
Hydalgo

Hideaki (Japanese) A clever man; having wisdom
Hideakie, Hideaky, Hideakey, Hideakee, Hideakea

Hieronim (Polish) Form of Jerome, meaning "of the sacred name"
Hieronym, Hieronymos, Hieronimos, Heronim, Heronym, Heronymos, Heronimos

Hietamaki (Finnish) From
the sand hill
*Hietamakie, Hietamaky,
Hietamakey, Hietamakee,
Hietamakea*

Hieu (Vietnamese) A
pious man

Hikmat (Islamic) Filled
with wisdom
Hykmat

Hildefuns (German) One
who is ready for battle
*Hildfuns, Hyldefuns,
Hyldfuns*

Hillel (Hebrew) One who
is praised
*Hyllel, Hillell, Hyllell, Hilel,
Hylel, Hilell, Hylell*

Hiranmay (Indian) The
golden one
*Hiranmaye, Hiranmai,
Hiranmae, Hyranmay,
Hyranmaye, Hyranmai,
Hyranmae*

Hiroshi (Japanese) A gen-
erous man
*Hiroshie, Hiroshy,
Hiroshey, Hiroshee,
Hiroshea, Hyroshi,
Hyroshie, Hyroshey*

Hirsi (African) An amulet
*Hirsie, Hirsy, Hirsey,
Hirsee, Hirsea*

Hisoka (Japanese) One
who is secretive
*Hysoka, Hisokie, Hysokie,
Hisoki, Hysoki, Hisokey,
Hysokey, Hisoky*

Hitakar (Indian) One who
wishes others well
Hitakarin, Hitakrit

Hobart (American) Form
of Hubert, meaning "hav-
ing a shining intellect"
*Hobarte, Hoebart,
Hoebarte, Hobert, Hoberte,
Hoburt, Hoburte, Hobirt*

Hohberht (German) One
who is high and bright
*Hohbert, Hohburt, Hohbirt,
Hohbyrt, Hoh*

Holcomb (English) From
the deep valley
Holcom, Holcombe

Holden (English) From a
hollow in the valley
Holdan, Holdyn, Holdon

Holland (American) From
the Netherlands
*Hollend, Hollind, Hollynd,
Hollande, Hollende,
Hollinde, Hollynde*

Hollis (English) From the
holly tree
*Hollys, Holliss, Hollyss,
Hollace, Hollice, Holli,
Hollie, Holly*

Holman (English) A man from the valley
Holmann, Holmen, Holmin, Holmyn, Holmon, Holmun

Holt (English) From the forest
Holte, Holyt, Holyte, Holter, Holtur, Holtor, Holtur, Holtir

Honaw (Native American) Resembling a bear
Honawe, Honau

Hondo (African) A warring man
Hondoh, Honda, Hondah

Honesto (Spanish) One who is honest
Honestio, Honestiyo, Honesteo, Honesteyo, Honestoh

Honon (Native American) Resembling a bear
Honun, Honen, Honan, Honin, Honyn

Honovi (Native American) Having great strength
Honovie, Honovy, Honovey, Honovee, Honovea

Honza (Czech) A gift from God

Horsley (English) From the horse meadow
Horsly, Horslea, Horsleah, Horslee, Horsleigh, Horsli, Horslie

Horst (German) From the thicket
Horste, Horsten, Horstun, Horstin, Horstyn, Horston, Horstun, Horstman

Hoshi (Japanese) Resembling a star
Hoshiko, Hoshyko, Hoshie, Hoshee, Hoshea, Hoshy, Hoshey

Hototo (Native American) One who whistles; a warrior spirit that sings

Houston (Gaelic/English) From Hugh's town, from the town on the hill
Huston, Houstyn, Hustin, Husten, Hustin, Houstun

Howard (English) The guardian of the home
Howerd, Howord, Howurd, Howird, Howyrd, Howi, Howie, Howy

Howi (Native American) Resembling a turtle dove

Hrothgar (Anglo-Saxon) A king
Hrothgarr, Hrothegar, Hrothegarr, Hrothgare, Hrothegare

Hubert (German) Having a shining intellect
Hobart, Huberte, Huburt, Huburte, Hubirt, Hubirte, Hubyrt, Hubyrte, Hubie, Uberto

Hudson (English) The son of Hugh; from the river
Hudsun, Hudsen, Hudsan, Hudsin, Hudsyn

Hugin (Norse) A thoughtful man
Hugyn, Hugen, Hugan, Hugon, Hugun

Humam (Arabic) A generous and brave man

Hungan (Haitian) A spirit master or priest
Hungen, Hungon, Hungun, Hungin, Hungyn

Hungas (Irish) A vigorous man

Hunter (English) A great huntsman and provider
Huntar, Huntor, Huntur, Huntir, Huntyr, Hunte, Hunt, Hunting

Husky (American) A big man; a manly man
Huski, Huskie, Huskey, Huskee, Huskea, Husk, Huske

Huslu (Native American) Resembling a hairy bear
Huslue, Huslou

Husto (Spanish) A righteous man
Hustio, Husteo, Hustiyo, Husteyo

Huynh (Vietnamese) An older brother

I

Iakovos (Hebrew) Form of Jacob, meaning "he who supplants"
Iakovus, Iakoves, Iakovas, Iakovis, Iakovys

Ian (Gaelic) Form of John, meaning "God is gracious"
Iain, Iaine, Iayn, Iayne, Iaen, Iaene, Iahn

Iavor (Bulgarian) From the sycamore tree
Iaver, Iavur, Iavar, Iavir, Iavyr

Ibrahim (Arabic) Form of Abraham, meaning "father of a multitude; father of nations"
Ibraheem, Ibraheim, Ibrahiem, Ibraheam, Ibrahym

Ichabod (Hebrew) The glory has gone
Ikabod, Ickabod, Icabod, Ichavod, Ikavod, Icavod, Ickavod, Icha

Ichtaca (Nahuatl) A secretive man
Ichtaka, Ichtacka

Ida (Anglo-Saxon) A king
Idah

Idi (African) Born during the holiday of Idd
Idie, Idy, Idey, Idee, Idea

Ido (Arabic / Hebrew) A mighty man / to evaporate
Iddo, Idoh, Iddoh

Idris (Welsh) An eager lord
Idrys, Idriss, Idrisse, Idryss, Idrysse

Iefan (Welsh) Form of John, meaning "God is gracious"
Iefon, Iefen, Iefin, Iefyn, Iefun, Ifan, Ifon, Ifen

Ifor (Welsh) An archer
Ifore, Ifour, Ifoure

Igasho (Native American) A wanderer
Igashoe, Igashow, Igashowe

Ignatius (Latin) A fiery man; one who is ardent
Ignac, Ignace, Ignacio, Ignacius, Ignatious, Ignatz, Ignaz, Ignazio

Igor (Scandinavian / Russian) A hero / Ing's soldier
Igoryok

Ihit (Indian) One who is honored
Ihyt, Ihitt, Ihytt

Ihsan (Arabic) A charitable man
Ihsann, Ihsen, Ihsin, Ihsyn, Ihson, Ihsun

Ike (Hebrew) Form of Isaac, meaning "full of laughter"
Iki, Ikie, Iky, Ikey, Ikee, Ikea

Iker (Basque) A visitor
Ikar, Ikir, Ikyr, Ikor, Ikur

Ilario (Italian) A cheerful man
Ilareo, Ilariyo, Ilareyo, Ilar, Ilarr, Ilari, Ilarie, Ilary

Ilhuitl (Nahuatl) Born during the daytime

Illanipi (Native American) An amazing man
Illanipie, Illanipy, Illanipey, Illanipee, Illanipea

Iluminado (Spanish) One who shines brightly
Illuminado, Iluminato, Illuminato, Iluminados, Iluminatos, Illuminados, Illuminatos

Imaran (Indian) Having great strength
Imaren, Imaron, Imarun, Imarin, Imaryn

Inaki (Basque) An ardent man
Inakie, Inaky, Inakey, Inakee, Inakea, Inacki, Inackie, Inackee

Ince (Hungarian) One who is innocent
Inse

Indiana (English) From
the land of the Indians;
from the state of Indiana
*Indianna, Indyana,
Indyanna*

Ingemar (Scandinavian)
The son of Ing
*Ingamar, Ingemur, Ingmar,
Ingmur, Ingar, Ingemer,
Ingmer*

Inger (Scandinavian) One
who is fertile
Inghar, Ingher

Ingo (Scandinavian /
Danish) A lord / from the
meadow
Ingoe, Ingow, Ingowe

Ingram (Scandinavian) A
raven of peace
*Ingra, Ingrem, Ingrim, Ingrym,
Ingrum, Ingrom, Ingraham,
Ingrahame, Ingrams*

Iniko (African) Born dur-
ing troubled times
*Inicko, Inico, Inyko, Inycko,
Inyco*

Iranga (Sri Lankan) One
who is special

Irenbend (Anglo-Saxon)
From the iron bend
Ironbend

Irwin (English) A friend of
the wild boar
*Irwinn, Irwinne, Irwyn,
Irwynne, Irwine, Irwen,
Irwenn, Irwenne*

*ᵀ**Isaac** (Hebrew) Full of
laughter
*Ike, Isaack, Isaak, Isac,
Isacco, Isak, Issac, Itzak*

*ᵀ**Isaiah** (Hebrew) God is
my salvation
*Isa, Isaia, Isais, Isia, Isiah,
Issiah, Izaiah, Iziah*

Iseabail (Hebrew) One
who is devoted to God
*Iseabaile, Iseabayl, Iseabyle,
Iseabael, Iseabaele*

Isham (English) From the
iron one's estate
*Ishem, Ishom, Ishum,
Ishim, Ishym, Isenham*

Isidore (Greek) A gift of
Isis
*Isador, Isadore, Isidor,
Isidoro, Isidorus, Isidro*

Iskander (Arabic) Form
of Alexander, meaning
"a helper and defender of
mankind"
*Iskinder, Iskandar,
Iskindar, Iskynder,
Iskyndar, Iskender, Iskendar*

Israel (Hebrew) God per-
severes
*Israeli, Israelie, Isreal,
Izrael*

Istvan (Hungarian) One
who is crowned
*Istven, Istvin, Istvyn, Istvon,
Istvun*

Iulian (Romanian) A youthful man
Iulien, Iulio, Iuleo

Ivan (Slavic) Form of John, meaning "God is gracious"
Ivann, Ivanhoe, Ivano, Iwan, Iban, Ibano, Ivanti, Ivantie

Ives (Scandinavian) The archer's bow; of the yew wood
Ivair, Ivar, Iven, Iver, Ivo, Ivon, Ivor, Ivaire

Ivy (English) Resembling the evergreen vining plant
Ivee, Ivey, Ivie, Ivi, Ivea

Iyai (Hebrew) Surrounded by light
Iyyar, Iyer, Iyyer

j

Ja (Korean / African) A handsome man / one who is magnetic

Jabari (African) A valiant man
Jabarie, Jabary, Jabarey, Jabaree, Jabarea

Jabbar (Indian) One who consoles others
Jabar

Jabin (Hebrew) God has built; one who is perceptive

Jabon (American) A fiesty man
Jabun, Jabin, Jabyn, Jaben, Jaban

Jace (Hebrew) God is my salvation
Jacen, Jacey, Jacian, Jacy, Jaice, Jayce, Jaece, Jase

Jacinto (Spanish) Resembling a hyacinth
Jacynto, Jacindo, Jacyndo, Jacento, Jacendo, Jacenty, Jacentey, Jacentee

•**Jack** (English) Form of John, meaning "God is gracious"
Jackie, Jackman, Jacko, Jacky, Jacq, Jacqin, Jak, Jaq

•**Jackson** (English) The son of Jack or John
Jacksen, Jacksun, Jacson, Jakson, Jaxen, Jaxon, Jaxun, Jaxson

•ᵀ**Jacob** (Hebrew) He who supplants
Jake, James, Kuba, Iakovos, Yakiv, Yankel, Yaqub, Jaco, Jacobo, Jacobi, Jacoby, Jacobie, Jacobey, Jacobo

^**Jacoby** (Hebrew) Form of Jacob, meaning he who supplants

Jadal (American) One who is punctual
Jadall, Jadel, Jadell

Jade (Spanish) Resembling the green gemstone
Jadee, Jadie, Jayde, Jaden

*†**Jaden** (Hebrew / English) One who is thankful to God; God has heard / form of Jade, meaning "resembling the green gemstone"
*Jaiden, Jadyn, Jaeden, Jaidyn, **Jayden**, Jaydon*

Jagan (English) One who is self-confident
Jagen, Jagin, Jagyn, Jagon, Jagun, Jago

Jahan (Indian) Man of the world
Jehan, Jihan, Jag, Jagat, Jagath

Jaidayal (Indian) The victory of kindness
Jadayal, Jaydayal, Jaedayal

Jaime (Spanish) Form of James, meaning "he who supplants"
Jamie, Jaime, Jaimee, Jaimey, Jaimi, Jaimie, Jaimy, Jamee

Jaimin (French) One who is loved
Jaimyn, Jamin, Jamyn, Jaymin, Jaymyn, Jaemin, Jaemyn

Jairdan (American) One who enlightens others
Jardan, Jayrdan, Jaerdan, Jairden, Jarden, Jayrden, Jaerden

Jaja (African) A gift from God

Jajuan (American) One who loves God

*†**Jake** (English) Form of Jacob, meaning "he who supplants"
Jaik, Jaike, Jayk, Jayke, Jakey, Jaky

Jakome (Basque) Form of James, meaning "he who supplants"
Jackome, Jakom, Jackom, Jacome

Jalen (American) One who heals others; one who is tranquil
Jaylon, Jaelan, Jalon, Jaylan, Jaylen, Jalan

Jamal (Arabic) A handsome man
Jamail, Jahmil, Jam, Jamaal, Jamy, Jamar

Jamar (American) Form of Jamal, meaning "a handsome man"
Jamarr, Jemar, Jemarr, Jimar, Jimarr, Jamaar, Jamari, Jamarie

*¹**James** (Hebrew) Form of
Jacob, meaning "he who
supplants"
*Jaimes, Jaymes, Jame,
Jaym, Jaim, Jaem, Jaemes,
Jamese, Jim, Jaime, Diego,
Hagop, Hemi, Jakome*

Jameson (English) The
son of James
*Jaimison, Jamieson,
Jaymeson, Jamison,
Jaimeson, Jaymison,
Jaemeson, Jaemison*

Jamin (Hebrew) The right
hand of favor
*Jamian, Jamiel, Jamon,
Jaymin, Jaemin, Jaymon*

Janesh (Hindi) A leader of
the people
Janeshe

Japa (Indian) One who
chants
Japeth, Japesh, Japendra

Japheth (Hebrew) May he
expand; in the Bible, one
of Noah's sons
*Jaypheth, Jaepheth,
Jaipheth, Jafeth, Jayfeth*

Jarah (Hebrew) One who
is as sweet as honey
Jarrah, Jara, Jarra

Jared (Hebrew) of the
descent; descending
*Jarad, Jarod, Jarrad, Jarryd,
Jarred, Jarrod, Jaryd, Jerod,
Jerrad, Jered*

Jarman (German) A man
from Germany
Jarmann, Jerman, Jermann

Jaron (Israeli) A song of
rejoicing
*Jaran, Jaren, Jarin, Jarran,
Jarren, Jarrin, Jarron, Jaryn*

Jaroslav (Slavic) Born with
the beauty of spring
Jaroslaw

Jarrett (English) One who
is strong with the spear
*Jaret, Jarret, Jarrott, Jerett,
Jarritt, Jaret*

***Jason** (Hebrew / Greek)
God is my salvation / a
healer; in mythology, the
leader of the Argonauts
*Jucen, Jaisen, Jaison, Jasen,
Jasin, Jasun, Jayson, Jaysen*

Jasper (Persian) One who
holds the treasure
*Jaspar, Jaspir, Jaspyr,
Jesper, Jespar, Jespir, Jespyr*

Jatan (Indian) One who is
nurturing

Javan (Hebrew) Man from
Greece; in the Bible,
Noah's grandson
*Jayvan, Jayven, Jayvon,
Javon, Javern, Javen*

Javier (Spanish) the owner
of a new house
Javiero

Jay (Latin / Sanskrit)
Resembling a jaybird /
one who is victorious
*Jae, Jai, Jaye, Jayron,
Jayronn, Jey*

Jean (French) Form of
John, meaning "God is gra-
cious"
*Jeanne, Jeane, Jene,
Jeannot, Jeanot*

Jedidiah (Hebrew) One
who is loved by God
*Jedadiah, Jedediah, Jed,
Jedd, Jedidiya, Jedidiyah,
Jedadia, Jedadiya*

Jeffrey (English) A man of
peace
Jeff, Geoffrey, Jeffery, Jeffree

Jehu (Hebrew) He is God
*Jayhu, Jahu, Jehue, Jeyhu,
Jeyhue, Jayhue, Jahue, Jehew*

Jelani (African) One who is
mighty; strong
*Jelanie, Jelany, Jelaney,
Jelanee, Jelanea*

Jennett (Hindi) One who
is heaven-sent
*Jenett, Jennet, Jenet, Jennitt,
Jenitt, Jennit, Jenit*

Jerald (English) Form of
Gerald, meaning "one
who rules with the spear"
*Jeraldo, Jerold, Jerrald,
Jerrold*

•**Jeremiah** (Hebrew) One
who is exalted by the Lord
*Jeremia, Jeremias, Jeremija,
Jeremiya, Jeremyah,
Jeramiah, Jeramia, Jerram,
Geremia*

Jeremy (Hebrew) Form of
Jeremiah, meaning "one
who is exalted by the lord"
*Jeramey, Jeramie, Jeramy,
Jerami, Jereme, Jeromy*

Jermaine (French / Latin)
A man from Germany /
one who is brotherly
*Jermain, Jermane,
Jermayne, Jermin, Jermyn,
Jermayn, Jermaen,
Jermaene*

Jerome (Greek) Of the
sacred name
*Jairome, Jeroen, Jeromo,
Jeronimo, Jerrome, Jerom,
Jerolyn, Jerolin, Hieronim*

Jerram (Hebrew) Form of
Jeremiah, meaning "one
who is exalted by the Lord"
*Jeram, Jerrem, Jerem,
Jerrym, Jerym*

Jesimiel (Hebrew) The
Lord establishes
Jessimiel

Jesse (Hebrew) God exists; a
gift from God; God sees all
*Jess, Jessey, Jesiah, Jessie,
Jessy, Jese, Jessi, Jessee*

***Jesus** (Hebrew) God is my salvation
*Jesous, Jesues, **Jesús**, Xesus*

Jett (English) Resembling the jet-black lustrous gemstone
Jet, Jette

Jibril (Arabic) Refers to the archangel Gabriel
Jibryl, Jibri, Jibrie, Jibry, Jibrey, Jibree

Jim (English) Form of James, meaning "he who supplants"
Jimi, Jimmee, Jimmey, Jimmie, Jimmy, Jimmi, Jimbo

Jimoh (African) Born on a Friday
Jymoh, Jimo, Jymo

Jivan (Hindi) A giver of life
Jivin, Jiven, Jivyn, Jivon

Joab (Hebrew) The Lord is my father
Joabb, Yoav

Joachim (Hebrew) One who is established by God; God will judge
Jachim, Jakim, Joacheim, Joaquim, Joaquin, Josquin, Joakim, Joakeen

Joe (English) Form of Joseph, meaning "God will add"
Jo, Joemar, Jomar, Joey, Joie, Joee, Joeye

Joel (Hebrew) Jehovah is God; God is willing

^**Johan** (German) Form of John, meaning "God is gracious"

*†**John** (Hebrew) God is gracious; in the Bible, one of the Apostles
*Sean, **Jack**, **Juan**, Ian, Ean, **Evan**, Giovanni, Hanna, Hovannes, Iefan, Ivan, Jean, Xoan, Yochanan, Yohan, Johnn, Johnny, Jhonny*

***Jonathan** (Hebrew) A gift of God
Johnathan, Johnathon, Jonathon, Jonatan, Jonaton, Jonathen, Johnathen, Jonaten, Yonatan

*†**Jordan** (Hebrew) Of the down-flowing river; in the Bible, the river where Jesus was baptized
Johrdan, Jordain, Jordaine, Jordane, Jordanke, Jordann, Jorden, Jordaen

Jonah (Hebrew) Resembling a dove; in the Bible, the man swallowed by a whale

^**Jonas** (Greek) Form of Jonah, meaning "resembling a dove"

Jorge (Spanish) Form of George, meaning "one who works the earth; a farmer"

•**Jose** (Spanish) Form of
Joseph, meaning "God
will add"
José, Joseito, Joselito

•†**Joseph** (Hebrew) God
will add
*Joe, Guiseppe, Yosyp, Jessop,
Jessup, Joop, Joos, **José**, Jose,
Josef, Joseito*

•†**Joshua** (Hebrew) God is
salvation
*Josh, Joshuah, Josua, Josue,
Joushua, Jozua, Joshwa,
Joshuwa*

•**Josiah** (Hebrew) God will
help
*Josia, Josias, Joziah, Jozia,
Jozias*

Journey (American) One
who likes to travel
*Journy, Journi, Journie,
Journee, Journye, Journea*

•**Juan** (Spanish) Form of
John, meaning "God is
gracious"
Juanito, Juwan, Jwan

Judah (Hebrew) One who
praises God
*Juda, Jude, Judas, judsen,
Judson, Judd, Jud*

^**Jude** (Latin) Form of
Judah, meaning one who
praises God.

•**Julian** (Greek) The child of
Jove; one who is youthful
*Juliano, Julianus, Julien,
Julyan, Julio, Jolyon,
Jullien, Julen*

Julius (Greek) One who is
youthful
Juleus, Yuliy

Juma (African) Born on a
Friday
Jumah

Jumbe (African) Having
great strength
*Jumbi, Jumbie, Jumby,
Jumbey, Jumbee*

Jumoke (African) One who
is dearly loved
Jumok, Jumoak

Jun (Japanese) One who is
obedient

Junaid (Arabic) A warrior
Junaide, Junayd, Junayde

Jung (Korean) A righteous
man

Jurgen (German) Form of
George, meaning "one who
works the earth; a farmer"
Jorgen, Jurgin, Jorgin

Justice (English) One who
upholds moral rightness
and fairness
*Justyce, Justiss, Justyss,
Justis, Justus, Justise*

*ᴛ**Justin** (Latin) One who is just and upright
Joost, Justain, Justan, Just, Juste, Justen, Justino, Justo

Justinian (Latin) An upright ruler
Justinien, Justinious, Justinius, Justinios, Justinas, Justinus

k

Kabir (Indian) A spiritual leader
Kabeer, Kabear, Kabier, Kabeir, Kabyr, Kabar

Kabonesa (African) One who is born during difficult times

Kacancu (African) The firstborn child
Kacancue, Kakancu, Kakancue, Kacanku, Kacankue

Kacey (Irish) A vigilant man; one who is alert
Kacy, Kacee, Kacea, Kaci, Kacie, Kasey, Kasy, Kasi

Kachada (Native American) A white-skinned man

•**Kaden** (Arabic) A beloved companion
Kadan, Kadin, Kadon, Kaidan, Kaiden, Kaidon, Kaydan, Kayden

Kadmiel (Hebrew) One who stands before God
Kamiell

Kaemon (Japanese) Full of joy; one who is right-handed
Kamon, Kaymon, Kaimon

Kagen (Irish) A fiery man; a thinker
Kaigen, Kagan, Kaigan, Kaygen, Kaygan, Kaegen, Kaegan

Kahoku (Hawaiian) Resembling a star
Kahokue, Kahokoo, Kahokou

Kai (Hawaiian / Welsh / Greek) Of the sea, the keeper of the keys / of the earth
Kye

Kaimi (Hawaiian) The seeker
Kaimie, Kaimy, Kaimey, Kaimee, Kaimea

Kalama (Hawaiian) A source of light
Kalam, Kalame

ʌ**Kale** (English) Form of Charles, meaning "one who is manly and strong / a free man"

Kaleb (Hebrew)
Resembling an aggressive
dog
*Kaileb, Kaeleb, Kayleb,
Kalob, Kailob, Kaelob*

Kalidas (Hindi) A poet or
musician; a servant of Kali
Kalydas

Kalki (Indian) Resembling
a white horse
*Kalkie, Kalky, Kalkey,
Kalkee, Kalkea*

Kalkin (Hindi) The tenth-
born child
*Kalkyn, Kalken, Kalkan,
Kalkon, Kalkun*

Kamden (English) From
the winding valley
*Kamdun, Kamdon,
Kamdan, Kamdin, Kamdyn*

^**Kane** (Gaelic) The little
warrior
*Kayn, Kayne, Kaen, Kaene,
Kahan, Kahane*

Kang (Korean) A healthy
man

Kano (Japanese) A powerful man
Kanoe, Kanoh

Kantrava (Indian)
Resembling a roaring
animal

Kaper (American) One
who is capricious
Kahper, Kapar, Kahpar

Kapono (Hawaiian) A
righteous man

Karcsi (French) A strong,
manly man
*Karcsie, Karcsy, Karcsey,
Karcsee, Karcsea*

Karl (German) A free man
*Carl, Karel, Karlan, Karle,
Karlens, Karli, Karlin,
Karlo, Karlos*

Karman (Gaelic) The lord
of the manor
*Karmen, Karmin, Karmyn,
Karmon, Karmun*

^**Karson** (Scottish) Form of
Carson, meaning son of a
marsh dweller
Karsen

Kasem (Asian) Filled with
joy

Kasen (Basque) Protected
by a helmet
*Kasin, Kasyn, Kason,
Kasun, Kasan*

Kashvi (Indian) A shining
man
*Kashvie, Kashvy, Kashvey,
Kashvee, Kashvea*

Kasib (Arabic) One who is
fertile
*Kaseeb, Kaseab, Kasieb,
Kaseib, Kasyb*

Kasim (Arabic) One who is divided
Kassim, Kaseem, Kasseem, Kaseam, Kasseam, Kasym, Kassym

Kasimir (Slavic) One who demands peace
Kasimeer, Kasimear, Kasimier, Kasimeir, Kasimyr, Kaz, Kazimierz

Katzir (Hebrew) The harvester
Katzyr, Katzeer, Katzear, Katzier, Katzeir

Kaushal (Indian) One who is skilled
Kaushall, Koshal, Koshall

Kazim (Arabic) An eventempered man
Kazeem, Kazeam, Kaziem, Kazeim, Kazym

Keahi (Hawaiian) Of the flames
Keahie, Keahy, Keahey, Keahee, Keahea

Kealoha (Hawaiian) From the bright path
Keeloha, Kieloha

Kean (Gaelic / English) A warrior / one who is sharp
Keane, Keen, Keene, Kein, Keine, Keyn, Keyne, Kien

Keandre (American) One who is thankful
Kiandre, Keandray, Kiandray, Keandrae, Kiandrae, Keandrai, Kiandrai

Keanu (Hawaiian) Of the mountain breeze
Keanue, Kianu, Kianue, Keanoo, Kianoo, Keanou

Keaton (English) From the town of hawks
Keatun, Keeton, Keetun, Keyton, Keytun

Kedar (Arabic) A powerful man
Keder, Kedir, Kedyr, Kadar, Kader, Kadir, Kadyr

Kefir (Hebrew) Resembling a young lion
Kefyr, Kefeer, Kefear, Kefier, Kefeir

Keegan (Gaelic) A small and fiery man
Kegan, Keigan, Keigan, Keagan, Keagen, Keegen

Keith (Scottish) Man from the forest
Keithe, Keath, Keathe, Kieth, Kiethe, Keyth, Keythe, Keithen

Kellach (Irish) One who suffers strife during battle
Kelach, Kellagh, Kelagh, Keallach

^**Kellen** (Gaelic/German)
One who is slender/from
the swamp
*Kellan, Kellon, Kellun,
Kellin*

Kelley (Celtic / Gaelic) A
warrior / one who defends
*Kelly, Kelleigh, Kellee,
Kellea, Kelleah, Kelli, Kellie*

Kendi (African) One who
is much loved
*Kendie, Kendy, Kendey,
Kendee, Kendea*

Kendrick (English /
Gaelic) A royal ruler / the
champion
*Kendric, Kendricks,
Kendrik, Kendrix,
Kendryck, Kenrick, Kenrik,
Kenricks*

Kenley (English) From the
king's meadow
*Kenly, Kenlee, Kenleigh,
Kenlea, Kenleah, Kenli,
Kenlie*

Kenn (Welsh) Of the
bright waters

Kennedy (Gaelic) A hel-
meted chief
*Kennedi, Kennedie,
Kennedey, Kennedee,
Kennedea, Kenadie, Kenadi,
Kenady*

Kenneth (Irish) Born of
the fire; an attractive man
*Kennet, Kennett, Kennith,
Kennit, Kennitt*

Kent (English) From the
edge or border
Kentt, Kennt, Kentrell

Kenton (English) From the
king's town
*Kentun, Kentan, Kentin,
Kenten, Kentyn*

Kenyon (Gaelic) A blond-
haired man
*Kenyun, Kenyan, Kenyen,
Kenyin*

Kepler (German) One who
makes hats
*Keppler, Kappler, Keppel,
Keppeler*

Kerbasi (Basque) A warrior
*Kerbasie, Kerbasee,
Kerbasea, Kerbasy, Kerbasey*

Kershet (Hebrew) Of the
rainbow

Kesler (American) An
energetic man; one who is
independent
*Keslar, Keslir, Keslyr, Keslor,
Keslur*

Keung (Chinese) A universal spirit

***Kevin** (Gaelic) A beloved
and handsome man
*Kevyn, Kevan, Keven,
Keveon, Kevinn, Kevion,
Kevis, Kevon*

Khairi (Swahili) A kingly man
*Khairie, Khairy, Khairey,
Khairee, Khairea*

Khalon (American) A
strong warrior
*Khalun, Khalen, Khalan,
Khalin, Khalyn*

Khayri (Arabic) One who is
charitable
*Khayrie, Khayry, Khayrey,
Khayree, Khayrea*

Khouri (Arabic) A spiritual
man; a priest
*Khourie, Khoury, Khourey,
Khouree, Kouri, Kourie,
Koury, Kourey*

Khushi (Indian) Filled
with happiness
*Khushie, Khushey, Khushy,
Khushee*

Kibbe (Native American) A
nocturnal bird
Kybbe

Kibo (African) From the
highest moutain peak
*Keybo, Keebo, Keabo, Keibo,
Kiebo*

Kidd (English) Resembling
a young goat
Kid, Kydd, Kyd

Kiefer (German) One who
makes barrels
*Keefer, Keifer, Kieffer,
Kiefner, Kieffner, Kiefert,
Kuefer, Kueffner*

Kildaire (Irish) From coun-
ty of Kildare
*Kyldaire, Kildare, Kyldare,
Kildair, Kyldair, Killdaire,
Kylldaire, Kildayr*

Kim (Vietnamese) As precious as gold
Kym

Kimoni (African) A great
man
*Kimonie, Kimony, Kimoney,
Kimonee, Kymoni, Kymonie,
Kymony, Kymoney*

Kincaid (Celtic) The leader
during battle
*Kincade, Kincayd,
Kincayde, Kincaide,
Kincaed, Kincaede,
Kinkaid, Kinkaide*

Kindin (Basque) The fifth-
born child
*Kinden, Kindan, Kindyn,
Kindon, Kindun*

Kindle (American) To set
aflame
Kindel, Kyndle, Kyndel

King (English) The royal ruler
Kyng

^Kingston (English) From
the king's town
Kingstun, Kinston, Kindon

Kinnard (Irish) From the
tall hill
*Kinard, Kinnaird, Kinaird,
Kynnard, Kynard,
Kynnaird, Kynaird*

Kinsey (English) The victorious prince
Kynsey, Kinsi, Kynsi, Kinsie, Kynsie, Kinsee, Kynsee, Kinsea

Kione (African) One who has come from nowhere

Kioshi (Japanese) One who is quiet
Kioshe, Kioshie, Kioshy, Kioshey, Kioshee, Kyoshi, Kyoshe, Kyoshie

Kipp (English) From the small pointed hill
Kip, Kipling, Kippling, Kypp, Kyp, Kiplyng, Kipplyng, Kippi

Kiri (Vietnamese) Resembling the mountains
Kirie, Kiry, Kirey, Kiree, Kirea

Kirk (Norse) A man of the church
Kyrk, Kerk, Kirklin, Kirklyn

Kirkland (English) From the church's land
Kirklan, Kirklande, Kyrkland, Kyrklan, Kyrklande

Kirkley (English) From the church's meadow
Kirkly, Kirkleigh, Kirklea, Kirkleah, Kirklee, Kirkli, Kirklie

Kit (English) Form of Christopher, meaning "one who bears Christ inside"
Kitt, Kyt, Kytt

Kitchi (Native American) A brave young man
Kitchie, Kitchy, Kitchey, Kitchee, Kitchea

Kitoko (African) A handsome man
Kytoko

Kivi (Finnish) As solid as stone
Kivie, Kivy, Kivey, Kivee, Kivea

Knight (English) A noble solidier
Knights

Knoton (Native American) Of the wind
Knotun, Knotan, Knoten, Knotin, Knotyn

Knud (Danish) A kind man
Knude

^**Kobe** (African / Hungarian) Tortoise / Form of Jacob, meaning he who supplants
Kobi, Koby

Kody (English) One who is helpful
Kodey, Kodee, Kodea, Kodi, Kodie

Koen (German) An honest advisor
Koenz, Kunz, Kuno

Kohana (Native American / Hawaiian) One who is swift / the best

Kohler (German) One who mines coal
Koler

Kojo (African) Born on a Monday
Kojoe, Koejo, Koejoe

Koka (Hawaiian) A man from Scotland

^**Kolton** (American) Form of Colton, meaning from the coal town
Kolten, Koltan

Konane (Hawaiian) Born beneath the bright moon
Konain, Konaine, Konayn, Konayne, Konaen, Konaene

Konnor (English) A wolf lover; one who is strong-willed
Konnur, Konner, Konnar, Konnir, Konnyr

Koofrey (African) Remember me
Koofry, Koofri, Koofrie, Koofree

Kordell (English) One who makes cord
Kordel, Kord, Kordale

Koresh (Hebrew) One who digs in the earth; a farmer
Koreshe

Kory (Irish) From the hollow; of the churning waters
Korey, Kori, Korie, Koree, Korea, Korry, Korrey, Korree

Kozma (Greek) One who is decorated
Kozmah

Kozue (Japanese) Of the tree branches
Kozu, Kozoo, Kozou

Kraig (Gaelic) From the rocky place; as solid as a rock
Kraige, Krayg, Krayge, Kraeg, Kraege, Krage

Kramer (German) A shop-keeper
Kramar, Kramor, Kramir, Kramur, Kramyr, Kraymer, Kraimer, Kraemer

Krany (Czech) A man of short stature
Kraney, Kranee, Kranea, Krani, Kranie

Krikor (Armenian) A vigilant watchman
Krykor, Krikur, Krykur

Kristian (Scandinavian) An annointed Christian
Kristan, Kristien, Krist, Kriste, Krister, Kristar, Khristian, Khrist

Kristopher (Scandinavian)
A follower of Christ
*Khristopher, Kristof,
Kristofer, Kristoff, Kristoffer,
Kristofor, Kristophor, Krystof*

Kuba (Polish) Form of
Jacob, meaning "he who
supplants"
Kubas

Kuckunniwi (Native
American) Resembling a
little wolf
Kukuniwi

Kuleen (Indian) A high-
born man
*Kulin, Kulein, Kulien,
Kulean, Kulyn*

Kumar (Indian) A prince;
a male child

Kuri (Japanese) Resembling
a chestnut
*Kurie, Kury, Kurey, Kuree,
Kurea*

Kuron (African) One who
gives thanks
*Kurun, Kuren, Kuran,
Kurin, Kuryn*

Kurt (German) A brave
counselor
Kurte

Kushal (Indian) A talented
man; adroit
Kushall

Kwaku (African) Born on a
Wednesday
*Kwakue, Kwakou, Kwako,
Kwakoe*

Kwan (Korean) Of a bold
character
Kwon

Kwintyn (Polish) The fifth-
born child
*Kwentyn, Kwinton,
Kwenton, Kwintun,
Kwentun, Kwintan,
Kwentan, Kwinten*

*T**Kyle** (Gaelic) From the
narrow channel
*Kile, Kiley, Kye, Kylan,
Kyrell, Kylen, Kily, Kili*

Kylemore (Gaelic) From
the great wood
Kylmore, Kylemor, Kylmor

Kyrone (English) Form of
Tyrone, meaning "from
Owen's land"
*Kyron, Keirohn, Keiron,
Keirone, Keirown, Kirone*

Lacey (French) Man from
Normandy; as delicate as
lace
Lacy, Laci, Lacie, Lacee, Lacea

Lachlan (Gaelic) From the land of lakes
Lachlen, Lachlin, Lachlyn, Locklan, Locklen, Locklin, Locklyn, Loklan

Lachman (Gaelic) A man from the lake
Lachmann, Lockman, Lockmann, Lokman, Lokmann, Lakman, Lakmann

Ladan (Hebrew) One who is alert and aware
Laden, Ladin, Ladyn, Ladon, Ladun

Ladd (English) A servant; a young man
Lad, Laddey, Laddie, Laddy, Laddi, Laddee, Laddea, Ladde

Ladislas (Slavic) A glorious ruler
Lacko, Ladislaus, Laslo, Laszlo, Lazlo, Ladislav, Ladislauv, Ladislao

Lagrand (American) A majestic man
Lagrande

Laibrook (English) One who lives on the road near the brook
Laebrook, Laybrook, Laibroc, Laebroc, Laybroc, Laibrok, Laebrok, Laybrok

Laird (Scottish) The lord of the manor
Layrd, Laerd, Lairde, Layrde, Laerde

Laken (American) Man from the lake
Laike, Laiken, Laikin, Lakin, Lakyn, Lakan, Laikyn, Laeken

Lalam (Indian) The best
Lallam, Lalaam, Lallaam

Lam (Vietnamese) Having a full understanding

Laman (Arabic) A bright and happy man
Lamaan, Lamann, Lamaann

Lamar (German / French) From the renowned land / of the sea
Lamarr, Lamarre, Lemar, Lemarr

Lambert (Scandinavian) The light of the land
Lambart, Lamberto, Lambirt, Landbert, Lambirto, Lambrecht, Lambret, Lambrett

Lambi (Norse) In mythology, the son of Thorbjorn
Lambie, Lamby, Lambey, Lambe, Lambee

Lameh (Arabic) A shining man

Lamorak (English) In Arthurian legend, the brother of Percival
Lamerak, Lamurak, Lamorac, Lamerac, Lamurac, Lamorack, Lamerack, Lamurack

Lance (English) Form of Lancelot, meaning an attendant, a knight of the Round Table

Lander (English) One who owns land
Land, Landers, Landis, Landiss, Landor, Lande, Landry, Landri

*ᵀᐱ**Landon** (English) From the long hill
Landyn, Landan, Landen, Landin, Lando, Langdon, Langden, Langdan

Lane (English) One who takes the narrow path
Laine, Lain, Laen, Laene, Layne, Layn

Langhorn (English) Of the long horn
Langhorne, Lanhorn, Lanhorne

Langilea (Polynesian) Having a booming voice, like thunder
Langileah, Langilia, Langiliah

Langston (English) From the tall man's town
Langsten, Langstun, Langstown, Langstin, Langstyn, Langstan, Langton, Langtun

Langundo (Native American / Polynesian) A peaceful man / one who is graceful

Langworth (English) One who lives near the long paddock
Langworthe, Lanworth, Lanworthe

Lanier (French) One who works with wool

Lantos (Hungarian) One who plays the lute
Lantus

Lapidos (Hebrew) One who carries a torch
Lapydos, Lapidot, Lapydot, Lapidoth, Lapydoth, Lapidus, Lapydus

Laquinton (American) Form of Quinton, meaning "from the queen's town or settlement"
Laquinntan, Laquinnten, Laquinntin, Laquinnton, Laquintain, Laquintan, Laquintyn, Laquintynn

Lar (Anglo-Saxon) One who teaches others

Larson (Scandinavian) The
son of Lawrence
*Larsan, Larsen, Larsun,
Larsin, Larsyn*

Lasalle (French) From the
hall
Lasall, Lasal, Lasale

Lashaun (American) An
enthusiastic man
*Lashawn, Lasean, Lashon,
Lashond*

Lassit (American) One
who is open-minded
Lassyt, Lasset

Lathan (American) Form
of Nathan, meaning "a
gift from God"
*Lathen, Lathun, Lathon,
Lathin, Lathyn, Latan,
Laten, Latun*

Latimer (English) One who
serves as an interpreter
*Latymer, Latimor, Latymor,
Latimore, Latymore,
Lattemore, Lattimore*

Latty (English) A generous
man
*Lattey, Latti, Lattie, Lattee,
Lattea*

Laurian (English) One who
lives near the laurel trees
*Laurien, Lauriano, Laurieno,
Lawrian, Lawrien, Lawriano,
Lawrieno*

Lave (Italian) Of the burning rock
Lava

Lawford (English) From
the ford near the hill
*Lawforde, Lawferd,
Lawferde, Lawfurd,
Lawfurde*

Lawler (Gaelic) A soft-
spoken man; one who
mutters
*Lauler, Lawlor, Loller,
Lawlar, Lollar, Loller,
Laular, Laulor*

Lawley (English) From the
meadow near the hill
*Lawly, Lawli, Lawlie,
Lawleigh, Lawlee, Lawlea,
Lawleah*

Lawrence (Latin) Man
from Laurentum; crowned
with laurel
*Larance, Laranz, Larenz,
Larrance, Larrence, Larrens,
Larrey, Larry*

Laziz (Arabic) One who is
pleasant
*Lazeez, Lazeaz, Laziez,
Lazeiz, Lazyz*

Leaman (American) A
powerful man
*Leeman, Leamon, Leemon,
Leamond, Leamand*

Lear (Greek) Of the royalty
Leare, Leer, Leere

Leather (American) As tough as hide
Lether

Leavitt (English) A baker
Leavit, Leavytt, Leavyt, Leavett, Leavet

Leben (English) Filled with hope

Lech (Slavic) In mythology, the founder of the Polish people
Leche

Ledyard (Teutonic) The protector of the nation
Ledyarde, Ledyerd, Ledyerde

Lee (English) From the meadow
Leigh, Lea, Leah, Ley

Leeto (African) One who embarks on a journey
Leato, Leito, Lieto

Legend (American) One who is memorable
Legende, Legund, Legunde

Leighton (English) From the town near the meadow
Leightun, Layton, Laytun, Leyton, Leytun

Lekhak (Hindi) An author
Lekhan

Lema (African) One who is cultivated
Lemah, Lemma, Lemmah

Lemon (American) Resembling the fruit
Lemun, Lemin, Lemyn, Limon, Limun, Limin, Limyn, Limen

Len (Native American) One who plays the flute

Lencho (African) Resembling a lion
Lenchos, Lenchio, Lenchiyo, Lencheo, Lencheyo

Lennon (English) Son of love
Lennan

Lennor (English) A courageous man

Lennox (Scottish) One who owns many elm trees
Lenox, Lenoxe, Lennix, Lenix, Lenixe

Lensar (English) One who stays with his parents
Lenser, Lensor, Lensur

Lenton (American) A pious man
Lentin, Lentyn, Lentun, Lentan, Lenten, Lent, Lente

Leo (Latin) Having the strength of a lion
Lio, Lyo, Leon

Leonard (German) Having the strength of a lion
Len, Lenard, Lenn, Lennard, Lennart, Lennerd, Leonardo

Leor (Latin) One who listens well
Leore

Lerato (Latin) The song of my soul
Leratio, Lerateo

Leron (French / Arabic) The circle / my song
Lerun, Leran, Leren, Lerin, Leryn

Leroy (French) The king
Leroi, Leeroy, Leeroi, Learoy, Learoi

Levi (Hebrew) We are united as one; in the Bible, one of Jacob's sons
Levie, Levin, Levyn, Levy, Levey, Levee

Li (Chinese) Having great strength

•Liam (Gaelic) From of William, meaning "the determined protector"

Lian (Chinese) Of the willow

Liang (Chinese) A good man
Lyang

Lidmann (Anglo-Saxon) A man of the sea; a sailor
Lidman, Lydmann, Lydman

Lif (Scandinavian) An energetic man; lively

Lihau (Hawaiian) A spirited man

Like (Asian) A soft-spoken man
Lyke

Lilo (Hawaiian) One who is generous
Lylo, Leelo, Lealo, Leylo, Lielo, Leilo

Lincoln (English) from the village near the lake
Lincon, Lyncon, Linc, Lynk, Lync

Lindford (English) From the linden-tree ford
Linford, Lindforde, Linforde, Lyndford, Lynford, Lyndforde, Lynforde

Lindhurst (English) From the village by the linden trees
Lyndhurst, Lindenhurst, Lyndenhurst, Lindhirst, Lindherst, Lyndhirst, Lyndherst, Lindenhirst

Lindley (English) From the meadow of linden trees
Lindly, Lindleigh, Lindlea, Lindleah, Lindlee, Lindli

Lindman (English) One who lives near the linden trees
Lindmann, Lindmon

Line (English) From the bank

Lipût (Hungarian) A brave young man

Lisimba (African) One who has been attacked by a lion
Lisymba, Lysimba, Lysymba

Liu (Asian) One who is quiet; peaceful

Llewellyn (Welsh) Resembling a lion
Lewellen, Lewellyn, Llewellen, Llewelyn, Llwewellin, Llew, Llewe, Llyweilun

Lochan (Hindi / Irish) The eyes / one who is lively

*›***Logan** (Gaelic) From the little hollow
Logann, Logen, Login, Logyn, Logenn, Loginn, Logynn

Lolonyo (African) The beauty of love
Lolonyio, Lolonyeo, Lolonio, Lolonea

Loman (Gaelic) One who is small and bare
Lomann, Loeman, Loemann

Lombard (Latin) One who has a long beard
Lombardi, Lombardo, Lombardie, Lombardy, Lombardey, Lombardee

London (English) From the captial of England
Lundon, Londen, Lunden

Lonzo (Spanish) One who is ready for battle
Lonzio, Lonzeo

Lootah (Native American) Refers to the color red
Loota, Loutah, Louta, Lutah, Luta

Lorcan (Irish) The small fierce one
Lorcen, Lorcin, Lorcyn, Lorcon, Lorcun, Lorkan, Lorken, Lorkin

Lord (English) One who has authority and power
Lorde, Lordly, Lordley, Lordlee, Lordlea, Lordleigh, Lordli, Lordlie

Lore (Basque / English) Resembling a flower / form of Lawrence, meaning "man from Laurentum; crowned with laurel"
Lorea

Lorimer (Latin) One who makes harnesses
Lorrimer, Lorimar, Lorrimar, Lorymar, Lorrymar, Lorymer, Lorrymer

Louis (German) A famous warrior
*Lew, Lewes, Lewis, Lodewick, Lodovico, Lou, Louie, Lucho, **Luis***

Luba (Yugoslavian) One who loves and is loved
Lubah

Lucas (English) A man
from Lucania
*Lukas, Loucas, Loukas,
Luckas, Louckas, Lucus,
Lukus, Ghoukas*

Lucian (Latin) Surrounded
by light
*Luciano, Lucianus, Lucien,
Lucio, Lucjan, Lukianos,
Lukyan, Luce*

Lucky (English) A fortu-
nate man
*Luckey, Luckee, Luckea,
Lucki, Luckie*

Ludlow (English) The
ruler of the hill
Ludlowe

Luis (Spanish) Form of
Louis, meaning "a famous
warrior"
Luiz

Luke (Greek) A man
from Lucania
Luc, Luken

Lunt (Scandinavian) From
the grove
Lunte

Luthando (Latin) One who
is dearly loved

Luther (German) A soldier
of the people
*Louther, Luter, Luthero,
Lutero, Louthero, Luthus,
Luthas, Luthos*

Lux (Latin) A man of the light
*Luxe, Luxi, Luxie, Luxee,
Luxea, Luxy, Luxey*

Ly (Vietnamese) A reasonable man

Lynn (English) A man of
the lake
Linn, Lyn, Lynne, Linne

m

Maahes (Egyptian)
Resembling a lion

Mac (Gaelic) The son
of Mac (Macarthur,
Mackinley, etc.)
*Mack, Mak, Macky, Macky,
Macki, Mackie, Mackee,
Mackea*

Macadam (Gaelic) The
son of Adam
*Macadhamh, MacAdam,
McAdam, MacAdhamh*

Macallister (Gaelic) The
son of Alistair
*MacAlister, McAlister,
McAllister, Macalister*

Macardle (Gaelic) The son
of great courage
*MacArdle, McCardle,
Macardell, MacArdell,
McCardell*

Macartan (Gaelic) The son
of Artan
*MacArtan, McArtan,
Macarten, McArten,
McArten*

Macarthur (Gaelic) The
son of Arthur
*MacArthur, McArthur,
Macarther, MacArther,
McArther*

Macauslan (Gaelic) The
son of Absalon
*MacAuslan, McAuslan,
Macauslen, MacAuslen,
McAuslen*

Maccoll (Gaelic) The son
of Coll
McColl, Maccoll, MacColl

Maccrea (Gaelic) The son
of grace
*McCrea, Macrae, MacCrae,
MacCray, MacCrea*

Macedonio (Greek) A
man from Macedonia
*Macedoneo, Macedoniyo,
Macedoneyo*

Macgowan (Gaelic) The
son of a blacksmith
*MacGowan, Magowan,
McGowan, McGowen,
McGown, MacCowan,
MacCowen*

Machau (Hebrew) A gift
from God

Machenry (Gaelic) The
son of Henry
MacHenry, McHenry

Machk (Native American)
Resembling a bear

Macintosh (Gaelic) The
son of the thane
*MacIntosh, McIntosh,
Macintoshe, MacIntoshe,
McIntoshe, Mackintosh,
MacKintosh*

Mackay (Gaelic) The son
of fire
*MacKay, McKay, Mackaye,
MacKaye, McKaye*

Mackinley (Gaelic) The
son of the white warrior
*MacKinley, McKinley,
MacKinlay, McKinlay,
Mackinlay, Mackinlie,
MacKinlie*

Macklin (Gaelic) The son
of Flann
*Macklinn, Macklyn,
Macklynn, Macklen,
Macklenn*

Maclaine (Gaelic) The son
of John's servant
*MacLaine, Maclain,
MacLain, Maclayn,
McLaine, McLain,
Maclane, MacLane*

Macleod (Gaelic) The son
of the ugly one
*MacLeod, McLeod,
McCloud, MacCloud*

Macmurray (Gaelic) The
son of Murray
*MacMurray, McMurray,
Macmurra, MacMurra*

Macnab (Gaelic) The son
of the abbot
MacNab, McNab

Macon (English / French)
To make / from the city in
France
*Macun, Makon, Makun,
Maken, Mackon, Mackun*

Macqueen (Gaelic) The
son of the good man
MacQueen, McQueen

Macrae (Gaelic) The son
of Ray
*MacRae, McRae, Macray,
MacRay, McRay, Macraye,
MacRaye, McRaye*

Madden (Pakistani) One
who is organized; a plan-
ner
*Maddon, Maddan, Maddin,
Maddyn, Maddun, Maden,
Madon, Madun*

Maddox (Welsh) The son
of the benefactor
Madox, Madocks, Maddocks

Madhur (Indian) A sweet
man

Magee (Gaelic) The son of
Hugh
*MacGee, McGee, MacGhee,
Maghee*

Maguire (Gaelic) The son
of the beige one
*Magwire, MacGuire,
McGuire, MacGwire,
McGwire*

Magus (Latin) A sorcerer
*Magis, Magys, Magos,
Magas, Mages*

Mahan (American) A
cowboy
*Mahahn, Mahen, Mayhan,
Maihan, Maehan, Mayhen,
Maihen, Maehen*

Mahant (Indian) Having a
great soul
Mahante

Mahatma (Hindi) Of great
spiritual development

Mahfouz (Arabic) One
who is protected
*Mafouz, Mahfooz, Mafooz,
Mahfuz, Mafuz*

Mahkah (Native
American) Of the earth
Mahka, Makah, Maka

Mahmud (Arabic) One
who is praiseworthy
*Mahmood, Mahmoud,
Mehmood, Mehmud,
Mehmoud*

Mailhairer (French) An ill-fated man

Maimon (Arabic) One who is dependable; having good fortune
Maymon, Maemon, Maimun, Maymun, Maemun, Mamon, Mamun

Maitland (English) From the meadow land
Maytland, Maetland, Maitlande, Maytlande, Maetlande

Majdy (Arabic) A glorious man
Majdey, Majdi, Majdie, Majdee, Majdea

Makaio (Hawaiian) A gift from God

Makena (Hawaiian) Man of abundance
Makenah

Makin (Arabic) Having great strength
Makeen, Makean, Makein, Makien, Makyn

Makis (Hebrew) A gift from God
Madys, Makiss, Makyss, Makisse, Madysse

Malachi (Hebrew) A messenger of God
Malachie, Malachy, Malaki, Malakia, Malakie, Malaquias, Malechy, Maleki

Malawa (African) A flourishing man

Malcolm (Gaelic) Follower of St. Columbus
Malcom, Malcolum, Malkolm, Malkom, Malkolum

Mali (Indian) A ruler; the firstborn son
Malie, Maly, Maley, Malee, Malea

Mamoru (Japanese) Of the earth
Mamorou, Mamorue, Mamorew, Mamoroo

Manchester (English) From the city in England
Manchestar, Manchestor, Manchestir, Manchestyr, Manchestur

Mandan (Native American) A tribal name
Manden, Mandon, Mandun, Mandin, Mandyn

Mandhatri (Indian) A prince; born to royalty
Mandhatrie, Mandhatry, Mandhatrey, Mandhatree, Mandhatrea

Mani (African) From the mountain
Manie, Many, Maney, Manee, Manea

Manjit (Indian) A conqueror of the mind; having great knowledge
Manjeet, Manjeat, Manjeit, Manjiet, Manjyt

Manley (English) From the man's meadow; from the hero's meadow
Manly, Manli, Manlie, Manlea, Manleah, Manlee, Manleigh

Manmohan (Indian) A handsome and pleasing man
Manmohen, Manmohin, Manmohyn

Mannheim (German) From the hamlet in the swamp
Manheim

Mano (Hawaiian) Resembling a shark
Manoe, Manow, Manowe

Manohar (Indian) A delightful and captivating man
Manoharr, Manohare

Mansel (English) From the clergyman's house
Mansle, Mansell, Mansele, Manselle, Manshel, Manshele, Manshell, Manshelle

Mansfield (English) From the field near the small river
Mansfeld, Maunfield, Maunfeld

Manton (English) From the man's town; from the hero's town
Mantun, Manten, Mannton, Manntun, Munnten

Manu (African) The second-born child
Manue, Manou, Manoo

Manuel (Spanish) Form of Emmanuel, meaning "God is with us"
Manuelo, Manuello, Manolito, Manolo, Manollo, Manny, Manni

Manya (Indian) A respected man
Manyah

Manzo (Japanese) The third son with ten-thousand-fold strength

Mar (Spanish) Of the sea
Marr, Mare, Marre

Marcel (French) The little warrior
Marceau, Marcelin, Marcellin, Marcellino, Marcell, Marcello, Marcellus, Marcelo

Marcus (Latin) Form of Mark, meaning "dedicated to Mars, the god of war"
Markus, Marcas, Marco, Markos

Mariatu (African) One who is pure; chaste
Mariatue, Mariatou, Mariatoo

Marid (Arabic) A rebellious man
Maryd

Mario (Latin) A manly man
Marius, Marios, Mariano, Marion, Mariun, Mareon

ᴛ**Mark** (Latin) Dedicated to Mars, the god of war
Marc, Markey, Marky, Marki, Markie, Markee, Markea, Markov

Marmion (French) Our little one
Marmyon, Marmeon

Marsh (English) From the marshland
Marshe

Marshall (French / English) A caretaker of horses / a steward
Marchall, Marischal, Marischall, Marschal, Marshal, Marshell, Marshel, Marschall

Marston (English) From the town near the marsh
Marstun, Marsten, Marstin, Marstyn, Marstan

Martin (Latin) Dedicated to Mars, the god of war
Martyn, Mart, Martel, Martell, Marten, Martenn, Marti, Martie

Marvin (Welsh) A friend of the sea
Marvinn, Marvinne, Marven, Marvenn, Marvenne, Marvyn, Marvynn, Marvynne, Mervin

Maryland (English) Honoring Queen Mary; from the state of Maryland
Mariland, Maralynd, Marylind, Marilind

Masanao (Japanese) A good man

Masao (Japanese) A righteous man

*ᴛ**Mason** (English) One who works with stone
Masun, Masen, Masan, Masin, Masyn, Masson, Massun, Massen

Masselin (French) A young Thomas
Masselyn, Masselen, Masselan, Masselon, Masselun, Maselin, Maselyn, Maselon

Masura (Japanese) A good destiny
Masoura

Mataniah (Hebrew) A gift
from God
Matania, Matanya,
Matanyahu, Mattania,
Mattaniah, Matanyah

Matata (African) One who
causes trouble

Matin (Arabic) Having
great strength
Maten, Matan, Matyn,
Maton, Matun

Matisse (French) One who
is gifted
Matiss, Matysse, Matyss,
Matise, Matyse

Matlock (American) A
rancher
Matlok, Mulloc

Matoskah (Native
American) Resembling a
white bear
Matoska

*ᵀ**Matthew** (Hebrew) A gift
from God
Matt, Mathew, Matvey,
Mateas, Mattix, Madteos,
Matthias, Mat, Mateo,
Matteo, Mateus

Matunde (African) One
who is fruitful
Matundi, Matundie

Matvey (Russian) Form of
Matthew, meaning "a gift
from God"
Matvy, Matvee, Matvea,
Matvi, Matvie, Motka,
Mutvlyko

Matwau (Native
American) The enemy

Maurice (Latin) A dark-
skinned man; Moorish
Maurell, Maureo, Mauricio,
Maurids, Maurie, Maurin,
Maurio, Maurise, Baurice

Maverick (English) An
independent man; a non-
conformist
Maveric, Maverik, Mavrick,
Mavric, Mavrik

Mawulol (African) One
who gives thanks to God

^**Maximilian** (Latin) The
greatest
Max, Macks, Maxi, Maxie,
Maxy, Maxey, Maxee,
*Maxea, **Maximus***

Maxfield (English) From
Mack's field
Mackfield, Maxfeld,
Macksfeld

ᵀ**Maxwell** (English) From
Mack's spring
Maxwelle, Mackswell,
Maxwel, Mackswel,
Mackwelle, Maxwill,
Maxwille, Mackswill

Mayer (Latin / German / Hebrew) A large man / a farmer / one who is shining bright
Maier, Mayar, Mayor, Mayir, Mayur, Meyer, Meir, Myer

Mayfield (English) From the strong one's field
Mayfeld, Maifield, Maifeld, Maefield, Maefeld

Mayo (Gaelic) From the yew tree plain
Mayoe, Maiyo, Maeyo, Maiyoe, Maeyoe, Mayoh, Maioh

Mccoy (Gaelic) The son of Coy
McCoy

McKenna (Gaelic) The son of Kenna; to ascend
McKennon, McKennun, McKennen, McKennan

Mckile (Gaelic) The son of Kyle
McKile, Mckyle, McKyle, Mackile, Mackyle, MacKile, MacKyle

Medad (Hebrew) A beloved friend
Meydad

Medgar (German) Having great strength
Medgarr, Medgare, Medgard, Medárd

Medwin (German) A strong friend
Medwine, Medwinn, Medwinne, Medwen, Medwenn, Medwenne, Medwyn, Medwynn

Meged (Hebrew) One who has been blessed with goodness

Mehdi (Arabian) One who is guided
Mehdie, Mehdy, Mehdey, Mehdee, Mehdea

Mehetabel (Hebrew) One who is favored by God
Mehetabell, Mehitabel, Mehitabell, Mehytabel, Mehytabell

Meilyr (Welsh) A regal ruler

Meinrad (German) A strong counselor
Meinred, Meinrod, Meinrud, Meinrid, Meinryd

Meka (Hawaiian) Of the eyes
Mekah

Melancton (Greek) Resembling a black flower
Melankton, Melanctun, Melanktun, Melancten, Melankten, Melanchton, Melanchten, Melanchthon

Mele (Hawaiian) One who is happy

Melesio (Spanish) An attentive man; one who is careful
Melacio, Melasio, Melecio, Melicio, Meliseo, Milesio

Meletius (Greek) A cautious man
Meletios, Meletious, Meletus, Meletos

Meli (Native American) One who is bitter
Melie, Mely, Meley, Melee, Melea, Meleigh

Melker (Swedish) A king
Melkar, Melkor, Melkur, Melkir, Melkyr

Melton (English) From the mill town
Meltun, Meltin, Meltyn, Melten, Meltan

Melville (English) From the mill town
Melvill, Melvil, Melvile, Melvylle, Melvyll, Melvyl, Melvyle

Melvin (English) A friend who offers counsel
Melvinn, Melvinne, Melven, Melvenn, Melvenne, Melvyn, Melvynn, Melvynne, Belvin

Memphis (American) From the city in Tennessee
Memfis, Memphys, Memfys, Memphus, Memfus

Menachem (Hebrew) One who provides comfort
Menaheim, Menahem, Menachim, Menachym, Menahim, Menahym, Machum, Machem

Menassah (Hebrew) A forgetful man
Menassa, Menass, Menas, Menasse, Menasseh

Menefer (Egyptian) Of the beautiful city
Menefar, Menefir, Menefyr, Menefor, Menefur

Menelik (African) The son of a wise man
Menelick, Menelic, Menelyk, Menelyck, Menelyc

Merewood (English) From the forest with the lake
Merwood, Merewode, Merwode

Merlin (Welsh) Of the sea fortress; in Arthurian legend, the wizard and mentor of King Arthur
Merlyn, Merlan, Merlon, Merlun, Merlen, Merlinn, Merlynn, Merlonn

Merrill (English) Of the shining sea
Meril, Merill, Merrel, Merrell, Merril, Meryl, Merryll, Meryll

Merton (English) From
the town near the lake
*Mertun, Mertan, Merten,
Mertin, Mertyn, Murton,
Murtun, Murten*

Mervin (Welsh) Form of
Marvin, meaning "a friend
of the sea"
*Mervinn, Mervinne,
Mervyn, Mervynn,
Mervynne, Merven,
Mervenn, Mervenne*

Meshach (Hebrew) An
enduring man
*Meshack, Meshac, Meshak,
Meeshach, Meeshack,
Meeshak, Meeshac*

Mhina (African) One who
is delightful
*Mhinah, Mheena,
Mheenah, Mheina,
Mheinah, Mhienah,
Mhienah, Mhyna*

*Michael (Hebrew) Who
is like God?
*Makai, Micael, Mical, Micha,
Michaelangelo, Michail,
Michal, Micheal,* **Miguel,** *Mick*

Micah (Hebrew) Form of
Michael, meaning "who is
like God?"
Mica, Mycah

Mick (English) Form of
Michael, meaning "who is
like God?"
*Micke, Mickey, Micky,
Micki, Mickie, Mickee,
Mickea, Mickel*

Mieko (Japanese) A bright
man

Miguel (Portuguese /
Spanish) Form of Michael,
meaning "who is like God?"
Migel, Myguel

Milan (Latin) An eager and
hardworking man
Mylan

Miles (German / Latin)
One who is merciful / a
soldier
*Myles, Miley, Mily, Mili,
Milie, Milee*

Milford (English) From
the mill's ford
*Millford, Milfurd, Millfurd,
Milferd, Millferd, Milforde,
Millforde, Milfurde*

Miller (English) One who
works at the mill
*Millar, Millor, Millur, Millir,
Millyr, Myller, Millen,
Millan*

^Milo (German) Form of
Miles, meaning one who
is merciful
Mylo

Milson (English) The son
of Miles
*Milsun, Milsen, Milsin,
Milsyn, Milsan*

Mimir (Norse) In mythology, a giant who guarded the well of wisdom
Mymir, Mimeer, Mimyr, Mymeer, Mymyr, Meemir, Meemeer, Meemyr

Miner (Latin / English) One who works in the mines / a youth
Minor, Minar, Minur, Minir, Minyr

Mingan (Native American) Resembling a gray wolf
Mingen, Mingin, Mingon, Mingun, Mingyn

Minh (Vietnamese) A clever man

Minster (English) Of the church
Mynster, Minstar, Mynstar, Minstor, Mynstor, Minstur, Mynstur, Minstir

Miracle (American) An act of God's hand
Mirakle, Mirakel, Myracle, Myrakle

Mirage (French) An illusion
Myrage

Mirumbi (African) Born during a period of rain
Mirumbie, Mirumby, Mirumbey, Mirumbee, Mirumbea

Missouri (Native American) From the town of large canoes; from the state of Missouri
Missourie, Mizouri, Mizourie, Missoury, Mizoury, Missuri, Mizuri, Mizury

Mitchell (English) Form of Michael, meaning "who is like God?"
Mitch, Mitchel, Mytch, Mitchum, Mytchill, Mitcham

Mitsu (Japanese) Of the light
Mytsu, Mitsue, Mytsue

Mochni (Native American) Resembling a talking bird
Mochnie, Mochny, Mochney, Mochnee, Mochnea

Modesty (Latin) One who is without conceit
Modesti, Modestie, Modestee, Modestus, Modestey, Modesto, Modestio, Modestine

Mogens (Dutch) A powerful man
Mogen, Mogins, Mogin, Mogyns, Mogyn, Mogan, Mogans

Mohajit (Indian) A charming man
Mohajeet, Mohajeat, Mohajeit, Mohajiet, Mohajyt

Mohammed (Arabic) One who is greatly praised; the name of the prophet and founder of Islam
Mahomet, Mohamad, Mohamed, Mohamet, Mohammad, Muhammad, Muhammed, Mehmet

Mohave (Native American) A tribal name
Mohav, Mojave

Mojag (Native American) One who is never quiet

Molan (Irish) The servant of the storm
Molen

Momo (American) A warring man

Mona (African) A jealous man
Monah

Mongo (African) A well-known man
Mongoe, Mongow, Mongowe

Mongwau (Native American) Resembling an owl

Monroe (Gaelic) From the mouth of the river Roe
Monro, Monrow, Monrowe, Munro, Munroe, Munrow, Munrowe

Montenegro (Spanish) From the black mountain

Montgomery (French) From Gomeric's mountain
Monty, Montgomerey, Montgomeri, Montgomerie, Montgomeree, Montgomerea

Monty (English) Form of Montgomery, meaning "from Gomeric's mountain"
Montey, Monti, Montie, Montee, Montea, Montes, Montez

Moon (American) Born beneath the moon; a dreamer

Mooney (Irish) A wealthy man
Moony, Mooni, Moonie, Maonaigh, Moonee, Moonea, Moone

Moose (American) Resembling the animal; a big, strong man
Moos, Mooze, Mooz

Moran (Irish) A great man
Morane, Morain, Moraine, Morayn, Morayne, Moraen, Moraene

Morathi (African) A wise man
Morathie, Morathy, Morathey, Morathee, Morathea

Moreland (English) From the moors
Moorland, Morland

Morley (English) From the meadow on the moor
Morly, Morleigh, Morlee, Morlea, Morleah, Morli, Morlie, Moorley

Morpheus (Greek) In mythology, the god of dreams
Morfeus, Morphius, Mofius

Mortimer (French) Of the still water; of the dead sea
Mortymer, Morty, Mortey, Morti, Mortie, Mortee, Mortea, Mort, Morte

Moses (Hebrew) A savior; in the Bible, the leader of the Israelites; drawn from the water
Mioshe, Mioshye, Mohsen, Moke, Moise, Moises, Mose, Moshe

Mostyn (Welsh) From the mossy settlement
Mostin, Mosten, Moston, Mostun, Mostan

Moswen (African) A light-skinned man
Moswenn, Moswenne, Moswin, Moswinn, Moswinne, Moswyn, Moswynn, Moswynne

Moubarak (Arabian) One who is blessed
Mubarak, Moobarak

Mounafes (Arabic) A rival

Muhannad (Arabic) One who wields a sword
Muhanned, Muhanad, Muhaned, Muhunnad, Muhunud, Muhanned, Muhaned

Mukhtar (Arabic) The chosen one
Muktar

Mukisa (Ugandan) Having good fortune
Mukysa

Mulcahy (Irish) A war chief
Mulcahey, Mulcahi, Mulcahie, Mulcahee, Mulcahea

Mundhir (Arabic) One who cautions others
Mundheer, Mundhear, Mundheir, Mundhier, Mundhyr

Murdock (Scottish) From the sea
Murdok, Murdoc, Murdo, Murdoch, Murtagh, Murtaugh, Murtogh, Murtough

Murfain (American) Having a warrior spirit
Murfaine, Murfayn, Murfayne, Murfaen, Murfaene, Murfane

Muriel (Gaelic) Of the shining sea
Muryel, Muriell, Muryell, Murial, Muriall, Muryal, Muryall, Murell

Murphy (Gaelic) A warrior of the sea
Murphey, Murphee, Murphea, Murphi, Murphie, Murfey, Murfy, Murfee

Murray (Gaelic) The lord of the sea
Murrey, Murry, Murri, Murrie, Murree, Murrea, Murry

Murron (Celtic) A bitter man
Murrun, Murren, Murran, Murrin, Murryn

Murtadi (Arabic) One who is content
Murtadie, Murtady, Murtadey, Murtadee, Murtadea

Musad (Arabic) One who is lucky
Musaad, Mus'ad

Mushin (Arabic) A charitable man
Musheen, Mushean, Mushein, Mushien, Mushyn

Muskan (Arabic) One who smiles often
Musken, Muskon, Muskun, Muskin, Muskyn

Muslim (Arabic) An adherent of Islam
Muslym, Muslem, Moslem, Moslim, Moslym

Mustapha (Arabic) The chosen one
Mustafa, Mostapha, Mostafa, Moustapha, Moustafa

Muti (Arabic) One who is obedient
Mutie, Muty, Mutey, Mutee, Mutea, Muta

Myron (Greek) Refers to myrrh, a fragrant oil
Myrun, Myran, Myren, Myrin, Myryn, Miron, Mirun, Miran

Mystique (French) A man with an air of mystery
Mystic, Mistique, Mysteek, Misteek, Mystiek, Mistiek, Mysteeque, Misteeque

n

Nabendu (Indian) Born beneath the new moon
Nabendue, Nabendoo, Nabendou

Nabhi (Indian) The best
*Nabhie, Nabhy, Nabhey,
Nabhee, Nabhea*

Nabhomani (Indian) Of
the sun
*Nabhomanie, Nabhomany,
Nabhomaney,
Nabhomanee, Nabhomanea*

Nabil (Arabic) A highborn
man
*Nabeel, Nabeal, Nabeil,
Nabiel, Nabyl*

Nabu (Babylonian) In
mythology, the god of
writing and wisdom
*Nabue, Naboo, Nabo, Nebo,
Nebu, Nebue, Neboo*

Nachshon (Hebrew) An
adventurous man; one
who is daring
Nachson

Nadav (Hebrew) A generous man
Nadaav

Nadif (African) One who
is born between seasons
*Nadeef, Nadief, Nadeif,
Nadyf, Nadeaf*

Nadim (Arabic) A beloved
friend
*Nadeem, Nadeam, Nadiem,
Nadeim, Nadym*

Naftali (Hebrew) A strug-
gling man; in the Bible,
one of Jacob's sons
*Naphtali, Naphthali,
Neftali, Nefthali, Nephtali,
Nephthali, Naftalie,
Naphtalie*

Nagel (German) One who
makes nails
*Nagle, Nagler, Naegel,
Nageler, Nagelle, Nagele,
Nagell*

Nahir (Hebrew) A clear-
headed and bright man
*Naheer, Nahear, Naheir,
Nahier, Nahyr, Naher*

Nahum (Hebrew) A com-
passionate man
*Nahom, Nahoum, Nuhoom,
Nahuem*

Naji (Arabic) One who is
safe
*Najea, Naje, Najee, Najie,
Najy, Najey, Nanji, Nanjie*

Najib (Arabic) Of noble
descent; a highborn man
*Najeeb, Najeab, Najeib,
Najieb, Najyb, Nageeb,
Nageab, Nagyb*

Nally (Irish) A poor man
*Nalley, Nalli, Nallie, Nallee,
Nallea, Nalleigh*

Namir (Israeli) Resembling
a leopard
*Nameer, Namear, Namier,
Nameir, Namyr*

Nandan (Indian) One who is pleasing
Nanden, Nandin, Nandyn, Nandon, Nandun

Naotau (Indian) Our new son
Naotou

Napier (French / English) A mover / one who takes care of the royal linens
Neper

Napoleon (Italian / German) A man from Naples / son of the mists
Napolean, Napolion, Napoleone, Napoleane, Napolione

Narcissus (Greek) Resembling a daffodil; self-love; in mythology, a youth who fell in love with his reflection
Narciso, Narcisse, Narkissos, Narses, Narcisus, Narcis, Narciss

Naresh (Indian) A king
Nareshe, Natesh, Nateshe

Nasih (Arabic) One who advises others
Nasyh

Natal (Spanish) Born at Christmastime
Natale, Natalino, Natalio, Natall, Natalle, Nataleo, Natica

*◦***Nathan** (Hebrew) Form of Nathaniel, meaning "a gift from God"
Nat, Natan, Nate, Nathen, Nathon, Nathin, Nathyn, Nathun, Lathan

*◦***Nathaniel** (Hebrew) A gift from God
Nathan, Natanael, Nataniel, Nathanael, Nathaneal, Nathanial, Nathanyal, Nathanyel, Nethanel

Nature (American) An outdoorsy man
Natural

Navarro (Spanish) From the plains
Navaro, Navarrio, Navario, Navarre, Navare, Nabaro, Nabarro

Naveed (Persian) Our best wishes
Navead, Navid, Navied, Naveid, Navyd

Nazim (Arabian) Of a soft breeze
Nazeem, Nazeam, Naziem, Nazeim, Nazym

Nebraska (Native American) From the flat water land; from the state of Nebraska

Neckarios (Greek) Of the nectar; one who is immortal
Nectaire, Nectarios, Nectarius, Nektario, Nektarius, Nektarios, Nektaire

Neelotpal (Indian) Resembling the blue lotus
Nealotpal, Nielotpal, Neilotpal, Nilothpal, Neelothpal

Negm (Arabian) Resembling a star

Nehal (Indian) Born during a period of rain
Nehall, Nehale, Nehalle

Nehemiah (Hebrew) God provides comfort
Nehemia, Nechemia, Nechemiah, Nehemya, Nehemyah, Nechemya, Nechemyah

Neil (Gaelic) The champion
Neal, Neale, Neall, Nealle, Nealon, Neel, Neilan, Neile

Neirin (Irish) Surrounded by light
Neiryn, Neiren, Neerin, Neeryn, Neeren

Nelek (Polish) Resembling a horn
Nelec, Neleck

Nelson (English) The son of Neil; the son of a champion
Nealson, Neilson, Neillson, Nelsen, Nilson, Nilsson, Nelli, Nellie

Neptune (Latin) In mythology, god of the sea
Neptun, Neptoon, Neptoone, Neptoun, Neptoune

Neroli (Italian) Resembling an orange blossom
Nerolie, Neroly, Neroley, Neroleigh, Nerolea, Nerolee

Nevan (Irish) The little saint
Naomhan

Neville (French) From the new village
Nev, Nevil, Nevile, Nevill, Nevylle, Nevyl, Nevyle, Nevyll

Newcomb (English) From the new valley
Newcom, Newcome, Newcombe, Neucomb, Neucombe, Neucom, Neucome

Newlin (Welsh) From the new pond
Newlinn, Newlyn, Newlynn, Neulin, Neulinn, Neulyn, Neulynn

Newman (English) A newcomer
Newmann, Neuman, Neumann

Nhat (Vietnamese) Having a long life
Nhatt, Nhate, Nhatte

Niaz (Persian) A gift
Nyaz

Nibaw (Native American)
One who stands tall
Nybaw, Nibau, Nybau

Nicholas (Greek) Of the
victorious people
*Nick, Nicanor, Niccolo,
Nichol, Nicholai, Nicholaus,
Nikolai, Nicholl, Nichols,
Colin, Nicolas, Nico*

Nick (English) Form of
Nicholas, meaning "of the
victorious people"
*Nik, Nicki, Nickie, Nickey,
Nicky, Nickee, Nickea, Niki*

Nickler (American) One
who is swift
*Nikler, Nicler, Nyckler,
Nykler, Nycler*

Nicomedes (Greek) One
who thinks of victory
*Nikomedes, Nicomedo,
Nikomedo*

Nihal (Indian) One who is
content
*Neehal, Neihal, Niehal,
Neahal, Neyhal, Nyhal*

Nihar (Indian) Covered
with the morning's dew
*Neehar, Niehar, Neihar,
Neahar, Nyhar*

Nikan (Persian) One who
brings good things
*Niken, Nikin, Nikyn,
Nikon, Nikun*

Nikshep (Indian) One who
is treasured
Nykshep

Nikunja (Indian) From the
grove of trees

Nino (Italian / Spanish)
God is gracious / a young
boy
Ninoshka

Nirad (Indian) Of the
clouds
Nyrad

Niran (Thai) The eternal
one
*Nyran, Niren, Nirin, Niryn,
Niron, Nirun, Nyren, Nyrin*

Nirav (Indian) One who
is quiet
Nyrav

Nirbheet (Indian) A fear-
less man
*Nirbhit, Nirbhyt, Nirbhay,
Nirbhaye, Nirbhai, Nirbhae*

Niremaan (Arabic) One
who shines as brightly as
fire
*Nyremaan, Nireman,
Nyreman*

Nishan (Armenian) A sign
or symbol

Nishok (Indian) Filled
with happiness
Nyshok, Nishock, Nyshock

Nissan (Hebrew) A miracle child
Nisan

Niyol (Native American) Of the wind

Njord (Scandinavian) A man from the north
Njorde, Njorth, Njorthe

*ᴛ**Noah** (Hebrew) A peaceful wanderer
Noa

Nodin (Native American) Of the wind
Nodyn, Noden, Nodan, Nodon, Nodun

Nolan (Gaelic) A famous and noble man; a champion of the people
Nolen, Nolin, Nolon, Nolun, Nolyn, Noland, Nolande

North (English) A man from the north
Northe

Northcliff (English) From the northern cliff
Northcliffe, Northclyf, Northclyff, Northclyffe

Norval (Scottish) From the northern valley
Norvall, Norvale, Norvail, Norvaile, Norvayl, Norvayle, Norvael, Norvaele

Norward (English) A guardian of the north
Norwarde, Norwerd, Norwerde, Norwurd, Norwurde

Noshi (Native American) A fatherly man
Noshie, Noshy, Noshey, Noshee, Noshea, Nosh, Noshe

Notaku (Native American) Resembling a growling bear
Notakou, Notakue, Notakoo

Nuhad (Arabic) A brave young man
Nuehad, Nouhad, Neuhad

Nukpana (Native American) An evil man
Nukpanah, Nukpanna, Nukpannah, Nuckpana, Nucpana

Nulte (Irish) A man from Ulster
Nulti, Nultie, Nulty, Nultey, Nultee, Nultea

Nuncio (Spanish) A messenger
Nunzio

Nuriel (Hebrew) God's light
Nuriell, Nuriele, Nurielle, Nuryel, Nuryell, Nuryele, Nuryelle, Nooriel

Nuru (African) My light
Nurue, Nuroo, Nurou, Nourou, Nooroo

Nyack (African) One who is persistent
Niack, Nyak, Niak, Nyac, Niac

Nye (English) One who lives on the island
Nyle, Nie, Nile

O

Obedience (American) A well-behaved man
Obediance, Obedyence, Obedeynce

Oberon (German) A royal bear; having the heart of a bear
Oberron

Obert (German) A wealthy and bright man
Oberte, Oberth, Oberthe, Odbart, Odbarte, Odbarth, Odbarthe, Odhert

Ochi (African) Filled with laughter
Ochie, Ochee, Ochea, Ochy, Ochey

Odam (English) A son-in-law
Odom, Odem, Odum

Ode (Egyptian / Greek) Traveler of the road / a lyric poem

Oded (Hebrew) One who is supportive and encouraging

Oder (English) From the river
Odar, Odir, Odyr, Odur

Odin (Norse) In mythology, the supreme deity
Odyn, Odon, Oden, Odun

Odinan (Hungarian) One who is wealthy and powerful
Odynan, Odinann, Odynann

Odion (African) The first-born of twins
Odiyon, Odiun, Odiyun

Odissan (African) A wanderer; traveler
Odyssan, Odisan, Odysan, Odissann, Odyssann, Odisann, Odysann

Ofir (Hebrew) The golden son
Ofeer, Ofear, Ofyr, Ofier, Ofeir, Ofer

Ogaleesha (Native American) A man wearing a red shirt
Ogaleasha, Ogaleisha, Ogaleysha, Ogalesha, Ogaliesha, Ogalisha

Oghe (Irish) One who rides horses
Oghi, Oghie, Oghee, Oghea, Oghy, Oghey

Oguz (Hungarian) An arrow
Oguze, Oguzz, Oguzze

Ohanko (Native American) A reckless man
Ohankio, Ohankiyo

Ojaswit (Indian) A powerful and radiant man
Ojaswyt, Ojaswin, Ojaswen, Ojaswyn, Ojas

Okal (African) To cross
Okall

Okan (Turkish) Resembling a horse
Oken, Okin, Okyn

Okapi (African) Resembling an animal with a long neck
Okapie, Okapy, Okapey, Okapee, Okapea, Okape

Okechuku (African) Blessed by God

Oki (Japanese) From the center of the ocean
Okie, Oky, Okey, Okee, Okea

Oklahoma (Native American) Of the red people; from the state of Oklahoma

Oktawian (African) The eighth-born child
Oktawyan, Oktawean, Octawian, Octawyan, Octawean

Olaf (Scandinavian) The remaining of the ancestors
Olay, Ole, Olef, Olev, Oluf, Uolevi

Olafemi (African) A lucky young man
Olafemie, Olafemy, Olafemey, Olafemee, Olafemea

Oleg (Russian) One who is holy
Olezka

Oliver (Latin) From the olive tree
Oliviero, Olivero, Olivier, Oliviero, Olivio, Ollie

Olney (English) From the loner's field
Olny, Olnee, Olnea, Olni, Olnie, Ollaneg, Olaneg

Olujimi (African) One who is close to God
Olujimie, Olujimy, Olujimey, Olujimee, Olujimea

Olumide (African) God has arrived
Olumidi, Olumidie, Olumidy, Olumidey, Olumidee, Olumidea, Olumyde, Olumydi

Omar (Arabic) A flourishing man; one who is well-spoken
Omarr, Omer

Omeet (Hebrew) My light
Omeete, Omeit, Omeite, Omeyt, Omeyte, Omit, Omeat, Omeate

Omega (Greek) The last great one; the last letter of the Greek alphabet
Omegah

Onaona (Hawaiian) Having a pleasant scent

Ond (Hungarian) The tenth-born child
Onde

Ondrej (Czech) A manly man
Ondrejek, Ondrejec, Ondrousek, Ondravsek

Onkar (Indian) The purest one
Onckar, Oncar, Onkarr, Onckarr, Oncarr

Onofrio (Italain) A defender of peace
Onofre, Onofrius, Onophrio, Onophre, Onfrio, Onfroi

Onslow (Arabic) From the hill of the enthusiast
Onslowe, Ounslow, Ounslowe

Onyebuchi (African) God is in everything
Onyebuchie, Onyebuchy, Onyebuchey, Onyebuchee, Onyebuchea

Oqwapi (Native American) Resembling a red cloud
Oqwapie, Oqwapy, Oqwapey, Oqwapee, Oqwapea

Oram (English) From the enclosure near the river-bank
Oramm, Oraham, Orahamm, Orham, Orhamm

Ordell (Latin) Of the beginning
Ordel, Ordele, Ordelle, Orde

Ordway (Anglo-Saxon) A fighter armed with a spear
Ordwaye, Ordwai, Ordwae

Oren (Hebrew / Gaelic) From the pine tree / a pale-skinned man
Orenthiel, Orenthiell, Orenthiele, Orenthielle, Orenthiem, Orenthium, Orin

Orleans (Latin) The golden child
Orlean, Orleane, Orleens, Orleen, Orleene, Orlins, Olryns, Orlin

Orly (Hebrew) Surrounded by light
Orley, Orli, Orlie, Orlee, Orleigh, Orlea

Ormod (Anglo-Saxon) A sorrowful man

Ormond (English) One who defends with a spear / from the mountain of bears
Ormonde, Ormund, Ormunde, Ormemund, Ormemond, Ordmund, Ordmunde, Ordmond

Ornice (Irish / Hebrew) A pale-skinned man / from the cedar tree
Ornyce, Ornise, Orynse, Orneice, Orneise, Orniece, Orniese, Orneece

Orris (Latin) One who is inventive
Orriss, Orrisse, Orrys, Orryss, Orrysse

Orson (Latin) Resembling a bear; raised by a bear
Orsen, Orsin, Orsini, Orsino, Orsis, Orsonio, Orsinie, Orsiny

Orth (English) An honest man
Orthe

Orton (English) From the settlement by the shore
Ortun, Oraton, Oratun

Orville (French) From the gold town
Orvell, Orvelle, Orvil, Orvill, Orvele, Orvyll, Orvylle, Orvyl

Orwel (Welsh) Of the horizon
Orwell, Orwele, Orwelle

Os (English) The divine

Osborn (Norse) A bear of God
Osborne, Osbourn, Osbourne, Osburn, Osburne

Oscar (English / Gaelic) A spear of the gods / a friend of deer
Oskar, Osker, Oscer, Osckar, Oscker, Oszkar, Oszcar

Osher (Hebrew) A man of good fortune

Osias (Greek) Salvation
Osyas

Osileani (Polynesian) One who talks a lot
Osileanie, Osileany, Osileaney, Osileanee, Osileanea

Oswald (English) The power of God
Oswalde, Osvald, Osvaldo, Oswaldo, Oswell, Osvalde, Oswallt, Osweald

Oswin (English) A friend of God
Oswinn, Oswinne, Oswen, Oswenn, Oswenne, Oswyn, Oswynn, Oswynne

Othniel (Hebrew) God's
lion
*Othniell, Othnielle,
Othniele, Othnyel, Othnyell,
Othnyele, Othnyelle*

Otmar (Teutonic) A
famous warrior
*Otmarr, Othmar, Othmarr,
Otomar, Ottomar*

Otoahhastis (Native
American) Resembling a
tall bull

Ottokar (German) A spir-
ited warrior
*Otokar, Otokarr, Ottokarr,
Ottokars, Otokars, Ottocar,
Otocar, Ottocars*

Ouray (Native American)
The arrow
Ouraye, Ourae, Ourai

Ourson (French)
Resembling a little bear
*Oursun, Oursoun, Oursen,
Oursan, Oursin, Oursyn*

Ovid (Latin) A shepherd;
an egg
*Ovyd, Ovidio, Ovido,
Ovydio, Ovydo, Ovidiu,
Ovydiu, Ofydd*

Owen (Welsh / Gaelic)
Form of Eugene, mean-
ing "a well-born man" / a
youthful man
*Owenn, Owenne, Owin,
Owinn, Owinne, Owyn,
Owynn, Owynne*

Oxton (English) From the
oxen town
*Oxtun, Oxtown, Oxnaton,
Oxnatun, Oxnatown*

Oz (Hebrew) Having great
strength
*Ozz, Ozzi, Ozzie, Ozzy,
Ozzey, Ozzee, Ozzea, Ozi*

Ozni (Hebrew) One who
knows God
*Oznie, Ozny, Ozney,
Oznee, Oznea*

Ozuru (Japanese)
Resembling a stork
*Ozurou, Ozourou, Ozuroo,
Ozooroo*

p

Paavo (Finnish) Form of
Paul, meaning "a small or
humble man"
Paaveli

Pace (Hebrew / English)
Refers to Passover / a
peaceful man
*Paice, Payce, Paece, Pacey,
Pacy, Pacee, Paci, Pacie*

Pacho (Spanish) An independent man; one who
is free

Pachu'a (Native American) Resembling a water snake

Paco (Spanish) A man from France
Pacorro, Pacoro, Puquito

Padgett (French) One who strives to better himself
Padget, Padgette, Padgete, Padgeta, Padgetta, Padge, Paget, Pagett

Padman (Indian) Resembling the lotus
Padmann

Padruig (Scottish) Of the royal family

Paine (Latin) Man from the country; a peasant
Pain, Payn, Payne, Paen, Paene, Pane, Paien

Palamedes (English) In Arthurian legend, a knight
Palomydes, Palomedes, Palamydes, Palsmedes, Palsmydes, Pslomydes

Palban (Spanish) A blond-haired man
Palben, Palbin, Palbyn, Palbon, Palbun

Paley (English) Form of Paul, meaning "a small or humble man"
Paly, Pali, Palie, Palee, Palea

Palladin (Greek) Filled with wisdom
Palladyn, Palladen, Palladan, Paladin, Paladyn, Paladen, Paladan

Palmer (English) A pilgrim bearing a palm branch
Pullmer, Palmar, Pallmar, Palmerston, Palmiro, Palmeero, Palmeer, Palmire

Pan (Greek) In mythology, god of the shepherds
Pann

Panama (Spanish) From the canal

Pancho (Spanish) A man from France

Pankaj (Indian) Resembling the lotus flower

Panya (African) Resembling a mouse
Panyah

Panyin (African) The first-born of twins
Panyen

Paras (Hindi) A touchstone
Parasmani, Parasmanie, Parasmany, Parasmaney, Parasmanee

Parker (English) The keeper of the park
Parkar, Parkes, Parkman, Park

Parley (Scottish) A reluctant man
Parly, Parli, Parlie, Parlee, Parlea, Parle

Parmenio (Spanish) A studious man; one who is intelligent
Parmenios, Parmenius

Parounag (Armenian) One who is thankful

Parrish (Latin) Man of the church
Parish, Parrishe, Parishe, Parrysh, Parysh, Paryshe, Parryshe, Parisch

Parry (Welsh) The son of Harry
Parrey, Parri, Parrie, Parree, Parrea

Parthenios (Greek) One who is pure; chaste
Parthenius

Parthik (Greek) One who is pure; chaste
Parthyk, Parthick, Parthyck, Parthic, Parthyc

Pascal (Latin) Born during Easter
Pascale, Pascalle, Paschal, Paschalis, Pascoe, Pascual, Pascuale, Pasqual

Patamon (Native American) Resembling a tempest
Patamun, Patamen, Pataman, Patamyn, Patamin

Patch (American) Form of Peter, meaning "as solid and strong as a rock"
Pach, Patche, Patchi, Patchie, Patchy, Patchey, Patchee

•Patrick (Latin) A nobleman; patrician
Packey, Padric, Pat, Patrece, Patric, Patrice, Patreece, Patricio

Patton (English) From the town of warriors
Paten, Patin, Paton, Patten, Pattin, Paddon, Padden, Paddin

Patwin (Native American) A manly man
Patwinn, Patwinne, Patwyn, Patwynne, Patwynn, Patwen, Patwenn, Patwenne

Paul (Latin) A small or humble man
Pauley, Paulie, Pauly, Paley, Paavo

Paurush (Indian) A courageous man
Paurushe, Paurushi, Paurushie, Paurushy, Paurushey, Paurushee

Pavanjit (Indian) Resembling the wind
Pavanjyt, Pavanjeet, Pavanjeat, Pavanjete

^**Paxton** (English) From the peaceful town
Packston, Paxon, Paxten, Paxtun, Packstun, Packsten

Pazel (Hebrew) God's gold; treasured by God
Pazell, Pazele, Pazelle

Pearroc (English) Man of the forest
Pearoc, Pearrok, Pearok, Pearrock, Pearock

Pecos (American) From the river; a cowboy
Pekos, Peckos

Pedro (Spanish) Form of Peter, meaning "as solid and strong as a rock"
Pedrio, Pepe, Petrolino, Piero, Pietro

Pelham (English) From the house of furs; from Peola's home
Pellham, Pelam, Pellam

Pell (English) A clerk or one who works with skins
Pelle, Pall, Palle

Pelon (Spanish) Filled with joy
Pellon

Pelton (English) From the town by the lake
Pellton, Peltun, Pelltun, Peltan, Pelltan, Pelten, Pellten, Peltin

Penda (African) One who is dearly loved
Pendah, Penha, Penhah

Penley (English) From the enclosed meadow
Penly, Penleigh, Penli, Penlie, Penlee, Penlea, Penleah, Pennley

Penrod (German) A respected commander

Pentele (Hungarian) A merciful man
Pentelle, Pentel, Pentell

Penuel (Hebrew) The face of God
Penuell, Penuele, Penuelle

Percival (French) One who can pierce the vale"
Purcival, Percy, Percey, Perci, Percie, Percee, Percea, Persy, Persey, Persi

Peregrine (Latin) One who travels; a wanderer
Perry, Perree, Perrea, Perri, Perrie, Perregrino

Perez (Hebrew) To break through
Peretz

Pericles (Greek) One who is in excess of glory
Perricles, Perycles, Perrycles, Periclees, Perriclees, Peryclees, Perryclees, Periclez

Perk (American) One who is cheerful and jaunty
Perke, Perky, Perkey, Perki, Perkie, Perkee, Perkea

Perkinson (English) The son of Perkin; the son of Peter
Perkynson

Perseus (Greek) In mythology, son of Zeus who slew Medusa
Persius, Persyus, Persies, Persyes

Perth (Celtic) From the thorny thicket
Perthe, Pert, Perte

Perye (English) From the pear tree

Peter (Greek) As solid and strong as a rock
Peder, Pekka, Per, Petar, Pete, Peterson, Petr, Petre, Pierce, Patch, Pedro

Petuel (Hindi) The Lord's vision
Petuell, Petuele, Petuelle

Peyton (English) From the village of warriors
Payton, Peytun, Paytun, Peyten, Payten, Paiton, Paitun, Paiten

Pharis (Irish) A heroic man
Pharys, Pharris, Pharrys

Phex (American) A kind man
Phexx

Philemon (Hebrew) A loving man
Phylemon, Philimon, Phylimon, Philomon, Phylomon, Philamon, Phylamon

Philetus (Greek) A collector
Phyletus, Philetos, Phyletos

Phillip (Greek) One who loves horses
Phil, Philip, Felipe, Filipp, Phillie, Philly

Philo (Greek) One who loves and is loved

Phoebus (Greek) A radiant man
Phoibos

Phomello (African) A successful man
Phomelo

Phong (Vietnamese) Of the wind

Phuc (Vietnamese) One who is blessed
Phuoc

Picardus (Hispanic) An adventurous man
Pycardus, Picardos, Pycardos, Picardas, Pycardas, Picardis, Pycardis, Picardys

Pickworth (English) From the woodcutter's estate
Pikworth, Picworth, Pickworthe, Pikworthe, Picworthe

Pierce (English) Form of Peter, meaning "as solid and strong as a rock"
Pearce, Pears, Pearson, Pearsson, Peerce, Peirce, Pierson, Piersson

Pin (Vietnamese) Filled with joy
Pyn

Pio (Latin) A pious man
Pyo, Pios, Pius, Pyos, Pyus

Pirro (Greek) A red-haired man
Pyrro

Pitney (English) From the island of the stubborn man
Pitny, Pitni, Pitnie, Pitnee, Pitnea, Pytney, Pytny, Pytni

Pittman (English) A laborer
Pyttman, Pitman, Pytman

Plantagenet (French) Resembling the broom flower

Poetry (American) A romantic man
Poetrey, Poetri, Poetrie, Poetree, Poetrea, Poet, Poete

Pollux (Greek) One who is crowned
Pollock, Pollok, Polloc, Pollack, Polloch

Polo (African) Resembling an alligator
Poloe, Poloh

Ponce (Spanish) The fifth-born child
Ponse

Pongor (Hungarian) A mighty man
Pongorr, Pongoro, Pongorro

Poni (African) The second-born son
Ponni, Ponie, Ponnie, Pony, Ponny, Poney, Ponney, Ponee

Pons (Latin) From the bridge
Pontius, Ponthos, Ponthus

Poornamruth (Indian) Full of sweetness
Pournamruth

Poornayu (Indian) Full of life; blessed with a full life
Pournayu, Poornayou, Pournayou, Poornayue, Pournayue

Porat (Hebrew) A productive man

Porfirio (Greek) Refers to a purple coloring
Porphirios, Prophyrios, Porfiro, Porphyrios

Powhatan (Native American) From the chief's hill

Prabhakar (Hindu) Of the sun

Prabhat (Indian) Born during the morning

Pragun (Indian) One who is straightforward; honest

Pramod (Indian) A delightful young man

Pranit (Indian) One who is humble; modest
Pranyt, Praneet, Praneat

Prasad (Indian) A gift from God

Prashant (Indian) One who is peaceful; calm
Prashante, Prashanth, Prashanthe

Pratap (Hindi) A majestic man

Pravat (Thai) History

Prem (Indian) An affectionate man

Prentice (English) A student; an apprentice
Prentyce, Prentise, Prentyse, Prentiss, Prentis

Prescott (English) From the priest's cottage
Prescot, Prestcot, Prestcott, Preostcot

Preston (English) From the priest's town
Prestin, Prestyn, Prestan, Prestun, Presten, Pfeostun

Prewitt (French) A brave young one
Prewet, Prewett, Prewit, Pruitt, Pruit, Pruet, Pruett

Prine (English) One who surpasses others
Pryne

Prometheus (Greek) In mythology, he stole fire from the heavens and gave it to man
Promitheus, Promethius, Promithius

Prop (American) A fun-loving man
Propp, Proppe

Prosper (Latin) A fortunate man
Prospero, Prosperus

Pryderi (Celtic) Son of the sea
Pryderie, Prydery, Pryderey, Pryderee, Pryderea

Prydwen (Welsh) A handsome man
Prydwenn, Prydwenne, Prydwin, Prydwinne, Prydwinn, Prydwyn, Prydwynn, Prydwynne

Pullman (English) One who works on a train
Pulman, Pullmann, Pulmann

Pyralis (Greek) Born of fire
Pyraliss, Pyralisse, Pyralys, Pyralyss, Pyralysse, Pyre

q

Qabil (Arabic) An able-bodied man
Qabyl, Qabeel, Qabeal, Qabeil, Qabiel

Qadim (Arabic) From an ancient family
Qadeem, Qadiem, Qadeim, Qadym, Qadeam

Qaiser (Arabic) A king; a ruler
Qeyser

Qamar (Arabic) Born beneath the moon
Qamarr, Quamar, Quamarr

Qimat (Hindi) A highly valued man
Qymat

Qing (Chinese) Of the deep water
Qyng

Quaashie (American) An ambitious man
Quashie, Quashi, Quashy, Quashey, Quashee, Quashea, Quaashi, Quuashy

Quaddus (American) A bright man
Quadus, Quaddos, Quados

Quade (Latin) The fourth-born child
Quadrees, Quadres, Quadrys, Quadries, Quadreis, Quadreys, Quadreas, Quadrhys

Quaid (Irish) Form of Walter, meaning "the commander of the army"
Quaide, Quayd, Quayde, Quaed, Quaede

Quashawn (American) A tenacious man
Quashaun, Quasean, Quashon, Quashi, Quashie, Quashee, Quashea, Quashy

Qued (Native American) Wearing a decorated robe

Quentin (Latin) The fifth-born child
Quent, Quenten, Quenton, Quentun, Quentan, Quentyn, Quente, Qwentin

Quick (American) One who is fast; a witty man
Quik, Quicke, Quic

Quillan (Gaelic) Resembling a cub
Quilan, Quillen, Quilen, Quillon, Quilon

Quilliam (Gaelic) Form of William, meaning "the determined protector"
Quilhelm, Quilhelmus, Quilliams, Quilliamson

Quimby (Norse) From the woman's estate
Quimbey, Quimbee, Quimbea, Quimbi, Quimbie

Quincy (English) The fifth-born child; from the fifth son's estate
Quincey, Quinci, Quincie, Quincee, Quinncy, Quinnci, Quyncy, Quyncey

Quinlan (Gaelic) A strong and healthy man
Quindlan, Quinlen, Quindlen, Quinian, Quinlin, Quindlin, Quinlyn, Quindlyn

Quinn (Gaelic) One who provides counsel; an intelligent man
Quin, Quinne, Qwinn, Quynn, Qwin, Quiyn, Quyn, Qwinne

Quintavius (American) The fifth-born child
Quintavios, Quintavus, Quintavies

Quinto (Spanish) The fifth-born child
Quynto, Quintus, Quintos, Quinty, Quinti, Quintie

Quinton (Latin) From the queen's town or settlement
Laquinton

Quintrell (English) An elegant and dashing man
Quintrel, Quintrelle, Quyntrell, Quyntrelle, Quyntrel, Quyntrele, Quintrele

Quirinus (Latin) One who wields a spear
Quirinos, Quirynus, Quirynos, Quirinius, Quirynius

Quito (Spanish) A lively man
Quyto, Quitos, Quytos

Quoc (Vietnamese) A patriot
Quok, Quock

Qutub (Indian) One who is tall

r

Rabbaanee (African) An easygoing man

Rabbi (Hebrew) The master

Rach (African) Resembling a frog

Radames (Egyptian) A hero
Radamays, Radamayes, Radamais, Radamaise

Radford (English) From the red ford
Radforde, Radferd, Radfurd, Radferde, Radfurde

Rafael (Spanish) Form of Raphael, meaning "one who is healed by God"
Raphael, Raphaello, Rafaello

Rafe (Irish) A tough man
Raffe, Raff, Raf, Raif, Rayfe, Raife, Raef, Raefe

Rafi (Arabic) One who is exalted
Rafie, Rafy, Rafey, Rafea, Rafee, Raffi, Raffie, Raffy

Rafiki (African) A gentle friend
Rafikie, Rafikea, Rafikee, Rafiky, Rafikey

Rafiya (African) A dignified man
Rafeeya, Rafeaya, Rafeiya, Rafieya

Raghib (Arabic) One who is desired
Ragheb, Ragheeb, Ragheab, Raghyb, Ragheib, Raghieb

Ragnar (Norse) A warrior who places judgment
Ragnor, Ragner, Ragnir, Ragnyr, Ragnur, Regnar

Rahim (Arabic) A compassionate man
Rahym, Raheim, Rahiem, Raheem, Raheam

Raiden (Japanese) In mythology, the god of thunder and lightning
Raidon, Rayden, Raydon, Raeden, Raedon, Raden

Raimi (African) A compassionate man
Raimie, Raimy, Raimey, Raimee, Raimea

Rajab (African) A glorified man

Rajan (Indian) A king
Raj, Raja, Rajah

Rajarshi (Indian) The king's sage
Rajarshie, Rajarshy, Rajarshey, Rajarshee, Rajarshea

Rajesh (Hindi) The king's rule

Rajit (Indian) One who is decorated
Rajeet, Rajeit, Rajiet, Rajyt, Rajeat

Rajiv (Hindi) To be striped
Rajyv, Rajeev, Rajeav

Ralph (English) Wolf counsel
Ralf, Ralphe, Ralfe, Ralphi, Ralphie, Ralphee, Ralphea, Ralphy, Raoul

Ram (Hebrew / Sanskrit) A superior man / one who is pleasing
Rahm, Rama, Rahma, Ramos, Rahmos, Ram, Ramm

Rambert (German) Having great strength; an intelligent man
Ramberte, Ramberth, Ramberthe, Ramburt

Rami (Arabic) A loving man
Ramee, Ramea, Ramie, Ramy, Ramey

Ramiro (Portuguese) A famous counselor; a great judge
Ramyro, Rameero, Rameyro, Ramirez, Ramyrez, Rameerez

Ramsey (English) From the raven island; from the island of wild garlic
Ramsay, Ramsie, Ramsi, Ramsee, Ramsy, Ramsea, Ramzy, Ramzey

Rand (German) One who shields others
Rande

Randall (German) The wolf shield
Randy, Randal, Randale, Randel, Randell, Randl, Randle, Randon, Rendall

Randolph (German) The wolf shield
Randy, Randolf, Ranolf, Ranolph, Ranulfo, Randulfo, Randwulf, Ranwulf, Randwolf

Randy (English) Form of Randall or Randolph, meaning "the wolf shield"
Randey, Randi, Randie, Randee, Randea

Rang (English) Resembling a raven
Range

Rangey (English) From raven's island
Rangy, Rangi, Rangie, Rangee, Rangea

Rangle (American) A cowboy
Rangel

Ranjan (Indian) A delightful boy

Raoul (French) Form of Ralph, meaning "wolf counsel"
Raoule, Raul, Roul, Rowl, Raule, Roule, Rowle

Raqib (Arabic) A glorified man
Raqyb, Raqeeb, Raqeab, Rakib, Rakeeb, Rakeab, Rakyb

Rashard (American) A good-hearted man
Rasherd, Rashird, Rashurd, Rashyrd

Rashaun (American) Form of Roshan, meaning "born during the daylight"
Rashae, Rashane, Rashawn, Rayshaun, Rayshawn, Raishaun, Raishawn, Raeshaun

Ratul (Indian) A sweet man
Ratule, Ratoul, Ratoule, Ratool, Ratoole

Raulo (Spanish) One who is wise
Rawlo

Ravi (Hindi) From the sun
Ravie, Ravy, Ravey, Ravee, Ravea

Ravid (Hebrew) A wanderer; one who searches
Ravyd, Raveed, Ravead, Raviyd, Ravied, Raveid

Ravindra (Indian) The strength of the sun
Ravyndra

Ravinger (English) One who lives near the ravine
Ravynger

Rawlins (French) From the renowned land
Rawlin, Rawson, Rawlinson, Rawlings, Rawling, Rawls, Rawl, Rawle

Ray (English) Form of Raymond, meaning "a wise protector"
Rae, Rai, Rayce, Rayder, Rayse, Raye, Rayford, Raylen

Rayfield (English) From the field of roe deer
Rayfeld

Rayhurn (English) From the roe deer's stream
Rayhurne, Rayhorn, Rayhorne, Rayhourn, Rayhourne

Raymond (German) A wise protector
Ray, Raemond, Raemondo, Raimond, Raimondo, Raimund, Raimundo, Rajmund, Ramon

Rebel (American) An outlaw
Rebell, Rebele, Rebelle, Rebe, Rebbe, Rebbi, Rebbie, Rebbea

Redwald (English) Strong counsel
Redwalde, Raedwalde, Raedwald

Reeve (English) A bailiff
Reve, Reave, Reeford, Reeves, Reaves, Reves, Reaford

Regal (American) Born into royalty
Regall

Regan (Gaelic) Born into royalty; the little ruler
Raegan, Ragan, Raygan, Reganne, Regann, Regane, Reghan, Reagan

Regenfrithu (English) A peaceful raven

Reggie (Latin) Form of Reginald, meaning "the king's advisor"
Reggi, Reggy, Reggey, Reggea, Reggee, Reg

Reginald (Latin) The king's advisor
Reggie, Reynold, Raghnall, Rainault, Rainhold, Raonull, Raynald, Rayniero, Regin, Reginaldo

Regine (French) One who is artistic
Regeen, Regeene, Regean, Regeane, Regein, Regeine, Regien, Regiene

^**Reid** (English) A red-haired man; one who lives near the reeds
Read, Reade, Reed, Reede, Reide, Raed

Reilly (Gaelic) An outgoing man
Reilley, Reilli, Reillie, Reillee, Reilleigh, Reillea

Remington (English) From the town of the raven's family
Remyngton, Remingtun, Remyngtun

Renweard (Anglo-Saxon) The guardian of the house
Renward, Renwarden, Renwerd

Renzo (Japanese) The third-born son

Reuben (Hebrew) Behold, a son!
Reuban, Reubin, Reuven, Rouvin, Rube, Ruben, Rubin, Rubino

Rev (American) One who is distinct
Revv, Revin, Reven, Revan, Revyn, Revon, Revun

Rex (Latin) A king
Reks, Recks, Rexs

Rexford (English) From the king's ford
Rexforde, Rexferd, Rexferde, Rexfurd, Rexfurde

Reynold (English) Form of Reginald, meaning "the king's advisor"
Reynald, Reynaldo, Reynolds, Reynalde, Reynolde

Rhett (Latin) A well-spoken man
Rett, Rhet

Rhydderch (Welsh) Having reddish-brown hair

Richard (English) A powerful ruler
Rick, Rich, Ricard, Ricardo, Riccardo, Richardo, Richart, Richerd, Rickard, Rickert

Richmond (French / German) From the wealthy hill / a powerful protector
Richmonde, Richmund, Richmunde

Rick (English) Form of Richard, meaning "a powerful ruler"
Ric, Ricci, Ricco, Rickie, Ricki, Ricky, Rico, Rik

Rickward (English) A strong protector
Rickwerd, Rickwood, Rikward, Ricward, Rickweard, Rikweard, Ricweard

Riddock (Irish) From the smooth field
Ridock, Riddoc, Ridoc, Ryddock, Rydock, Ryddoc, Rydoc, Ryddok

Ridgeway (English) One who lives on the road near the ridge
Rydgeway, Rigeway, Rygeway

Rigg (English) One who lives near the ridge
Rig, Ridge, Rygg, Ryg, Rydge, Rige, Ryge, Riggs

Riley (English) From the rye clearing
Ryly, Ryli, Rylie, Rylee, Ryleigh, Rylea, Ryleah

Riordain (Irish) A bright man
Riordane, Riordayn, Riordaen, Reardain, Reardane, Reardayn, Reardaen

Riordan (Gaelic) A royal poet; a bard or minstrel
Riorden, Rearden, Reardan, Riordon, Reardon

Ripley (English) From the noisy meadow
Riply, Ripleigh, Ripli, Riplie, Riplea, Ripleah, Riplee, Rip

Rishley (English) From the untamed meadow
Rishly, Rishli, Rishlie, Rishlee, Rishlea, Rishleah, Rishleigh

Rishon (Hebrew) The first-born son
Ryshon, Rishi, Rishie, Rishea, Rishee, Rishy, Rishey

Risley (English) From the brushwood meadow
Risly, Risli, Rislie, Risleigh, Rislea, Risleah, Rislee

Riston (English) From the brushwood settlement
Ryston, Ristun, Rystun

Ritter (German) A knight
Rytter, Ritt, Rytt

^**River** (American) From the river
Ryver, Rivers, Ryvers

Roald (Norse) A famous ruler
Roal

Roam (American) One who wanders, searches
Roami, Roamie, Roamy, Roamey, Roamea, Roamee

Roark (Gaelic) A champion
Roarke, Rorke, Rourke, Rork, Rourk, Ruark, Ruarke

•**Robert** (German) One who is bright with fame
Bob, Rupert, Riobard, Roban, Robers, Roberto, Robertson, Robartach

Rochester (English) From the stone fortress

Rockford (English) From the rocky ford
Rockforde, Rokford, Rokforde, Rockferd, Rokferd, Rockfurd, Rokfurd

Roderick (German) A famous ruler
Rod, Rodd, Roddi, Roddie, Roddy, Roddee, Roddea

Rodney (German / English) From the famous one's island / from the island's clearing
Rodny, Rodni, Rodnie

Rogelio (Spanish) A famous soldier
Rogelo, Rogeliyo, Rogeleo, Rogeleyo, Rojelio, Rojeleo

Roland (German) From the renowned land
Roeland, Rolando, Roldan, Roley, Rollan, Rolland, Rollie, Rollin

Roman (Latin) A citizen of Rome
Romain, Romaine, Romeo

Ronald (Norse) The king's advisor
Ranald, Renaldo, Ronal, Ronaldo, Rondale, Roneld, Ronell, Ronello

Ronan (Gaelic) Resembling a little seal

Rong (Chinese) Having glory

Rook (English) Resembling a raven
Rooke, Rouk, Rouke, Ruck, Ruk

Rooney (Gaelic) A red-haired man
Roony, Rooni, Roonie, Roonca, Roonee, Roon, Roone

Roosevelt (Danish) From the field of roses
Rosevelt

Roper (English) One who makes rope
Rapere

Rory (Gaelic) A red-haired man
Rori, Rorey, Rorie, Rorea, Roree, Rorry, Rorrey, Rorri

Roshan (Hindi) Born during the daylight
Rashaun

Roslin (Gaelic) A little red-haired boy
Roslyn, Rosselin, Rosslyn, Rozlin, Rozlyn, Rosling, Rozling

Roswald (German) Of the mighty horses
Rosswald, Roswalt, Rosswalt

Roswell (English) A fascinating man
Rosswell, Rozwell, Roswel, Rozwel

Roth (German) A red-haired man
Rothe

Rousseau (French) A little red-haired boy
Roussell, Russo, Rousse, Roussel, Rousset, Rousskin

Rowdy (English) A boisterous man
Rowdey, Rowdi, Rowdie, Rowdee, Rowdea

Roy (Gaelic / French) A red-haired man / a king
Roye, Roi, Royer, Ruy

Royce (German / French) A famous man / son of the king
Roice, Royse, Roise

Ruadhan (Irish) A red-haired man; the name of a saint
Ruadan, Ruadhagan, Ruadagan

Ruarc (Irish) A famous ruler
Ruarck, Ruarcc, Ruark, Ruarkk, Ruaidhri, Ruaidri

Rubio (Spanish) Resembling a ruby

Rudeger (German) A friendly man
Rudegar, Rudger, Rudgar, Rudiger, Rudigar

Rudolph (German) A famous wolf
Rodolfo, Rodolph, Rodolphe, Rodolpho, Rudy, Rudey, Rudi, Rudie

Rudyard (English) From the red paddock

Rufus (Latin) A red-haired man
Ruffus, Rufous, Rufino

Ruiz (Spanish) A good friend

Rujul (Indian) An honest man
Rujool, Rujoole, Rujule, Rujoul, Rujoule

Rumford (English) From the broad ford
Rumforde, Rumferd, Rumferde, Rumfurd

Rupert (English) Form of Robert, meaning "one who is bright with fame"
Ruprecht

Rushford (English) From the ford with rushes
Rusheford, Rushforde, Rusheforde, Ryscford

Russell (French) A little red-haired boy
Russel, Roussell, Russ, Rusel, Rusell

Russom (African) The chief; the boss
Rusom, Russome, Rusome

Rusty (English) One who has red hair or a ruddy complexion
Rustey, Rusti, Rustie, Rustee, Rustea, Rust, Ruste, Rustice

Rutherford (English) From the cattle's ford
Rutherfurd, Rutherferd, Rutherforde, Rutherfurde

^⚦**Ryan** (Gaelic) The little ruler; little king
Rian, Rien, Rion, Ryen, Ryon, Ryun, Rhyan, Rhyen

Ryder (English) An accomplished horseman
Rider, Ridder, Ryden, Rydell, Rydder

^**Ryker** (Danish) Form of Richard, meaning "a powerful ruler"
Riker

Rylan (English) form of Ryland, meaning "from the place where rye is grown"
Ryelan, Ryle

S

Saarik (Hindi) Resembling a small songbird
Saarick, Saaric, Sarik, Sarick, Saric, Saariq, Sareek, Sareeq

Saber (French) Man of the sword
Sabere, Sabr, Sabre

Sabir (Arabic) One who is patient
Sabyr, Sabeer, Sabear, Sabeir, Sabier, Sabri, Sabrie, Sabree

Saddam (Arabic) A powerful ruler; the crusher
Saddum, Saddim, Saddym

Sadiq (Arabic) A beloved friend
Sadeeq, Sadyq, Sadeaq, Sadeek, Sadeak, Sadyk, Sadik

Saga (American) A storyteller
Sago

Sagar (Indian / English) A king / one who is wise
Saagar, Sagarr, Saagarr

Sagaz (Spanish) One who is clever
Sagazz

Sagiv (Hebrew) Having great strength
Sagev, Segiv, Segev

Sahaj (Indian) One who is natural

Saieshwar (Hindi) A well-known saint
Saishwar

Sailor (American) Man who sails the seas
Sailer, Sailar, Saylor, Sayler, Saylar, Saelor

Saith (English) One who is well-spoken
Saithe, Sayth, Saythe, Saeth, Saethe, Sath, Sathe

Sajal (Indian) Resembling a cloud
Sajall, Sajjal, Sajjall

Sajan (Indian) One who is dearly loved
Sajann, Sajjan, Sajjann

Saki (Japanese) One who is cloaked
Sakie, Saky, Sakey, Sakee, Sakea

Salaam (African) Resembling a peach

Salehe (African) A good man
Suleh, Salih

Salim (Arabic) One who is peaceful
Saleem, Salem, Selim

Salute (American) A patriotic man
Saloot, Saloote, Salout

Salvador (Spanish) A savior
Sal, Sally, Salvadore, Xalvador

Samanjas (Indian) One who is proper

Samarth (Indian) A powerful man; one who is efficient
Samarthe

Sameen (Indian) One who is treasured
Samine, Sameene, Samean, Sameane, Samyn, Samyne

Sami (Arabic) One who has been exalted
Samie, Samy, Samey, Samee, Samea

Sammohan (Indian) An attractive man

Sampath (Indian) A wealthy man
Sampathe, Sampat

Samson (Hebrew) As bright as the sun; in the Bible, a man with extraordinary strength
Sampson, Sansom, Sanson, Sansone

⋆Samuel (Hebrew) God has heard
Sam, Sammie, Sammy, Samuele, Samuello, Samwell, Samuelo, Sammey

Samuru (Japanese) The name of God

Sandburg (English) From the sandy village
Sandbergh, Sandberg, Sandburgh

Sandon (English) From the sandy hill
Sanden, Sandan, Sandun, Sandyn, Sandin

Sanford (English) From the sandy crossing
Sandford, Sanforde, Sandforde, Sanfurd, Sanfurde, Sandfurd, Sandfurde

Sang (Vietnamese) A bright man
Sange

Sanjiro (Japanese) An admirable man
Sanjyro

Sanjiv (Indian) One who lives a long life
Sanjeev, Sanjyv, Sanjeiv, Sanjiev, Sanjeav, Sanjivan

Sanorelle (American) An honest man
Sanorell, Sanorel, Sanorele

Santana (Spanish) A saintly man
Santanna, Santanah, Santannah, Santa

Santo (Italian) A holy man
Sante, Santino, Santos, Santee, Santi, Santie, Santea, Santy

Santiago (Spanish) refers to St. James

Sapan (Indian) A dream or vision
Sapann

Sar (Anglo-Saxon) One who inflicts pain
Sarlic, Sarlik

Sarbajit (Indian) The con-
querer
*Sarbajeet, Sarbajyt,
Sarbajeat, Sarbajet,
Sarvajit, Sarvajeet,
Sarvajyt, Sarvajeat*

Sarojin (Hindu)
Resembling a lotus
Saroj

Sarosh (Persian) One who
prays
Saroshe

Satayu (Hindi) In
Hinduism, the brother of
Amavasu and Vivasu
Satayoo, Satayou, Satayue

Satoshi (Japanese) Born
from the ashes
*Satoshie, Satoshy, Satoshey,
Satoshee, Satoshea*

Satparayan (Indian) A
good-natured man

Saturn (Latin) In mythology, the god of agriculture
Saturnin, Saturno, Saturnino

Satyankar (Indian) One
who speaks the truth
Satyancar, Satyancker

Saville (French) From the
willow town
*Savil, Savile, Savill, Savyile,
Savylle, Savyle, Sauville,
Sauvile*

Savir (Indian) A great
leader
*Savire, Saveer, Saveere,
Savear, Saveare, Savyr,
Savyre*

Sawyer (English) One who
works with wood
Sayer, Saer

Saxon (English) A swords-
man
*Saxen, Saxan, Saxton,
Saxten, Saxtan*

Sayad (Arabic) An accomplished hunter

Scadwielle (English) From
the shed near the spring
*Scadwyelle, Scadwiell,
Scadwyell, Scadwiel,
Scadwyel, Scadwiele,
Scadwyele*

Scand (Anglo-Saxon) One
who is disgraced
*Scande, Scandi, Scandie,
Scandee, Scandea*

Sceotend (Anglo-Saxon)
An archer

Schaeffer (German) A
steward
*Schaffer, Shaeffer, Shaffer,
Schaeffur, Schaffur,
Shaeffur, Shaffur*

Schelde (English) From
the river
Shelde

Schneider (German) A tailor
Shneider, Sneider, Snider, Snyder

Schubert (German) One who makes shoes
Shubert, Schuberte, Shuberte, Schubirt, Shubirt, Schuburt, Shuburt

Scirocco (Italian) Of the warm wind
Sirocco, Scyrocco, Syrocco

Scott (English) A man from Scotland
Scot, Scottie, Scotto, Scotty, Scotti, Scottey, Scottee, Scottea

Scowyrhta (Anglo-Saxon) One who makes shoes

Seabury (English) From the village by the sea
Seaburry, Sebury, Seburry, Seaberry, Seabery, Seberry

Seaman (English) A mariner

•Sean (Irish) Form of John, meaning "God is gracious"
Shaughn, Shawn, Shaun, Shon, Shohn, Shonn, Shaundre, Shawnel

Seanachan (Irish) One who is wise

Seanan (Hebrew / Irish) A gift from God / an old, wise man
Sinon, Senen, Siobhan

•Sebastian (Greek) The revered one
Sabastian, Seb, Sebastiano, Sebastien, Sebestyen, Sebo, Sebastyn, Sebestyen

Sedgwick (English) From the place of sword grass
Sedgewick, Sedgewyck, Sedgwyck, Sedgewic, Sedgewik, Sedgwic, Sedgwik, Sedgewyc

Seerath (Indian) A great man
Seerathe, Searath, Searathe

Sef (Egyptian) Son of yesterday
Sefe

Seferino (Greek) Of the west wind
Seferio, Sepherino, Sepherio, Seferyno, Sepheryno

Seignour (French) Lord of the house

Selas (African) Refers to the Trinity
Selassi, Selassie, Selassy, Selassey, Selassee, Selassea

Selestino (Spanish) One who is heaven-sent
Selestyno, Selesteeno, Selesteano

Sellers (English) One who dwells in the marshland
Sellars, Sellurs, Sellirs, Sellyrs

Seminole (Native American) A tribal name
Semynole

Seppanen (Finnish) A blacksmith
Sepanen, Seppenen, Sepenen, Seppanan, Sepanan

September (American) Born in the month of September
Septimber, Septymber, Septemberia, Septemberea

Septimus (Latin) The seventh-born child
Septymus

Seraphim (Hebrew) The burning ones; heavenly winged angels
Sarafino, Saraph, Serafin, Serafino, Seraph, Seraphimus, Serafim

Sereno (Latin) One who is calm; tranquil

Serfati (Hebrew) A man from France
Sarfati, Serfatie, Sarfatie, Serfaty, Sarfaty, Serfatey, Sarfatey, Serfatee

Sergio (Latin) An attendant; a servant
Seargeoh, Serge, Sergei, Sergeo, Sergey, Sergi, Sergios, Sergiu

Seth (Hebrew) One who has been appointed
Sethe, Seath, Seathe, Zeth

Seung (Korean) A victorious successor

Seven (American) Refers to the number; the seventh-born child
Sevin, Sevyn

Sewati (Native American) Resembling a bear claw
Sewatie, Sewaty, Sewatey, Sewatee, Sewatea

Sexton (English) The church's custodian
Sextun, Sextan, Sextin, Sextyn

Seymour (French) From the French town of Saint Maur
Seamore, Seamor, Seamour, Seymore

Shaan (Hebrew) A peaceful man

Shade (English) A secretive man
Shaid, Shaide, Shayd, Shayde, Shaed, Shaede

Shadi (Persian / Arabic) One who brings happiness and joy / a singer
Shadie, Shady, Shadey

Shadrach (Hebrew) Under the command of the moon god Aku
Shadrack, Shadrick, Shad

Shah (Persian) The king

Shai (Hebrew) A gift from God

Shail (Indian) A mountain rock
Shaile, Shayl, Shayle, Shael, Shaele, Shale

Shaka (African) A tribal leader
Shakah

Shakir (Arabic) One who is grateful
Shakeer, Shaqueer, Shakier, Shakeir, Shakear, Shakar, Shaker, Shakyr

Shane (English) Form of John, meaning "God is gracious"
Shayn, Shayne, Shaine, Shain

Shannon (Gaelic) Having ancient wisdom
Shanan, Shanen, Shannan, Shannen, Shanon

Shardul (Indian) Resembling a tiger
Shardule, Shardull, Shardulle

Shashi (Indian) Of the moonbeam
Shashie, Shashy, Shashey, Shashee, Shashea, Shashhi

Shavon (American) One who is open-minded
Shavaughn, Shavonne, Shavaun, Shovon, Shovonne, Shovaun

Shaw (English) From the woodland
Shawe

Shaykeen (American) A successful man
Shaykean, Shaykein, Shakeyn, Shakine

Shea (Gaelic) An admirable man / from the fairy fortress
Shae, Shai, Shay, Shaye, Shaylon, Shays

Sheen (English) A shining man
Sheene, Shean, Sheane

Sheffield (English) From the crooked field
Sheffeld

Sheldon (English) From the steep valley
Shelden, Sheldan, Sheldun, Sheldin, Sheldyn, Shel

Shelley (English) From the meadow's ledge
Shelly, Shelli, Shellie, Shellee, Shellea, Shelleigh, Shelleah

Shelton (English) From the farm on the ledge
Shellton, Sheltown, Sheltun, Shelten, Shelny, Shelney, Shelni, Shelnie

Shem (Hebrew) Having a well-known name

Shepherd (English) One who herds sheep
Shepperd, Shep, Shepard, Shephard, Shepp, Sheppard

Sheridan (Gaelic) A seeker
Sheredan, Sheridon, Sherridan, Seireadan, Sheriden, Sheridun, Sherard, Sherrard

Sherlock (English) A fair-haired man
Sherlocke, Shurlock, Shurlocke

Sherman (English) One who cuts wool cloth
Shermon, Scherman, Schermann, Shearman, Shermann, Sherm, Sherme

Sherrerd (English) From the open field
Shererd, Sherrard, Sherard

Shields (Gaelic) A faithful protector
Sheelds, Shealds

Shikha (Indian) A fiery man
Shykha

Shiloh (Hebrew) He who was sent
Shilo, Shyloh, Shylo

Shing (Chinese) A victorious man
Shyng

Shino (Japanese) A bamboo stem
Shyno

Shipton (English) From the ship town; from the sheep town

Shiro (Japanese) The fourth-born son
Shyro

Shorty (American) A man who is small in stature
Shortey, Shorti, Shortie, Shortee, Shortea

Shreshta (Indian) The best; one who is superior

Shubhang (Indian) A handsome man

Shuraqui (Arabic) A man from the east

Siamak (Persian) A bringer of joy
Syamak, Siamack, Syamack, Siamac, Syamac

Sidor (Russian) One who is talented
Sydor

Sierra (Spanish) From the jagged mountain range
Siera, Syerra, Syera, Seyera, Seeara

Sigehere (English) One who is victorious
Sygehere, Sigihere, Sygihere

Sigenert (Anglo-Saxon) A king
Sygenert, Siginert, Syginert

Sigmund (German) The victorious protector
Siegmund, Sigmond, Zsigmond, Zygmunt

Sihtric (Anglo-Saxon) A king
Sihtrik, Sihtrick, Syhtric, Syhtrik, Syhtrick, Sihtryc, Sihtryk, Sihtryck

Sik'is (Native American) A friendly man

Sikyahonaw (Native American) Resembling a yellow bear
Sikyahonau, Sykyahonaw, Sykyahonau

Silny (Czech) Having great strength
Silney, Silni, Silnie, Silnee, Silnea

Simbarashe (African) The power of God
Simbarashi, Simbarashie, Simbarashy, Simbarashey, Simbarashee

Simcha (Hebrew) Filled with joy
Symcha, Simha, Symha

Simmons (Hebrew) The son of Simon
Semmes, Simms, Syms, Simmonds, Symonds, Simpson, Symms, Simson

Simon (Hebrew) God has heard
Shimon, Si, Sim, Samien , Semyon, Simen, Simeon, Simone

Sinai (Hebrew) From the clay desert

Sinclair (English) Man from Saint Clair
Sinclaire, Sinclare, Synclair, Synclaire, Synclare

Singer (American) A vocalist
Synger

Sion (Armenian) From the fortified hill
Sionne, Syon, Syonne

Sirius (Greek) Resembling the brightest star
Syrius

Siyavash (Persian) One who owns black horses
Siyavashe

Skerry (Norse) From the rocky island
Skereye, Skerrey, Skerri, Skerrie, Skerree, Skerrea

Slade (English) Son of the valley
Slaid, Slaide, Slaed, Slaede, Slayd, Slayde

Sladkey (Slavic) A glorious man
Sladky, Sladki, Sladkie, Sladkee, Sladkea

Smith (English) A black-smith
Smyth, Smithe, Smythe, Smedt, Smid, Smitty, Smittee, Smittea

Snell (Anglo-Saxon) One who is bold
Snel, Snelle, Snele

Solange (French) An angel of the sun

Solaris (Greek) Of the sun
Solarise, Solariss, Solarisse, Solarys, Solaryss, Solarysse, Solstice, Soleil

Somer (French) Born during the summer
Somers, Sommer, Sommers, Sommar, Somar

Somerset (English) From the summer settlement
Sommerset, Sumerset, Summerset

Songaa (Native American) Having great strength
Songan

Sophocles (Greek) An ancient playwright
Sofocles

Sorley (Irish) Of the summer vikings
Sorly, Sorlee, Sorlea, Sorli, Sorlie

Soumil (Indian) A beloved friend
Soumyl, Soumille, Soumylle, Soumill, Soumyll

Southern (English) Man from the south
Sothern, Suthern

Sovann (Cambodian) The golden son
Sovan, Sovane

Spark (English / Latin) A gallant man / to scatter
Sparke, Sparki, Sparkie, Sparky, Sparkey, Sparkee, Sparkea

Spencer (English) One who dispenses provisions
Spenser

Squire (English) A knight's companion; the shield-bearer
Squier, Squiers, Squires, Squyre, Squyres

Stanford (English) From the stony ford
Standford, Standforde, Standforde, Stamford

Stanhope (English) From the stony hollow
Stanhop

Stanton (English) From the stone town
Stantown, Stanten, Staunton, Stantan, Stantun

Stark (German) Having great strength
Starke, Starck, Starcke

Stavros (Greek) One who is crowned

Steadman (English) One who lives at the farm
Stedman, Steadmann, Stedmann, Stedeman

Steed (English) Resembling a stallion
Steede, Stead, Steade

·Stephen (Greek) Crowned with garland
Staffan, Steba, Steben, Stefan, Stefano, Steffan, Steffen, Steffon, Steven, Steve

Sterling (English) One who is highly valued
Sterlyng, Stirling, Sterlyn

Stian (Norse) A voyager; one who is swift
Stig, Styg, Stygge, Stieran, Steeran, Steeren, Steeryn, Stieren

Stilwell (Anglo-Saxon) From the quiet spring
Stillwell, Stilwel, Stylwell, Styllwell, Stylwel, Stillwel

Stobart (German) A harsh man
Stobarte, Stobarth, Stobarthe

Stockley (English) From the meadow of tree stumps
Stockly, Stockli, Stocklie, Stocklee, Stockleigh

Storm (American) Of the tempest; stormy weather; having an impetuous nature
Storme, Stormy, Stormi, Stormie, Stormey, Stormee, Stormea

Stowe (English) A secretive man
Stow, Stowey, Stowy, Stowee, Stowea, Stowi, Stowie

Stratford (English) From the street near the river ford
Strafford, Stratforde, Straford, Strafforde, Straforde

Stratton (Scottish) A homebody
Straton, Stratten, Straten, Strattan, Stratan, Strattun, Stratun

Strider (English) A great warrior
Stryder

Striker (American) An aggressive man
Strike, Stryker, Stryke

Struthers (Irish) One who lives near the brook
Struther, Sruthair, Strother, Strothers

Stuart (English) A steward; the keeper of the estate
Steward, Stewart, Stewert, Stuert, Stu, Stew

Suave (American) A smooth and sophisticated man
Swave

Subhi (Arabic) Born during the early morning hours
Subhie, Subhy, Subhey, Subhee, Subhea

Suffield (English) From the southern field
Suffeld, Suthfeld, Suthfield

Sullivan (Gaelic) Having dark eyes
Sullavan, Sullevan, Sullyvan

Sully (English) From the southern meadow
Sulley, Sulli, Sullie, Sulleigh, Sullee, Sullea, Sulleah, Suthley

Sultan (African / American) A ruler / one who is bold
Sultane, Sulten, Sultun, Sulton, Sultin, Sultyn

Suman (Hindi) A wise man

Sundiata (African) Resembling a hungry lion
Sundyata, Soundiata, Soundyata, Sunjata

Sundown (American) Born at dusk
Sundowne

Su'ud (Arabic) One who has good luck
Suoud

Swahili (Arabic) Of the coastal people
Swahily, Swahiley, Swahilee, Swahiley, Swaheeli, Swaheelie, Swaheely, Swaheeley

Sylvester (Latin) Man from the forest
Silvester, Silvestre, Silvestro, Sylvestre, Sylvestro, Sly, Sevester, Seveste

Syon (Indian) One who is followed by good fortune

Szemere (Hungarian) A man of small stature
Szemir, Szemeer, Szemear, Szemyr

t

Tabari (Arabic) A famous historian
Tabarie, Tabary, Tabarey, Tabaree, Tabarea

Tabbai (Hebrew) A well-behaved boy
Tabbae, Tabbay, Tabbaye

Tabbart (German) A brilliant man
Tabbert, Tabart, Tabert, Tahbert, Tahberte

Tacari (African) As strong as a warrior
Tacarie, Tacary, Tacarey, Tacaree, Tacarea

Tadao (Japanese) One who is satisfied

Tadeusuz (Polish) One who is worthy of praise
Tadesuz

Tadi (Native American) Of the wind
Tadie, Tady, Tadey, Tadee, Tadea

Tadzi (American / Polish) Resembling the loon / one who is praised
Tadzie, Tadzy, Tadzey, Tadzee, Tadzea

Taft (French / English) From the homestead / from the marshes
Tafte

Taggart (Gaelic) Son of a priest
Taggert, Taggort, Taggirt, Taggyrt

Taghee (Native American) A chief
Taghea, Taghy, Taghey, Taghi, Taghie

Taheton (Native American) Resembling a hawk

Tahoe (Native American) From the big water
Taho

Tahoma (Native American) From the snowy mountain peak
Tehoma, Tacoma, Takoma, Tohoma, Tocoma, Tokoma, Tekoma, Tecoma

Taishi (Japanese) An ambitious man
Taishie, Taishy, Taishey, Taishee, Taishea

Taj (Indian) One who is crowned
Tahj, Tajdar

Tajo (Spanish) Born during the daytime

Taksony (Hungarian) One who is content; well-fed
Taksoney, Taksoni, Taksonie, Taksonee, Taksonea, Tas

Talasi (Native American) Resembling a cornflower
Talasie, Talasy, Talasey, Talasee, Talasea

Talford (English) From the high ford
Talforde, Tallford, Tallforde

Talfryn (Welsh) From the high hill
Talfrynn, Talfrin, Talfrinn, Talfren, Talfrenn, Tallfryn, Tallfrin, Tallfren

Talmai (Hebrew) From the furrows
Talmae, Talmay, Talmaye

Talmon (Hebrew) One who is oppressed
Talman, Talmin, Talmyn, Talmen

Talo (Finnish) From the homestead

Tam (Vietnamese / Hebrew) Having heart / one who is truthful

Taman (Hindi) One who is needed

Tamarius (American) A stubborn man
Tamarias, Tamarios, Tamerius, Tamerias, Tamerios

Tameron (American) Form of Cameron, meaning "having a crooked nose"
Tameren, Tameryn, Tamryn, Tamerin, Tamren, Tamrin, Bamron

Tammany (Native American) A friendly chief
Tammani, Tammanie, Tammaney, Tammanee, Tammanea

Tanafa (Polynesian) A drumbeat

Taneli (Hebrew) He will be judged by God
Tanelie, Tanely, Taneley, Tanelee, Tanelea

Tanish (Indian) An ambitious man
Tanishe, Taneesh, Taneeshe, Taneash, Taneashe, Tanysh, Tanyshe

Tanjiro (Japanese) The prized second-born son
Tanjyro

Tank (American) A man who is big and strong
Tankie, Tanki, Tanky, Tankey, Tankee, Tankea

Tanner (English) One who makes leather
Tannere, Tannor, Tannar, Tannir, Tannyr, Tannur, Tannis

Tannon (German) From the fir tree
Tannan, Tannen, Tannin, Tansen, Tanson, Tannun, Tannyn

Tano (Ghanese) From the river
Tanu

Tao (Chinese) One who will have a long life

Taos (Spanish) From the city in New Mexico

Tapani (Hebrew) A victorious man
Tapanie, Tapany, Tapaney, Tapanee, Tapanea

Tapko (American) Resembling an antelope

Tappen (Welsh) From the top of the cliff
Tappan, Tappon, Tappin, Tappyn, Tappun

Taran (Gaelic) Of the thunder
Taren, Taron, Tarin, Taryn, Tarun

Taranga (Indian) Of the waves

Taregan (Native American) Resembling a crane
Taregen, Taregon, Taregin, Taregyn

Tarit (Indian) Resembling lightning
Tarite, Tareet, Tareete, Tareat, Tareate, Taryt, Taryte

Tarn (Norse) From the mountain pool

Tarquin (Latin) One who is impulsive
Tarquinn, Tarquinne, Tarquen, Tarquenn, Tarquenne, Tarquyn, Tarquynn, Tarquynne

Tarrant (American) One who upholds the law
Tarrent, Tarrint, Tarrynt, Tarront, Tarrunt

Tarun (Indian) A youthful man
Taroun, Taroon, Tarune, Taroune, Taroone

Tashi (Tibetan) One who is prosperous
Tashie, Tashy, Tashey, Tashee, Tashea

Tate (English) A cheerful man; one who brings happiness to others
Tayt, Tayte, Tait, Taite, Taet, Taete

Tausiq (Indian) One who provides strong backing
Tauseeq, Tauseaq, Tausik, Tauseek, Tauseak

Tavaris (American) Of misfortune; a hermit
Tavarius, Tavaress, Tavarious, Tavariss, Tavarous, Tevarus, Tavorian, Tavarian

Tavas (Hebrew) Resembling a peacock

Tavi (Aramaic) A good man
Tavie, Tavy, Tavey, Tavee, Tavea

Tavin (German) Form of Gustav, meaning "of the staff of the gods"
Tavyn, Taven, Tavan, Tavon, Tavun, Tava, Tave

Tawa (Native American) Born beneath the sun
Tawah

Tay (Scottish) From the river
Taye, Tae, Tai

Teagan (Gaelic) A handsome man
Teegan, Teygan, Tegan, Teigan

Tecumseh (Native American) A traveler; resembling a shooting star
Tekumseh, Tecumse, Tekumse

Ted (English) Form of Theodore, meaning "a gift from God"
Tedd, Teddy, Teddi, Teddie, Teddee, Teddea, Teddey, Tedric

Tedmund (English) A protector of the land
Tedmunde, Tedmond, Tedmonde, Tedman, Theomund, Theomond, Theomunde, Theomonde

Teetonka (Native American) One who talks too much
Teitonka, Tietonka, Teatonka, Teytonka

Tegene (African) My protector
Tegeen, Tegeene, Tegean, Tegeane

Teiji (Japanese) One who is righteous
Teijo

Teilo (Welsh) A saintly man

Teka (African) He has replaced

Tekeshi (Japanese) A formidable and brave man
Tekeshie, Tekeshy, Tekeshey, Tekeshee, Tekeshea

Telly (Greek) The wisest man
Telley, Tellee, Tellea, Telli, Tellie

Temman (Anglo-Saxon) One who has been tamed

Temple (Latin) From the sacred place
Tempel, Templar, Templer, Templo

Teneangopte (Native American) Resembling a high-flying bird

Tennant (English) One who rents
Tennent, Tenant, Tenent

Tennessee (Native American) From the state of Tennessee
Tenese, Tenesee, Tenessee, Tennese, Tennesee, Tennesse

Teon (Anglo-Saxon) One who harms others

Terence (Latin) From an ancient Roman clan
Tarrants, Tarrance, Tarrence, Tarrenz, Terencio, Terrance, Terrence, Terrey, Terry

Teris (Irish) The son of Terence
Terys, Teriss, Teryss, Terris, Terrys, Terriss, Terryss

Terrian (American) One who is strong and ambitious
Terrien, Terriun, Terriyn

Terron (English) Form of Terence, meaning "from an ancient Roman clan"
Tarran, Tarren, Tarrin

Teshi (African) One who is full of laughter
Teshie, Teshy, Teshey, Teshee, Teshea

Tessema (African) One to whom people listen

Tet (Vietnamese) Born on New Year's

Teteny (Hungarian) A chieftain

Teva (Hebrew) A natural man
Tevah

Texas (Native American) One of many friends; from the state of Texas
Texus, Texis, Texes, Texos, Texys

Teyrnon (Celtic) A regal man
Teirnon, Tayrnon, Tairnon, Taernon, Tiarchnach, Tiarnach

Thabo (African) Filled with happiness

Thackary (English) Form of Zachary, meaning "the Lord remembers"
Thackery, Thakary, Thakery, Thackari, Thackarie, Thackarey, Thackaree, Thackarea

Thaddeus (Aramaic) Having heart
Tad, Tadd, Taddeo, Taddeusz, Thad, Thadd, Thaddaios, Thaddaos

Thandiwe (African) One who is dearly loved
Thandie, Thandi, Thandy, Thandey, Thandee, Thandea

Thang (Vietnamese) One who is victorious

Thanus (American) One who owns land

Thao (Vietnamese) One who is courteous

Thatcher (English) One who fixes roofs
Thacher, Thatch, Thatche, Thaxter, Thacker, Thaker, Thackere, Thakere

Thayer (Teutonic) Of the nation's army

Theodore (Greek) A gift from God
Ted, Teddy, Teddie, Theo, Theodor

Theron (Greek) A great hunter
Therron, Tharon, Theon, Tharron

Theseus (Greek) In mythology, hero who slew the Minotaur
Thesius, Thesyus

Thinh (Vietnamese) A prosperous man

·Thomas (Aramaic) One of twins
Tam, Tamas, Tamhas, Thom, Thomason, Thomson, Thompson, Tomas

Thor (Norse) In mythology, god of thunder
Thorian, Thorin, Thorsson, Thorvald, Tor, Tore, Turo, Thorrin

Thorburn (Norse) Thor's bear
Thorburne, Thorbern, Thorberne, Thorbjorn, Thorbjorne, Torbjorn, Torborg, Torben

Thormond (Norse) Protected by Thor
Thormonde, Thormund, Thormunde, Thurmond, Thurmonde, Thurmund, Thurmunde, Thormun

Thorne (English) From the thorn bush
Thorn

Thornycroft (English) From the field of thorn bushes
Thornicroft, Thorneycroft, Thorniecroft, Thorneecroft, Thorneacroft

Thuong (Vietnamese) One who loves tenderly

Thurston (English) From Thor's town; Thor's stone
Thorston, Thorstan, Thorstein, Thorsten, Thurstain, Thurstan, Thursten, Torsten

Thuy (Vietnamese) One who is kind

Tiassale (African) It has been forgotten

Tiberio (Italian) From the Tiber river
Tibero, Tyberio, Tybero, Tiberius, Tiberios, Tyberius, Tyberios

Tibor (Slavic) From the sacred place

Tiburon (Spanish) Resembling a shark

Tiernan (Gaelic) Lord of the manor
Tiarnan, Tiarney, Tierney, Tierny, Tiernee, Tiernea, Tierni, Tiernie

Tilian (Anglo-Saxon) One who strives to better himself
Tilien, Tiliun, Tilion

Tilon (Hebrew) A generous man
Tilen, Tilan, Tilun, Tilin, Tilyn

Tilton (English) From the fertile estate
Tillton, Tilten, Tillten, Tiltan, Tilltan, Tiltin, Tilltin, Tiltun

Timir (Indian) Born in the darkness
Timirbaran

Timothy (Greek) One who honors God
Tim, Timmo, Timmy, Timmothy, Timmy, Timo, Timofei, Timofeo

Tin (Vietnamese) A great thinker

Tino (Italian) A man of small stature
Teeno, Tieno, Teino, Teano, Tyno

Tip (American) A form of Thomas, meaning "one of twins"
Tipp, Tipper, Tippy, Tippee, Tippea, Tippey, Tippi, Tippie

Tisa (African) The ninth-born child
Tisah, Tysa, Tysah

^**Titus** (Greek / Latin) Of the giants / a great defender
Tito, Titos, Tytus, Tytos, Titan, Tytan, Tyto

Toa (Polynesian) A brave-hearted woman

Toan (Vietnamese) One who is safe
Toane

Tobias (Hebrew) The Lord is good
Toby

Todd (English) Resembling a fox
Tod

Todor (Bulgarian) A gift
from God
Todos, Todros

Tohon (Native American)
One who loves the water

Tokala (Native American)
Resembling a fox
Tokalo

Tomer (Hebrew) A man of
tall stature
*Tomar, Tomur, Tomir,
Tomor, Tomyr*

Tomi (Japanese / African)
A wealthy man / of the
people
*Tomie, Tomee, Tomea,
Tomy, Tomey*

Tonauac (Aztec) One who
possesses the light

Torger (Norse) The power
of Thor's spear
*Thorger, Torgar, Thorgar,
Terje, Therje*

Torht (Anglo-Saxon) A
bright man
Torhte

Torin (Celtic) One who
acts as chief
*Toran, Torean, Toren,
Torion, Torran, Torrian,
Toryn*

Tormaigh (Irish) Having
the spirit of Thor
*Tormey, Tormay, Tormaye,
Tormai, Tormae*

Torr (English) From the
tower
Torre

Torrence (Gaelic) From
the little hills
*Torence, Torrance, Torrens,
Torrans, Toran, Torran,
Torrin, Torn, Torry*

Torry (Norse / Gaelic)
Refers to Thor / form of
Torrence, meaning "from
the little hills"
*Torrey, Torree, Torrea,
Torri, Torrie, Tory, Torey,
Tori*

Toshiro (Japanese) One
who is talented and intelligent
Toshihiro

Tostig (English) A well-
known earl
Tostyg

Toviel (Hebrew) The Lord
is good
*Toviell, Toviele, Tovielle,
Tovi, Tovie, Tovee, Tovea,
Tovy*

Toyo (Japanese) A man of
plenty

Tracy (Gaelic) One who is
warlike
*Tracey, Traci, Tracie,
Tracee, Tracea, Treacy,
Trace, Tracen*

Travis (French) To cross over
Travys, Traver, Travers, Traviss, Trevis, Trevys, Travus, Traves

Treffen (German) One who socializes
Treffan, Treffin, Treffon, Treffyn, Treffun

Tremain (Celtic) From the town built of stone
Tramain, Tramaine, Tramayne, Tremaine, Tremayne, Tremaen, Tremaene, Tramaen

Tremont (French) From the three mountains
Tremonte, Tremount, Tremounte

Trenton (English) From the town near the rushing rapids
Trent, Trynt, Trenten, Trentyn

Trevin (English) From the fair town
Trevan, Treven, Trevian, Trevion, Trevon, Trevyn, Trevonn

Trevor (Welsh) From the large village
Trefor, Trevar, Trever, Treabhar, Treveur, Trevir, Trevur

Trey (English) The third-born child
Tre, Trai, Trae, Tray, Traye, Trayton, Treyton, Trayson

Trigg (Norse) One who is truthful
Trygg

Tripp (English) A traveler
Trip, Trypp, Tryp, Tripper, Trypper

Tripsy (American) One who enjoys dancing
Tripsey, Tripsee, Tripsea, Tripsi, Tripsie

Tristan (Celtic) A sorrowful man; in Arthurian legend, a knight of the Round Table
Trystan, Tris, Tristam, Tristen, Tristian, Tristin, Triston, Tristram

Trocky (American) A manly man
Trockey, Trocki, Trockie, Trockee, Trockea

Trong (Vietnamese) One who is respected

Troy (Gaelic) Son of a foot-soldier
Troye, Troi

Trumbald (English) A bold man
Trumbold, Trumbalde, Trumbolde

Trygve (Norse) One who wins with bravery

Tse (Native American) As solid as a rock

Tsidhqiyah (Hebrew) The Lord is just
Tsidqiyah, Tsidhqiya, Tsdqiya

Tsubasa (Japanese) A winged being
Tsubasah, Tsubase, Tsubaseh

Tucker (English) One who makes garments
Tuker, Tuckerman, Tukerman, Tuck, Tuckman, Tukman, Tuckere, Toukere

Tuketu (Native American) Resembling a running bear
Tuketue, Tuketoo, Tuketou, Telutci, Telutcie, Telutcy, Telutcey, Telutcee

Tulsi (Indian) A holy man
Tulsie, Tulsy, Tulsey, Tulsee, Tulsea

Tumaini (African) An optimist
Tumainie, Tumainee, Tumainy, Tumainey, Tumayni, Tumaynie, Tumaynee, Tumayney

Tunde (African) One who returns
Tundi, Tundie, Tundee, Tundea, Tundy, Tundey

Tunleah (English) From the town near the meadow
Tunlea, Tunleigh, Tunly, Tunley, Tunlee, Tunli, Tunlie

Tupac (African) A messenger warrior
Tupuck, Tupoc, Tupock

Turfeinar (Norse) In mythology, the son of Rognvald
Turfaynar, Turfaenar, Turfanar, Turfenar, Turfainar

Tushar (Indian) Of the snow
Tusharr, Tushare

Tusita (Chinese) One who is heaven-sent

Twrgadarn (Welsh) From the strong tower

Txanton (Basque) Form of Anthony, meaning "a flourishing man; of an ancient Roman family"
Txantony, Txantoney, Txantonee, Txantoni, Txantonie, Txantonea

Tybalt (Latin) He who sees the truth
Tybault, Tybalte, Tybaulte

Tye (English) From the fenced-in pasture
Tyg, Tyge, Tie, Tigh, Teyen

Tyfiell (English) Follower of the god Tyr
Tyfiel, Tyfielle, Tyfiele

*T**Tyler** (English) A tiler of roofs
Tilar, Tylar, Tylor, Tiler, Tilor, Ty, Tye, Tylere

Typhoon (Chinese) Of the great wind
Tiphoon, Tyfoon, Tifoon, Typhoun, Tiphoun, Tyfoun, Tifoun

Tyrone (French) From Owen's land
Terone, Tiron, Tirone, Tyron, Ty, Kyrone

Tyson (French) One who is high-spirited; fiery
Thyssen, Tiesen, Tyce, Tycen, Tyeson, Tyssen, Tysen, Tysan

U

U (Korean) A kind and gentle man

Uaithne (Gaelic) One who is innocent; green
Uaithn, Uaythne, Uaythn, Uathne, Uathn, Uaethne, Uaethn

Ualan (Scottish) Form of Valentine, meaning "one who is strong and healthy"
Ualane, Ualayn, Ualayne, Ualen, Ualon

Uba (African) One who is wealthy; lord of the house
Ubah, Ubba, Ubbah

Uberto (Italian) Form of Hubert, meaning "having a shining intellect"
Ulberto, Umberto

Udath (Indian) One who is noble
Udathe

Uddam (Indian) An exceptional man

Uddhar (Indian) One who is free; an independent man
Uddharr, Udhar, Udharr

Udell (English) From the valley of yew trees
Udale, Udel, Udall, Udayle, Udayl, Udail, Udaile, Udele

Udi (Hebrew) One who carries a torch
Udie, Udy, Udey, Udee, Udea

Udup (Indian) Born beneath the moon's light
Udupp, Uddup, Uddupp

Udyan (Indian) Of the garden
Uddyan, Udyann, Uddyann

Ugo (Italian) A great thinker

Uland (English) From the noble country
Ulande, Ulland, Ullande, Ulandus, Ullandus

Ulhas (Indian) Filled with happiness
Ulhass, Ullhas, Ullhass

Ull (Norse) Having glory; in mythology, god of justice and patron of agriculture
Ulle, Ul, Ule

Ulmer (German) Having the fame of the wolf
Ullmer, Ullmar, Ulmarr, Ullmarr, Ulfmer, Ulfmar, Ulfmaer

Ultman (Indian) A godly man
Ultmann, Ultmane

Umrao (Indian) One who is noble

Unai (Basque) A shepherd
Unay, Unaye, Unae

Unathi (African) God is with us
Unathie, Unathy, Unathey, Unathee, Unathea

Uncas (Native American) Resembling a fox
Unkas, Unckas

Ungus (Irish) A vigorous man
Unguss

Unique (American) Unlike others; the only one
Unikue, Unik, Uniqui, Uniqi, Uniqe, Unikque, Unike, Unicke

Uolevi (Finnish) Form of Olaf, meaning "the remaining of the ancestors"
Uolevie, Uolevee, Uolevy, Uolevey, Uolevea

Upchurch (English) From the upper church
Upchurche

Uranus (Greek) In mythology, the father of the Titans
Urainus, Uraynus, Uranas, Uraynas, Urainas, Uranos, Uraynos, Urainos

Uri (Hebrew) Form of Uriah, meaning "the Lord is my light"
Urie, Ury, Urey, Uree, Urea

Uriah (Hebrew) The Lord is my light
Uri, Uria, Urias, Urija, Urijah, Uriyah, Urjasz, Uriya

Urjavaha (Hindu) Of the Nimi dynasty

Urtzi (Basque) From the sky
*Urtzie, Urtzy, Urtzey,
Urtzee, Urtzea*

Usher (Latin) From the mouth of the river
*Ushar, Ushir, Ussher,
Usshar, Usshir*

Ushi (Chinese) As strong as an ox
*Ushie, Ushy, Ushey, Ushee,
Ushea*

Utah (Native American) People of the mountains; from the state of Utah

Utsav (Indian) Born during a celebration
*Utsavi, Utsave, Utsava,
Utsavie, Utsavy, Utsavey,
Utsavee, Utsavea*

Utt (Arabic) One who is kind and wise
Utte

Uzi (Hebrew) Having great power
*Uzie, Uzy, Uzey, Uzee,
Uzea, Uzzi, Uzzie, Uzzy*

Uzima (African) One who is full of life
*Uzimah, Uzimma,
Uzimmah, Uzyma*

Uzziah (Hebrew) The Lord is my strength
*Uzzia, Uziah, Uzia,
Uzzya, Uzzyah, Uzyah,
Uzya, Uzziel*

V

Vachel (French) Resembling a small cow
Vachele, Vachell

Vachlan (English) One who lives near water

Vadar (Dutch) A fatherly man
Vader, Vadyr

Vadhir (Spanish) Resembling a rose
Vadhyr, Vadheer

Vadim (Russian) A good-looking man
*Vadime, Vadym, Vadyme,
Vadeem, Vadeeme*

Vaijnath (Hindi) Refers to Lord Shiva
*Vaejnath, Vaijnathe,
Vaejnathe*

Valdemar (German) A well-known ruler
*Valdemarr, Valdemare,
Valto, Valdmar, Valdmarr,
Valdimar, Valdimarr*

Valentine (Latin) One who is strong and healthy
*Val, Valentin, Valentino,
Valentyne, Ualan*

Valerian (Latin) One who is strong and healthy
Valerien, Valerio, Valerius, Valery, Valeryan, Valere, Valeri, Valerii

Valin (Hindi) The monkey king

Valle (French) From the glen
Vallejo

Valri (French) One who is strong
Valrie, Valry, Valrey, Valree

Vance (English) From the marshland
Vanse

Vanderveer (Dutch) From the ferry
Vandervere, Vandervir, Vandervire, Vandervyr, Vandervyre

Vandy (Dutch) One who travels; a wanderer
Vandey, Vandi, Vandie, Vandee

Vandyke (Danish) From the dike
Vandike

Vanir (Norse) Of the ancient gods

Varante (Arabic) From the river

Vardon (French) From the green hill
Varden, Verdon, Verdun, Verden, Vurdun, Vardan, Verddun, Varddun

Varg (Norse) Resembling a wolf

Varick (German) A protective ruler
Varrick, Warick, Warrick

Varius (Latin) A versatile man
Varian, Varinius

Variya (Hindi) The excellent one

Vasava (Hindi) Refers to Indra

Vashon (American) The Lord is gracious
Vashan, Vashawn, Vashaun, Vashone, Vashane, Vashayn, Vashayne

Vasin (Indian) A great ruler
Vasine, Vaseen, Vaseene, Vasyn, Vasyne

Vasuki (Hindi) In Hinduism, a serpent king
Vasukie, Vasuky, Vasukey, Vasukee, Vasukea

Vasuman (Indian) Son born of fire

Vasyl (Slavic) A king
Vasil, Vassil, Wasyl

Vatsa (Indian) Our
beloved son
Vathsa

Vatsal (Indian) One who is
affectionate

Velimir (Croatian) One who
wishes for great peace
Velimeer, Velimyr, Velimire,
Velimeere, Velimyre

Velyo (Bulgarian) A great
man
Velcho, Veliko, Velin, Velko

Vere (French) From the
alder tree

Verge (Anglo-Saxon) One
who owns four acres

Vernon (French) From the
alder-tree grove
Vern, Vernal, Vernard,
Verne, Vernee, Vernen,
Verney, Vernin

Verrill (French) One who
is faithful
Verill, Verrall, Verrell,
Verroll, Veryl, Veryll, Verol,
Verall

Vibol (Cambodian) A man
of plenty
Viboll, Vibole, Vybol,
Vyboll, Vybole

Victor (Latin) One who is
victorious; the champion
Vic, Vick, Victoriano

Vidal (Spanish) A giver
of life
Videl, Videlio, Videlo,
Vidalo, Vidalio, Vidas

Vidar (Norse) Warrior of
the forest; in mythology, a
son of Odin
Vidarr

Vien (Vietnamese) One
who is complete; satisfied

Vincent (Latin) One who
prevails; the conquerer
Vicente, Vicenzio, Vicenzo,
Vin, Vince, Vincens,
Vincente, Vincentius

Viorel (Romanian)
Resembling the bluebell
Viorell, Vyorel, Vyorell

Vipin (Indian) From the
forest
Vippin, Vypin, Vypyn,
Vyppin, Vyppyn, Vipyn,
Vippyn

Vipul (Indian) A man of
plenty
Vypul, Vipull, Vypull,
Vipool, Vypool

Virag (Hungarian)
Resembling a flower

Virgil (Latin) The staff-
bearer
Verge, Vergil, Vergilio,
Virgilio, Vergilo, Virgilo,
Virgilijus

Virginius (Latin) One who is pure; chaste
Virginio, Virgino

Vitéz (Hungarian) A courageous warrior

Vito (Latin) One who gives life
Vital, Vitale, Vitalis, Vitaly, Vitas, Vitus, Vitali, Vitaliy, Vid

Vitus (Latin) Giver of life
Wit

Vladimir (Slavic) A famous prince
Vladamir, Vladimeer, Vladimyr, Vladimyre, Vladamyr, Vladamyre, Vladameer, Vladimer

Vladislav (Slavic) One who rules with glory

Volodymyr (Slavic) To rule with peace
Wolodymyr

Vulcan (Latin) In mythology, the god of fire
Vulkan, Vulckan

Vyacheslav (Russian) Form of Wenceslas, meaning "one who receives more glory"

W

Wade (English) To cross the river ford
Wayde, Waid, Waide, Waddell, Wadell, Waydell, Waidell, Waed

Wadley (English) From the meadow near the ford
Wadly, Wadlee, Wadli, Wadlie, Wadleigh

Wadsworth (English) From the estate near the ford
Waddsworth, Wadsworthe, Waddsworthe

Wafi (Arabic) One who is trustworthy
Wafie, Wafy, Wafey, Wafee, Wafiy, Wafiyy

Wahab (Indian) A big-hearted man

Wainwright (English) One who builds wagons
Wainright, Wainewright, Wayneright, Waynewright, Waynwright

Wakil (Arabic) A lawyer; a trustee
Wakill, Wakyl, Wakyle, Wakeel, Wakeele

Wakiza (Native American) A desperate fighter
Wakyza, Wakeza, Wakieza, Wakeiza

Walbridge (English) From the Welshman's bridge
Wallbridge, Walbrydge, Wallbrydge

Waljan (Welsh) The chosen one
Walljan, Waljen, Walljen, Waljon, Walljon

Walker (English) One who trods the cloth
Walkar, Walkir, Walkor

Walter (German) The commander of the army
Walther, Walt, Walte, Walder, Wat, Wouter, Wolter, Woulter, Galtero, Quaid

Wamblee (Native American) Resembling an eagle
Wambli, Wamblie, Wambly, Wambley, Wambleigh, Wamblea

Wanikiy (Native American) A savior
Wanikiya, Wanikie, Wanikey, Waniki, Wanikee

Wanjala (African) Born during a famine
Wanjalla, Wanjal, Wanjall

Warford (English) From the ford near the weir
Warforde, Weirford, Weirforde, Weiford, Weiforde

Warley (English) From the meadow near the weir
Warly, Warleigh, Warlee, Warlea, Warleah, Warli, Warlie, Weirley

Warner (German) Of the defending army
Werner, Wernher, Warnher, Worner, Wornher

Warra (Aboriginal) Man of the water
Warrah, Wara, Warah

Warrick (English) Form of Varick, meaning "a protective ruler"
Warrik, Warric, Warick, Warik, Waric, Warryck, Warryk, Warryc

Warrigal (Aboriginal) One who is wild
Warrigall, Warigall, Warigal, Warygal, Warygall

Warrun (Aboriginal) Of the sky
Warun

Warwick (English) From the farm near the weir
Warwik, Warwyck, Warwyk

Wasswa (African) The firstborn of twins
Waswa, Wasswah, Waswah

Wasyl (Ukranian) Form of Vasyl, meaning "a king"
Wasyle, Wasil, Wasile

Watson (English) The son of Walter
Watsin, Watsen, Watsan, Watkins, Watckins, Watkin, Watckin, Wattekinson

Wayne (English) One who builds wagons
Wain, Wanye, Wayn, Waynell, Waynne, Guwayne

Webster (English) A weaver
Weeb, Web, Webb, Webber, Weber, Webbestre, Webestre, Webbe

Wei (Chinese) A brilliant man; having great strength

Wenceslas (Polish) One who receives more glory
Wenceslaus, Wenzel, Vyacheslav

Wendell (German) One who travels; a wanderer
Wendel, Wendale, Wendall, Wendele, Wendal, Windell, Windel, Windal

Wesley (English) From the western meadow
Wes, Wesly, Wessley, Westleigh, Westley, Wesli, Weslie, Wesleigh

Westby (English) From the western farm
Westbey, Wesby, Wesbey, Westbi, Wesbi, Westbie, Wesbie, Westbee

Wharton (English) From the settlement near the weir
Warton, Wharten, Warten, Whartun, Wartun

Whit (English) A white-skinned man
White, Whitey, Whitt, Whitte, Whyt, Whytt, Whytte, Whytey

Whitby (English) From the white farm
Whitbey, Whitbi, Whitbie, Whitbee, Whytbcy, Whytby, Whytbi, Whytbie

Whitfield (English) From the white field
Whitfeld, Whytfield, Whytfeld, Witfield, Witfeld, Wytfield, Wytfeld

Whitley (English) From the white meadow
Whitly, Whitli, Whitlie, Whitlee, Whitleigh, Whytley, Whytly, Whytli

Whitman (English) A white-haired man
Whitmann, Witman, Witmann, Whitmane, Witmane, Whytman, Whytmane, Wytman

Wildon (English) From the wooded hill
Willdon, Wilden, Willden

Wiley (English) One who is crafty; from the meadow by the water
Wily, Wileigh, Wili, Wilie, Wilee, Wylie, Wyly, Wyley

Wilford (English) From the willow ford
Willford, Wilferd, Willferd, Wilf, Wielford, Weilford, Wilingford, Wylingford

William (German) The determined protector
Wilek, Wileck, Wilhelm, Wilhelmus, Wilkes, Wilkie, Wilkinson, Will, Guillaume, Quilliam

Willow (English) Of the willow tree
Willowe, Willo, Willoe

Wilmer (German) A strong-willed and well-known man
Wilmar, Wilmore, Willmar, Willmer, Wylmer, Wylmar, Wyllmer, Wyllmar

Winston (English) Of the joy stone; from the friendly town
Win, Winn, Winsten, Winstonn, Wynstan, Wynsten, Wynston, Winstan

Winthrop (English) From the friendly village
Winthrope, Wynthrop, Wynthrope, Winthorp, Wynthorp

Winton (English) From the enclosed pastureland
Wintan, Wintin, Winten, Wynton, Wyntan, Wyntin, Wynten

Wirt (Anglo-Saxon) One who is worthy
Wirte, Wyrt, Wyrte, Wurt, Wurte

Wit (Polish) Form of Vitus, meaning "giver of life"
Witt

Wlodzimierz (Polish) To rule with peace
Wlodzimir, Wlodzimerz

Wolfric (German) A wolf ruler
Wolfrick, Wolfrik, Wulfric, Wulfrick, Wulfrik, Wolfryk, Wolfryck, Wolfryc

Wolodymyr (Ukranian) Form of Volodymyr, meaning "to rule with peace"
Wolodimyr, Wolodimir, Wolodymeer, Wolodimeer

Woorak (Aboriginal) From the plains
Woorack, Woorac

Wyatt (English) Having
the strength of a warrior
*Wyat, Wyatte, Wyate, Wiatt,
Wiatte, Wiat, Wiate, Wyeth*

Wyndham (English) From
the windy village
Windham

Xakery (American) Form
of Zachery, meaning "the
Lord remembers"
*Xaccary, Xaccery, Xach,
Xacharie, Xachery, Xack,
Xackarey, Xackary*

Xalvador (Spanish) Form
of Salvador, meaning "a
savior"
*Xalvadore, Xalvadoro,
Xalvadorio, Xalbador,
Xalbadore, Xalbadorio,
Xalbadoro, Xabat*

Xannon (American) From
an ancient family
*Xanon, Xannen, Xanen,
Xannun, Xanun*

Xanthus (Greek) A blond-
haired man
Xanthos, Xanthe, Xanth

Xavier (Basque / Arabic)
Owner of a new house /
one who is bright
*Xaver, Xever, Xabier,
Xaviere, Xabiere, Xaviar,
Xaviare, Xavior*

Xenocrates (Greek) A foreign ruler

Xesus (Galician) Form of
Jesus, meaning "God is
my salvation"

Xoan (Galician) Form of
John, meaning "God is
gracious"
Xoane, Xohn, Xon

Xue (Chinese) A studious
young man

Yael (Israeli) Strength of
God
Yaele

Yagil (Hebrew) One who
rejoices, celebrates
Yagill, Yagyl, Yagylle

Yahto (Native American)
Having blue eyes; refers
to the color blue
Yahtoe, Yahtow, Yahtowe

Yahweh (Hebrew) Refers to God
Yahveh, Yaweh, Yaveh, Yehowah, Yehweh, Yehoveh

Yakiv (Ukranian) Form of Jacob, meaning "he who supplants"
Yakive, Yakeev, Yakeeve, Yackiv, Yackeev, Yakieve, Yakiev, Yakeive

Yakout (Arabian) As precious as a ruby

Yale (Welsh) From the fertile upland
Yayle, Yayl, Yail, Yaile

Yanai (Aramaic) God will answer
Yanae, Yana, Yani

Yankel (Hebrew) Form of Jacob, meaning "he who supplants"
Yankell, Yanckel, Yanckell, Yankle, Yanckle

Yaotl (Aztec) A great warrior
Yaotyl, Yaotle, Yaotel, Yaotyle

Yaphet (Hebrew) A handsome man
Yaphett, Yapheth, Yaphethe

Yaqub (Arabic) Form of Jacob, meaning "he who supplants"
Ya'qub, Yaqob, Yaqoub

Yardley (English) From the fenced-in meadow
Yardly, Yardleigh, Yardli, Yardlie, Yardlee, Yardlea, Yarley, Yarly

Yaromir (Russian) Form of Jaromir, meaning "from the famous spring"
Yaromire, Yaromeer, Yaromeere, Yaromyr, Yaromyre

Yas (Native American) Child of the snow

Yasahiro (Japanese) One who is peaceful and calm

Yasin (Arabic) A wealthy man
Yasine, Yaseen, Yaseene, Yasyn, Yasyne, Yasien, Yasiene, Yasein

Yasir (Arabic) One who is well-off financially
Yassir, Yasser, Yaseer, Yasr, Yasyr, Yassyr, Yasar, Yassar

Yegor (Russian) Form of George, meaning "one who works the earth; a farmer"
Yegore, Yegorr, Yegeor, Yeorges, Yeorge, Yeorgis

Yehonadov (Hebrew) A gift from God
Yehonadav, Yehonedov, Yehonedav, Yehoash, Yehoashe, Yeeshai, Yeeshae, Yishai

Yenge (African) A hard-working man
Yengi, Yengie, Yengy, Yengey, Yengee

Yeoman (English) A man-servant
Youman, Yoman

Yestin (Welsh) One who is just and fair
Yestine, Yestyn, Yestyne

Yigil (Hebrew) He shall be redeemed
Yigile, Yigyl, Yigyle, Yigol, Yigole, Yigit, Yigat

Yishachar (Hebrew) He will be rewarded
Yishacharr, Yishachare, Yissachar, Yissachare, Yisachur, Yisachare

Yiska (Native American) The night has gone

Yngve (Scandinavian) Refers to the god Ing

Yo (Cambodian) One who is honest

Yoav (Hebrew) Form of Joab, meaning "the Lord is my father"
Yoave, Yoavo, Yoavio

Yochanan (Hebrew) Form of John, meaning "God is gracious"
Yochan, Yohannan, Yohanan, Yochannan

Yohan (German) Form of John, meaning "God is gracious"
Yohanan, Yohann, Yohannes, Yohon, Yohonn, Yohonan

Yonatan (Hebrew) Form of Jonathan, meaning "a gift of God"
Yonaton, Yohnatan, Yohnaton, Yonathan, Yonathon, Yoni, Yonie, Yony

Yong (Korean) One who is courageous

York (English) From the yew settlement
Yorck, Yorc, Yorke

Yosyp (Ukranian) Form of Joseph, meaning "God will add"
Yosip, Yosype, Yosipe

Yovanny (English) Form of Giovanni, meaning "God is gracious"
Yovanni, Yovannie, Yovannee, Yovany, Yovani, Yovanie, Yovanee

Yukon (English) From the settlement of gold
Youkon, Yucon, Youcon, Yuckon, Youckon

Yuliy (Russian) Form of Julius, meaning "one who is youthful"
Yuli, Yulie, Yulee, Yuleigh, Yuly, Yuley, Yulika, Yulian

Yuudai (Japanese) A great hero
Yudai, Yuudae, Yudae, Yuuday, Yuday

Yves (French) A young archer
Yve, Yvo, Yvon, Yvan, Yvet, Yvete

Z

Zabian (Arabic) One who worships celestial bodies
Zabion, Zabien, Zaabian

Zabulon (Hebrew) One who is exalted
Zabulun, Zabulen

Zacchaeus (Hebrew) Form of Zachariah, meaning "The Lord remembers"
Zachaeus, Zachaios, Zaccheus, Zackaeus, Zacheus, Zackaios, Zaccheo

Zachariah (Hebrew) The Lord remembers
Zacaria, Zacarias, Zaccaria, Zaccariah, Zachaios, Zacharia, Zacharias, Zacherish

Zachary (Hebrew) Form of Zachariah, meaning "The Lord remembers"
Zaccary, Zaccery, Zach, Zacharie, Zachery, Zack, Zackarey, Zackary, Thackary, Xakery

Zaci (African) In mythology, the god of fatherhood

Zaden (Dutch) A sower of seeds
Zadin, Zadan, Zadon, Zadun, Zede, Zeden, Zedan

Zadok (Hebrew) One who is righteous; just
Zadoc, Zaydok, Zadock, Zaydock, Zaydoc, Zaidok, Zaidock, Zaidoc

Zador (Hungarian) An ill-tempered man
Zador, Zadoro, Zadorio

Zafar (Arabic) The conquerer; a victorious man
Zafarr, Zaffar, Zhafar, Zhaffar, Zafer, Zaffer

Zahid (Arabic) A pious man
Zahide, Zahyd, Zahyde, Zaheed, Zaheede, Zaheide, Zahiede, Zaheid

Zahir (Arabic) A radiant and flourishing man
Zahire, Zahireh, Zahyr, Zahyre, Zaheer, Zaheere, Zaheir, Zahier

Zahur (Arabic) Resembling
a flower
*Zahure, Zahureh, Zhahur,
Zaahur*

Zale (Greek) Having the
strength of the sea
*Zail, Zaile, Zayl, Zayle,
Zael, Zaele*

Zamir (Hebrew)
Resembling a songbird
*Zamire, Zameer, Zameere,
Zamyr, Zamyre, Zameir,
Zameire, Zamier*

Zander (Slavic) Form of
Alexander, meaning "a
helper and defender of
mankind"
*Zandros, Zandro, Zandar,
Zandur, Zandre*

Zane (English) form of
John, meaning "God is
gracious"
Zayne, Zayn, Zain, Zaine

Zareb (African) The pro-
tector; guardian
*Zarebb, Zaareb, Zarebe,
Zarreb, Zareh, Zaareh*

Zared (Hebrew) One who
has been trapped
*Zarede, Zarad, Zarade,
Zaared, Zaarad*

Zasha (Russian) A defend-
er of the people
*Zashah, Zosha, Zoshah,
Zashiya, Zoshiya*

^**Zayden** (Arabic) Form
of Zayd, meaning "To
become greater, to grow
Zaiden

Zeke (English) Form
of Ezekiel, meaning
"strengthened by God"
Zekiel, Zeek, Zeeke, Zeeq

Zene (African) A handsome man
Zeene, Zeen, Zein, Zeine

Zereen (Arabic) The gold-
en one
*Zereene, Zeryn, Zeryne,
Zerein, Zereine, Zerrin,
Zerren, Zerran*

Zeroun (Armenian) One
who is respected for his
wisdom
Zeroune, Zeroon, Zeroone

Zeth (English) Form of
Seth, meaning "one who
has been appointed"
Zethe

Zion (Hebrew) From the
citadel
Zionn, Zione, Zionne

Ziv (Hebrew) A radiant
man
*Zive, Ziiv, Zivi, Zivie,
Zivee, Zivy, Zivey*

Ziyad (Arabic) One who
betters himself; growth
Ziad

Zlatan (Croatian) The golden son
Zlattan, Zlatane, Zlatann, Zlatain, Zlatayn, Zlaten, Zlaton, Zlatin

Zoltan (Hungarian) A kingly man; a sultan
Zoltann, Zoltane, Zoltanne, Zsolt, Zsoltan

Zorion (Basque) Filled with happiness
Zorian, Zorien

Zoticus (Greek) Full of life
Zoticos, Zoticas

Zsigmond (Hungairan) Form of Sigmund, meaning "the victorious protector"
Zsigmund, Zsigmonde, Zsigmunde, Zsig, Zsiga

Zubair (Arabic) One who is pure
Zubaire, Zubayr, Zubayre, Zubar, Zubarr, Zubare, Zubaer

Zuberi (African) Having great strength
Zuberie, Zubery, Zuberey, Zuberee, Zubari, Zubarie, Zubary, Zubarey

Zubin (English) One with a toothy grin
Zubine, Zuben, Zuban, Zubun, Zubbin

Zuzen (Basque) One who is just and fair
Zuzenn, Zuzan, Zuzin

Zvonimir (Croatian) The sound of peace
Zvonimirr, Zvonimeer

Part 3

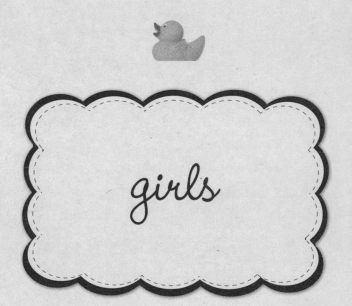

girls

a

Aadi (Hindi) Child of the beginning
Aadie, Aady, Aadey, Aadee, Aadea, Aadeah, Aadye

*****Aaliyah** (Arabic) An ascender, one having the highest social standing
Aaleyah, Aaliya, Aliyah, aliyah, Alliyah, Alieya, Aliyiah, Alliyia, Aleeya, Alee, Aleiya

Aaralyn (American) Woman with song
Aaralynn, Aaralin, Aaralinn, Aaralinne, Aralyn, Aralynn

Aba (African) Born on a Thursday
Abah, Abba, Abbah

Abarrane (Hebrew) Feminine form of Abraham; mother of a multitude; mother of nations
Abarrayne, Abarraine, Abarane, Abarayne, Abaraine, Abame, Abrahana

Abena (African) Born on a Tuesday
Abenah, Abeena, Abyna, Abina, Abeenah, Abynah, Abinah

Abertha (Welsh) One who is sacrificed
Aberthah

Abhilasha (Hindi) One who is desired
Abhilashah, Abhylasha, Abhylashah

Abiba (African) First child born after the grandmother has died
Abibah, Abeeba, Abyba, Abeebah, Abybah, Abeiba, Abeibah, Abieba

Abiela (Hebrew) My father is Lord
Abielah, Abiella, Abiellah, Abyela, Abyelah, Abyella, Abyellah

*****Abigail** (Hebrew) The source of a father's joy
Abbigail, Abigael, Abigale, Abbygail, Abygail, Abygayle, Abbygayle, Abbegale, Abby, Abbagail, Abbey, Abbie, Abbi, Abigayle

Abijah (Hebrew) My father is Lord
Abija, Abisha, Abishah, Abiah, Abia, Aviah, Avia

Abila (Spanish) One who is beautiful
Abilah, Abyla, Abylah

Abilene (American /
Hebrew) From a town in
Texas / resembling grass
*Abalene, Abalina, Abilena,
Abiline, Abileene, Abileen,
Abileena, Abilyn*

Abir (Arabic) Having a fra-
grant scent
*Abeer, Abyr, Abire, Abeere,
Abbir, Abhir*

Abira (Hebrew) A source of
strength; one who is strong
*Abera, Abyra, Abyrah,
Abirah, Abbira, Abeerah*

Abra (Hebrew / Arabic)
Feminine form of
Abraham; mother of a
multitude; mother of
nations / lesson; example
*Abri, Abrah, Abree, Abria,
Abbra, Abrah, Abbrah*

Academia (Latin) From
a community of higher
learning
*Akademia, Academiah,
Akademiah*

Acantha (Greek) Thorny;
in mythology, a nymph
who was loved by Apollo
*Akantha, Ackantha,
Acanthah, Akanthah,
Ackanthah*

Accalia (Latin) In mythol-
ogy, the foster mother of
Romulus and Remus
*Accaliah, Acalia, Accalya,
Acalya, Acca, Ackaliah,
Ackalia*

Adah (Hebrew) Ornament;
beautiful addition to the
family
Adda, Adaya, Ada

Adanna (African) Her
father's daughter; a father's
pride
*Adana, Adanah, Adannah,
Adanya, Adanyah*

Adanne (African) Her
mother's daughter; a
mother's pride
*Adane, Adayne, Adaine,
Adayn, Adain, Adaen,
Adaene*

Adaoma (Ibo) A good
woman

Adara (Greek / Arabic)
Beautiful girl / chaste one;
virgin
*Adair, Adare, Adaire,
Adayre, Adarah, Adarra,
Adaora, Adar*

Addin (Hebrew) One who
is adorned; voluptuous
Addine, Addyn, Addyne

Addison (English)
Daughter of Adam
*Addeson, Addyson, Adison,
Adisson, Addisyn*

Adeen (Irish) Little fire
shining brightly
*Adeene, Adean, Adeane,
Adein, Adeine, Adeyn,
Adeyne*

Adela (German) Of the nobility; serene; of good humor
Adele, Adelia, Adella, Adelle, Adelaid, Adelie, Adelina, Adali

Adeline (German) Form of Adela, meaning of the nobility
Adalyn, Adalynn, Adelyn, Adelynn

Adhelle (Teutonic) Lovely and happy woman
Adhella, Adhell, Adhele

Adianca (Native American) One who brings peace
Adianka, Adyanca, Adyanka

Adira (Hebrew / Arabic) Powerful, noble woman / having great strength
Adirah, Adeera, Adyra, Adeerah, Adyrah, Adeira, Adeirah, Adiera

Admina (Hebrew) Daughter of the red earth
Adminah, Admeena, Admyna, Admeenah, Admynah, Admeina

Adoración (Spanish) Having the adoration of all

Adra (Arabic) One who is chaste; a virgin

Adriana (Greek) Feminine form of Adrian; from the Adriatic Sea region; woman with dark features
Adria, Adriah, Adrea, Adreana, Adreanna, Adrienna, Adriane, Adriene, Adrie, Adrienne, Adriannu, Adrianne, Adriel

Adrina (Italian) Having great happiness
Adrinna, Adreena, Adrinah, Adryna, Adreenah, Adrynah

Aegea (Latin / Greek) From the Aegean Sea / in mythology, a daughter of the sun who was known for her beauty

Aegina (Greek) In mythology, a sea nymph
Aeginae, Aegyna, Aegynah

Aelfwine (English) A friend of the elves
Aelfwyne, Aethelwine, Aethelwyne

Aelwen (Welsh) Woman with a fair brow
Aelwenn, Aelwenne, Aelwin, Aelwinn, Aelwinne, Aelwyn, Aelwynn, Aelwynne

Aerwyna (English) A friend of the ocean

Afra (Hebrew / Arabic) Young doe / white; an earth color
Affra, Affrah, Afrah, Afrya, Afryah, Afria, Affery, Affrie

Afreda (English / Arabic)
Elf counselor / one who is
created
*Afredah, Afreeda, Aafreeda,
Afrida, Afridah, Aelfraed,
Afreedah, Afryda*

Afrodille (French) Daffodil;
showy and vivid
*Afrodill, Afrodil, Afrodile,
Afrodilla, Afrodila*

Afton (English) From the
Afton river

Agave (Greek) In mythology, a queen of Thebes

Agnes (Greek) One who is
pure; chaste
*Agneis, Agnese, Agness,
Agnies, Agnus, Agna, Agne,
Agnesa, Nessa, Oona*

Agraciana (Spanish) One
who forgives
*Agracianna, Agracyanna,
Agracyana, Agraciann,
Agraciane, Agracyann,
Agracyane, Agracianne*

Agrona (Celtic) In mythology, the goddess of war
and death
Agronna, Agronia, Agrone

Agurtzane (Basque) Refers
to the Virgin Mary; chaste;
pure
Aitziber

Ahelia (Hebrew) Breath; a
source of life
*Ahelie, Ahelya, Aheli,
Ahelee, Aheleigh, Ahelea,
Aheleah, Ahely*

Ahellona (Greek) Woman
who has masculine qualities
*Ahelona, Ahellonna,
Ahelonna*

Ahinoam (Hebrew) In the
Bible, one of David's wives

Ahuva (Hebrew) One who
is dearly loved
Ahuvah, Ahuda, Ahudah

Aiandama (Estonian)
Woman who gardens

Aida (English / French
/ Arabic) One who is
wealthy; prosperous / one
who is helpful / a returning
visitor
*Ayda, Aydah, Aidah, Aidee,
Aidia, Aieeda, Aaida*

Aidan (Gaelic) One who is
fiery; little fire
*Aiden, Adeen, Aden, Aideen,
Adan, Aithne, Aithnea, Ajthne*

Aiglentine (French)
Resembling the sweetbrier
rose
Aiglentina

Aiko (Japanese) Little one
who is dearly loved

Ailbhe (Irish) Of noble
character; one who is
bright

Aileen (Irish / Scottish)
Light bearer / from the
green meadow
*Ailean, Ailein, Ailene, Ailin,
Aillen, Ailyn, Alean, Aleane*

Ailis (Irish) One who is
noble and kind
*Ailish, Ailyse, Ailesh, Ailisu,
Ailise*

Ailna (German) One who
is sweet and pleasant; of
the nobility
Ailne

Ain (Irish / Arabic) In
mythology, a woman who
wrote laws to protect the
rights of women / pre-
cious eye

Aina (African) Child born
of a complicated delivery

Aine (Celtic) One who
brings brightness and joy

Aingeal (Irish) Heaven's
messenger; angel
Aingealag

Aionia (Greek) Everlasting
life
*Aioniah, Aionea, Aioneah,
Ayonia, Ayoniah, Ayonea,
Ayoneah*

Ainsley (Scottish) One's
own meadow
*Ainslie, Ainslee, Ainsly,
Ainslei, Aynslie, Aynslee,
Aynslie*

Airic (Celtic) One who is
pleasant and agreeable
*Airick, Airik, Aeric, Aerick,
Aerik*

Aisha (Arabic, African)
lively; womanly
Aiesha, Ayisha, Myisha

Aisling (Irish) A dream or
vision; an inspiration
*Aislin, Ayslin, Ayslinn,
Ayslyn, Ayslynn, Aislyn,
Aisylnn, Aislinn, Isleen*

Aitama (Estonian) One
who is helpful
*Aitamah, Aytama,
Aytamah*

Aitheria (Greek) Of the
wind
*Aitheriah, Aitherea,
Aithereah, Aytheria,
Aytheriah, Aytherea,
Aythereah*

Ajaya (Hindi) One who
is invincible; having the
power of a god
Ajay

Aka (Maori / Turkish)
Affectionate one / in
mythology, a mother god-
dess
Akah, Akka, Akkah

Akili (Tanzanian) Having
great wisdom
*Akilea, Akilee, Akilie,
Akylee, Akylie, Akyli,
Akileah*

Akilina (Latin) Resembling an eagle
Akilinah, Akileena, Akilyna, Akilinna, Ackilina, Acilina, Akylina, Akylyna

Aksana (Russian) Form of Oksana, meaning "hospitality"
Aksanna, Aksanah, Aksannah

Akua (African) Born on a Wednesday

Akuti (Indian) A princess; born to royalty
Akutie, Akutea, Akuteah, Akuty, Akutey, Akutee

Alaina (French) Beautiful and fair woman; dear child.
Alayna, Alaine, Alayne, Alainah, Alana, Alanah, Alanna, Alanis, Alyn, Alyna

Alair (French) One who has a cheerful disposition
Alaire, Allaire, Allair, Aulaire, Alayr, Alayre, Alaer

Alanza (Spanish) Feminine form of Alonzo; noble and ready for battle

Alaqua (Native American) Resembling the sweet gum tree

Alarice (German) Feminine form of Alaric; ruler of all
Alarise, Allaryce, Alarica, Alarisa, Alaricia, Alrica

Alcina (Greek) One who is strong-willed and opinionated
Alceena, Alcyna, Alsina, Alsyna, Alzina, Alcine, Alcinia, Alcyne

Alda (German, Spanish) Long-lived, old; wise; an elder
Aldah, Aldine, Aldina, Aldinah, Aldene, Aldona

Aldis (English) From the ancient house
Aldys, Aldiss, Aldisse, Aldyss, Aldysse

Aldonsa (Spanish) One who is kind and gracious
Aldonza, Aldonsia, Aldonzia

Aleah (Arabic) Exalted
Alea, Alia, Aliah, Aliana, Aleana

Aleen (Celtic) Form of Helen, meaning "the shining light"
Aleena, Aleenia, Alene, Alyne, Alena, Alenka, Alynah, Aleine

Alegria (Spanish) One who is cheerful and brings happiness to others
Alegra, Aleggra, Allegra, Alleffra, Allecra

Alera (Latin) Resembling an eagle
Alerra, Aleria, Alerya, Alerah, Alerrah

Alethea (Greek) One who is truthful
Altheia, Lathea, Lathey, Olethea

•**Alexa** (Greek) Form of Alexandra, meaning "helper and defender of mankind"
Aleka, Alexia

•**Alexandra** (Greek) Feminine form of Alexander; a helper and defender of mankind
Alexandria, Alexandrea, Alixandra, Alessandra, Alexis, Alondra, Aleksandra, Alejandra, Sandra, Sandrine, Sasha

•ᵀ**Alexis** (Greek) Form of Alexandra, meaning "helper and defender of mankind"
Alexus, Alexys, Alexia

Alhena (Arabic) A star in the constellation Gemini
Alhenah, Alhenna, Alhennah

ᵀ**Alice** (German) Woman of the nobility; truthful; having high moral character
Ally, Allie, Alyce, Alesia, Aleece

Alicia (Spanish) Form of Alice, meaning "woman of the nobility"
Alecia, Aleecia, Aliza, Aleesha, Alesha, Alisha

Alika (Hawaiian) One who is honest
Alicka, Alicca, Alyka, Alycka, Alycca

Alina (Arabic / Polish) One who is noble / one who is beautiful and bright
Aline

Alivia (Spanish) Form of Olivia, meaning of the olive tree

•**Allison** (English) Form of Alice, meaning "woman of the nobility, truthful / having high moral character"
Alisanne, Alison, Alicen, Alisen, Alisyn, Allyson, Alyson

Almira (English) A princess; daughter born to royalty
Almeera, Almeira, Almiera, Almyra, Almirah, Almeerah, Almeirah

Almodine (Latin) A highly prized stone
Almondyne, Almondeene, Almondeane, Almondeine

Almunda (Spanish) Refers to the Virgin Mary
Almundena, Almundina

Aloma (Spanish) Form of Paloma, meaning "dove-like"
Alomah, Alomma, Alommah

Alondra (Spanish) Form of Alexandra, meaning "helper and defender of mankind"

Alpha (Greek) The first-born child; the first letter of the Greek alphabet

Alphonsine (French) Feminine form of Alphonse; one who is ready for battle
Alphonsina, Alphonsyne, Alphonsyna, Alphonseene, Alphonseena, Alphonseane, Alphonseana, Alphonsiene

Alpina (Scottish) Feminine form of Alpin; blonde; white-skinned
Alpinah, Alpena, Alpeena, Alpyna, Alpeenah, Alpynah, Alpeina, Alpeinah

Altagracia (Spanish) The high grace of the Virgin Mary
Alta

Aludra (Arabic) A maiden; the name of a star in the constellation Canis Major
Aloodra

Alura (English) A divine counselor
Allura, Alurea, Alhraed

Alvera (Spanish) Feminine of Alvaro; guardian of all; speaker of the truth
Alveria, Alvara, Alverna, Alvernia, Alvira, Alvyra, Alvarita, Alverra

Alverdine (English) Feminine form of Alfred; one who counsels the elves
Alverdina, Alverdeene, Alverdeena, Alverdeane, Alverdeana, Alverdiene, Alverdiena, Alverdeine

•**Alyssa** (German) Form of Alice, meaning "woman of the nobility, truthful / having high moral character"
Alisa, Alissya, Alyssaya, Alishya, Alisia, Alissa, Allisa, Allyssa, Alysa, Alysse, Alyssia

Amada (Spanish) One who is loved by all
Amadia, Amadea, Amadita, Amadah

Amadea (Latin) Feminine form of Amedeo; loved by God
Amadya, Amadia, Amadine, Amadina, Amadika, Amadis

Amadi (African) One who rejoices
Amadie, Amady, Amadey, Amadye, Amadee, Amadea, Amadeah

Amalfi (Italian) From an Italian town overlooking the Gulf of Salerno
Amalfey, Amalfy, Amalfie, Amalfee, Amalfea, Amalfeah

Amalia (German) One who is industrius and hardworking
Amelia, Amalya, Amalie, Anulea, Amylia, Amyleah, Amilia, Neneca

Amalthea (Greek) One who soothes; in mythology, the foster mother of Zeus
Amaltheah, Amalthia, Amalthya

Amanda (Latin) One who is much loved
Amandi, Amandah, Amandea, Amandee, Amandey, Amande, Amandie, Amandy, Mandy

Amapola (Arabic) Resembling a poppy
Amapolah, Amapolla, Amapollah, Amapolia

Amara (Greek) One who will be forever beautiful
Amarah, Amarya, Amaira, Amaria, Amar

^**Amari** (African) Having great strength, a builder
Amaree, Amarie

Amaya (Japanese) Of the night rain
Amayah, Amaia, Amaiah

•**Amber** (French) Resembling the jewel; a warm honey color
Ambur, Ambar, Amberly, Amberlyn, Amberli, Amberlee, Ambyr, Ambyre

Ambrosia (Greek) Immortal; in mythology, the food of the gods
Ambrosa, Ambrosiah, Ambrosyna, Ambrosina, Ambrosyn, Ambrosine, Ambrozin, Ambrozyn

•**Amelia** (German) Form of Amalia or (Latin) form of Emily, meaning "one who is industrious and hardworking"
Amelie, Amelita, Amylia, Amely

America (Latin) A powerful ruler
Americus, Amerika, Amerikus

^**Amira** (Arabic) A princess; one who commands
Amirah, Ameera, Amyra, Ameerah, Amyrah, Ameira, Ameirah, Amiera

Amissa (Hebrew) One who is honest; a friend
Amisa, Amise, Amisia, Amiza, Amysa, Amysia, Amysya, Amyza

^**Amiyah** (American) Form of Amy, meaning "beloved."

Amlika (Indian) A nurturing woman; a mother
Amlikah, Amlyka, Amlykah

Amrita (Hindi) Having
immortality; full of
ambrosia
*Amritah, Amritta, Amryta,
Amrytta, Amrytte, Amritte,
Amryte, Amreeta*

Amser (Welsh) A period
of time

Amy (Latin) Dearly loved
*Aimee, Aimie, Aimi, Aimy,
Aimya, Aimey, Amice,
Amicia*

Anaba (Native American)
A woman returning from
battle
Anabah, Annaba, Annabah

Anabal (Gaelic) One who
is joyful
*Anaball, Annabal,
Annaball*

Anafa (Hebrew)
Resembling the heron
Anafah, Anapha, Anaphah

Anarosa (Spanish) A
graceful rose
Annarosa, Anarose, Annarose

Anastasia (Greek) One
who shall rise again
*Anastase, Anastascia,
Anastasha, Anastasie,
Stacia, Stasia, Stacy, Stacey*

Anasuya (Indian) One
who is charitable
Anasuyah, Annasuya

Ancina (Latin) Form of
Ann, meaning "a woman
graced with God's favor"
*Ancyna, Anncina,
Anncyna, Anceina,
Annceina, Anciena,
Annciena, Anceena*

•**Andrea** (Greek / Latin)
Courageous and strong /
feminine form of Andrew;
womanly
*Andria, Andrianna,
Andreia, Andreina,
Andreya, Andriana,
Andreana, Andera*

Aneira (Welsh) The golden
woman
*Aneera, Anyra, Aneirah,
Aneerah, Anyrah, Aniera,
Anierah, Aneara*

Angel (Greek) A heavenly
messenger

Angela (Greek) A heavenly
messenger; an angel
*Angelica, **Angelina**,
Angelique, Anjela, Anjelika,
Angella, Angelita, Angeline,
Angie, Angy*

•**Angelina** (Greek) Form of
Angela, meaning "a heav-
enly messenger, an angel"
*Angeline, Angelyn,
Angelene, Angelin*

Ani (Hawaiian) One who is
very beautiful
*Aneesa, Aney, Anie, Any,
Aany, Aanye, Anea, Aneah*

Aniceta (French) One who is unconquerable
Anicetta, Anniceta, Annicetta

Aniya (American) Form of Anna, meaning "a woman graced with God's favor
Aniyah

*★Anna** (Latin) A woman graced with God's favor
Annah, Ana, Ann, Anne, Anya, Ane, Annika, Anouche, Annchen, Ancina, Annie

Annabel (Italian) Graceful and beautiful woman
Annabelle, Annabell, Annabella, Annabele, Anabel, Anabell, Anabelle, Anabella

Annabeth (English) Graced with God's bounty
Anabeth, Annabethe, Annebeth, Anebeth, Anabethe

Annalynn (English) From the graceful lake
Analynn, Annalyn, Annaline, Annalin, Annalinn, Analyn, Analine, Analin

Annmarie (English) Filled with bitter grace
Annemarie, Annmaria, Annemaria, Annamarie, Annamaria, Anamarie, Anamaria, Anamari

Annora (Latin) Having great honor
Anora, Annorah, Anorah, Anoria, Annore, Annorya, Anorya, Annoria

Anona (English) Resembling a pineapple
Anonah, Annona, Annoniah, Annonya, Annonia

Anouhea (Hawaiian) Having a soft, cool fragrance

Ansley (English) From the noble's pastureland
Ansly, Anslie, Ansli, Anslee, Ansleigh, Anslea, Ansleah, Anslye

Antalya (Russian) Born with the morning's first light
Antaliya, Antalyah, Antaliyah, Antalia, Antaliah

Antea (Greek) In mythology, a woman who was scorned and committed suicide
Anteia, Anteah

Antje (German) A graceful woman

Antoinette (French) Praiseworthy
Toinette

Anuradha (Hindi) In Hinduism, goddess of good fortune
Anurada

Anwen (Welsh) A famed beauty
Anwin, Anwenne, Anwinne, Anwyn, Anwynn, Anwynne, Anwenn, Anwinn

Anya (Russian) Form of Anna, meaning "a woman graced with God's favor"

Aolani (Hawaiian) Cloud from heaven
Aolaney, Aolanee, Aolaniah, Aolanie, Aolany, Aolanya, Aolania, Aolanea

Apala (African) One who creates religious music
Apalla, Appalla, Appala, Apalah, Apallah, Appallah, Appalah

Apara (Yoruban) One who doesn't remain in one place
Aparra, Apparra, Appara, Aparah, Aparrah, Apparrah, Apparah

Aphrah (Hebrew) From the house of dust
Aphra

Aphrodite (Greek) Love; in mythology, the goddess of love and beauty
Afrodite, Afrodita, Aphrodita, Aphrodyte, Aphhrodyta, Aphrodytah

Aponi (Native American) Resembling a butterfly
Aponni, Apponni, Apponi

Apphia (Hebrew) One who is productive
Apphiah

Apple (American) Sweet fruit; one who is cherished
Appel, Aple, Apel

Apsaras (Indian) In mythology, nature spirits or water nymphs

Aquene (Native American) One who is peaceful
Aqueena, Aqueene, Aqueen

Arabella (Latin) An answered prayer; beautiful altar
Arabela, Arabel, Arabell

Araceli (Spanish) From the altar of heaven
Aracely, Aracelie, Areli, Arely

Aranka (Hungarian) The golden child

Ararinda (German) One who is tenacious
Ararindah, Ararynda, Araryndah

Arava (Hebrew) Resembling a willow; of an arid land
Aravah, Aravva, Aravvah

Arcadia (Greek / Spanish) Feminine form of Arkadios; woman from Arcadia / one who is adventurous
Arcadiah, Arkadia, Arcadya, Arkadya, Arckadia, Arckadya

Ardara (Gaelic) From the stronghold on the hill
Ardarah, Ardarra, Ardaria, Ardarrah, Ardariah

Ardel (Latin) Feminine form of Ardos; industrious and eager
Ardelle, Ardella, Ardele, Ardelia, Ardelis, Ardela, Ardell

Arden (Latin / English) One who is passionate and enthusiastic / from the valley of the eagles
Ardin, Ardeen, Ardena, Ardene, Ardan, Ardean, Ardine, Ardun

Ardra (Celtic / Hindi) One who is noble / the goddess of bad luck and misfortune

Argea (Greek) In mythology, the wife of Polynices
Argeia

Arglwyddes (Welsh) A distinguished lady

Argraff (Welsh) One who makes an impression
Argraffe, Argrafe

Aria (English) A beautiful melody
Ariah

·Ariana (Welsh / Greek) Resembling silver / one who is holy
*Ariane, Arian, **Arianna**, Arianne, Aerian, Aerion, Arianie, Arieon*

Ariel (Hebrew) A lionness of God
Arielle, Ariele, Airial, Ariela, Ariella, Aryela, Arial, Ari

Arietta (Italian) A short but beautiful melody
Arieta, Ariete, Ariet, Ariett, Aryet, Aryeta, Aryetta, Aryette

Arin (English) Form of Erin, meaning "woman of Ireland"
Aryn

Arisje (Danish) One who is superior

Arissa (Greek) One who is superior
Arisa, Aris, Aryssa, Arysa, Arys

Arizona (Native American) From the little spring / from the state of Arizona

Arnette (English) A little eagle
Arnett, Arnetta, Arnete, Arneta, Arnet

Aroha (Maori) One who loves and is loved

Arona (Maori) One who is colorful and vivacious
Aronah, Aronnah, Aronna

Arrosa (Basque) Sprinkled with dew from heaven; resembling a rose
Arrose

Arthurine (English)
Feminine form of Arthur;
as strong as a she-bear
*Arthurina, Arthuretta,
Arthuryne, Arthes, Arthene*

Artis (Irish / English /
Icelandic) Lofy hill; noble /
rock / follower of Thor
*Artisa, Artise, Artys, Artysa,
Artyse, Artiss, Arti, Artina*

Arusi (African) A girl born
during the time of a wedding
*Arusie, Arusy, Arusey,
Arusee, Arusea, Aruseah,
Arusye*

Arwa (Arabic) A female
mountain goat

Arya (Indian) One who is
noble and honored
*Aryah, Aryana, Aryanna,
Aryia*

Ascención (Spanish)
Refers to the Ascension

Aselma (Gaelic) One who
is fair-skinned
Aselmah

Asgre (Welsh) Having a
noble heart

Ashby (English) Home of
the ash tree
*Ashbea, Ashbie, Ashbeah,
Ashbey, Ashbi, Ashbee*

Asherat (Syrian) In mythology, goddess of the sea

Ashima (Hebrew) In the
Bible, a deity worshipped
at Hamath
*Ashimah, Ashyma,
Asheema, Ashimia,
Ashymah, Asheemah,
Asheima, Asheimah*

Ashira (Hebrew) One who
is wealthy; prosperous
*Ashyra, Ashyrah, Ashirah,
Asheera, Asheerah, Ashiera,
Ashierah, Asheira*

****Ashley** (English) From
the meadow of ash trees
*Ashlie, Ashlee, Ashleigh,
Ashly, Ashleye, Ashlya,
Ashala, Ashleay*

Ashlyn (American)
Combination of Ashley
and Lynn
Ashlynn, Ashlynne

Asia (Greek / English)
Resurrection / the rising
sun; in the Koran, the
woman who raised Moses;
a woman from the east
*Aysia, Asya, Asyah, Azia,
Asianne*

Asima (Arabic) One who
offers protection
*Asimah, Aseema, Azima,
Aseemah, Asyma, Asymah,
Asiema, Asiemah*

Asis (African) Of the sun
Asiss, Assis, Assiss

Asli (Turkish) One who is genuine and original
Aslie, Asly, Asley, Aslee, Asleigh, Aslea, Asleah, Alsye

Asma (Arabic) One of high status

Aspen (English) From the aspen tree
Aspin, Aspine, Aspina, Aspyn, Aspyna, Aspyne

Assana (Irish) From the waterfall
Assane, Assania, Assanna, Asanna, Asana

Assunta (Latin) One who is raised up
Assuntah, Asunta, Asuntah

Astra (Latin) Of the stars; as bright as a star
Astera, Astrea, Asteria, Astrey, Astara, Astraea, Astrah, Astree

Astrid (Scandinavian / German) One with divine strength
Astryd, Estrid

Asunción (Spanish) Refers to the Virgin Mary's assumption into heaven

Asura (African) Daughter born during the month of Ashur

Athena (Greek) One who is wise; in mythology, the goddess of war and wisdom
Athina, Atheena, Athene

Atthis (Greek) In mythology, the daughter of Cranaus who gave her name to Attica; a woman from Attica

Attracta (Irish) A virtuous woman; a saint
Athracht, Athrachta

•Aubrey (English) One who rules with elf-wisdom
Aubree, Aubrie, Aubry, Aubri, Aubriana

•^Audrey (English) Woman with noble strength
*Audree, Audry, Audra, Audrea, Adrey, Audre, Audray, Audrin, **Audrina***

Augusta (Latin) Feminine form of Augustus; venerable; majestic
Augustina, Agustina, Augustine, Agostina, Agostine, Augusteen, Augustyna, Agusta

Aulis (Greek) In mythology, a princess of Attica
Auliss, Aulisse, Aulys, Aulyss, Aulysse

Aurear (English) One who plays gentle music
Aureare, Auriar, Auriare

Aurora (Latin) Morning's first light; in mythology, the goddess of the dawn
Aurore, Aurea, Aurorette

˚ᵀAutumn (English) Born in the fall
Autum

˚ᵀAva (German / Iranian) A birdlike woman / from the water
Avah, Avalee, Avaleigh, Avali, Avalie, Avaley, Avelaine, Avelina

Avasa (Indian) One who is independent
Avasah, Avassa, Avasia, Avassah, Avasiah, Avasea, Avaseah

Avena (English) From the oat field
Avenah, Aviena, Avyna, Avina, Avinah, Avynah, Avienah, Aveinah

Avera (Hebrew) One who transgresses
Averah, Avyra, Avira

˚ᵀAvery (English) One who is a wise ruler; of the nobility
Avrie, Averey, Averie, Averi, Averee, Averea, Avereah

Aviana (Latin) Blessed with a gracious life
Avianah, Avianna, Aviannah, Aviane, Avianne, Avyana, Avyanna, Avyane

Aviva (Hebrew) One who is innocent and joyful; resembling springtime
Avivi, Avivah, Aviv, Avivie, Avivice, Avni, Avri, Avyva

Awel (Welsh) One who is as refreshing as a breeze
Awell, Awele, Awela, Awella

Awen (Welsh) A fluid essence; a muse; a flowing spirit
Awenn, Awenne, Awin, Awinn, Awinne, Awyn, Awynn, Awynne

Axelle (German / Latin / Hebrew) Source of life; small oak / axe / peace
Axella, Axell, Axele, Axl, Axela, Axelia, Axellia

Ayala (Hebrew) Resembling a gazelle
Ayalah, Ayalla, Ayallah

Ayla (Hebrew) From the oak tree
Aylah, Aylana, Aylanna, Aylee, Aylea, Aylene, Ayleena, Aylena

Aza (Arabic / African) One who provides comfort / powerful
Azia, Aiza, Aizia, Aizha

Azana (African) One who is superior
Azanah, Azanna, Azannah

Azar (Persian) One who is fiery; scarlet
Azara, Azaria, Azarah, Azarra, Azarrah, Azarr

Aznii (Chechen) A famed beauty
Azni, Aznie, Azny, Azney, Aznee, Aznea, Azneah

Azriel (Hebrew) God is my helper
Azrael, Azriell, Azrielle, Azriela, Azriella, Azruela

b

Baba (African) Born on a Thursday
Babah, Babba, Babbah, Baaba

Babette (French) Form of Barbara, meaning "a traveler from a foreign land; a stranger"; form of Elizabeth, meaning "my God is bountiful; God's promise"
Babett, Babete, Babet, Babbet, Babbett, Babbette, Babbete, Babita

Badia (Arabic) An elegant lady; one who is unique
Badiah, Badi'a, Badiya, Badea, Badya, Badeah

Badr (Arabic) Resembling the full moon
Badra, Badriyyah, Badriyah, Badriya, Badriyya, Badrya, Badria

Bahija (Arabic) A cheerful woman
Bahijah, Bahiga, Bahigah, Bahyja, Bahyjah, Bahyga, Bahygah

•Bailey (English) From the courtyard within castle walls; a public official
Bailee, Bayley, Baylee, Baylie, Baili, Bailie, Baileigh, Bayleigh

Baka (Indian) Resembling a crane
Bakah, Bakka, Backa, Bacca

Bakura (Hebrew) Resembling ripened fruit
Bakurah

Baldhart (German) A bold woman having great strength
Balhart, Baldhard, Balhard, Ballard, Balard, Balarde

Baligha (Arabic) One who is forever eloquent
Balighah, Baleegha, Balygha, Baliegha, Baleagha, Baleigha

Banba (Irish) In mythology, a patron goddess of Ireland

Bansuri (Indian) One who is musical
Bansurie, Bansari, Banseri, Bansurri, Bansury, Bansurey, Bansuree

Bara (Hebrew) One who is chosen
Barah, Barra, Barrah

Barbara (Latin) A traveler from a foreign land; a stranger
Barbra, Barbarella, Barbarita, Baibin, Babette, Bairbre, Barbary, Barb

Barika (African) A flourishing woman; one who is successful
Barikah, Baryka, Barikka, Barykka, Baricka, Barycka, Baricca, Barycca

Barr (English) A lawyer
Barre, Bar

Barras (English) From among the trees

Bathild (German) Heroine of a bold battle
Bathilde, Bathilda

Battseeyon (Hebrew) A daughter of Zion
Batseyon, Batseyonne, Battzion, Batzion

Beatha (Celtic) One who gives life
Betha, Beathah, Bethah

Beatrice (Latin) One who blesses others
Beatrix, Beatriz, Beatriss, Beatrisse, Bea, Beatrize, Beatricia, Beatrisa

Bebhinn (Irish) An accomplished singer
Bebhin, Bebhynn, Bebhyn, Bevin, Bevinne, Bevinn, Bevyn

Becky (English) Form of Rebecca, meaning "one who is bound to God"
Beckey, Becki, Beckie, Becca, Becka, Bekka, Beckee, Beckea

Bel (Indian) From the sacred wood

Belisama (Celtic) In mythology, a goddess of rivers and lakes
Belisamah, Belisamma, Belysama, Belisma, Belysma, Belesama

Bella (Italian) A woman famed for her beauty
Belle, Bela, Bell, Belita, Bellissa, Belia, Bellanca, Bellany

Bem (African) A peaceful woman
Berne

Bena (Native American) Resembling a pheasant
Benah, Benna, Bennah

Benigna (Spanish) Feminine form of Benigno; one who is kind; friendly

Benjamina (Hebrew)
Feminine form of
Benjamin; child of my
right hand
*Benjameena, Benyamina,
Benyameena, Benjameana,
Benyameana, Benjamyna,
Benyamyna*

Bennu (Egyptian)
Resembling an eagle

Beomia (Anglo-Saxon)
Battle maid
*Beomiya, Bemia, Beorhthilde,
Beorhthild, Beorhthilda,
Beomea, Beomeah*

Bernice (Greek) One who
brings victory
*Berenisa, Berenise, Berenice,
Bernicia, Bernisha, Berniss,
Bernyce, Bernys*

Bertha (German) One who
is famously bright and
beautiful
*Berta, Berthe, Berth, Bertina,
Bertyna, Bertine, Bertyne,
Birte*

Bertilda (English) A luminous battle maiden
Bertilde, Bertild

Bertrade (English) An
intelligent advisor
*Bertraide, Bertrayde,
Bertraed, Beorbtraed,
Bertraid, Bertrayd,
Bertraede*

Beryl (English) Resembling
the pale-green precious
stone
*Beryll, Berylle, Beril, Berill,
Berille*

Bess (English) Form of
Elizabeth, meaning "my
God is bountiful; God's
promise"
*Besse, Bessi, Bessie, Bessy,
Bessey, Bessee, Bessea*

Beth (English) Form of
Elizabeth, meaning "my
God is bountiful; God's
promise"
Bethe

Bethany (Hebrew) From
the house of figs
*Bethan, Bethani, Bethanie,
Bethanee, Bethaney,
Bethane, Bethann,
Bethanne*

Beyonce (American) One
who surpasses others
*Beyoncay, Beyonsay,
Beyonsai, Beyonsae,
Beyonci, Beyoncie,
Beyoncee, Beyoncea*

Bianca (Italian) A shining,
fair-skinned woman
Bianka, Byanca, Byanka

Bibiana (Italian) Form of
Vivian, meaning "lively
woman"
Bibiane, Bibianna

Bijou (French) As precious as a jewel

Bikita (African) Resembling an anteater
Bikitah, Bikyta, Bykita, Bykyta, Bikeyta, Bikeita

Billie (English) Feminine form of William; having a desire to protect
Billi, Billy, Billey, Billee, Billeigh, Billea, Billeah

Binga (German) From the hollow
Bingah, Bynga, Binge, Bynge, Bingeh, Byngeh

Bisgu (Anglo-Saxon) A compassionate woman
Bisgue, Bysgu, Bysgue

Bixenta (Basque) A victorious woman

Blaine (Scottish / Irish) A saint's servant / a thin woman
Blayne, Blane, Blain, Blayn, Blaen, Blaene

Blair (Scottish) From the field of battle
Blaire, Blare, Blayre, Blaer, Blaere, Blayr

Blake (English) A dark beauty
Blayk, Blayke, Blaik, Blaike, Blaek, Blaeke

Blimah (Hebrew) One resembling a blossom
Blima, Blime, Blyma, Blymah

Blondell (French) A fair-haired woman
Blondelle, Blondele, Blondene, Blondel, Blondela, Blondella

Blythe (English) Filled with happiness
Blyth, Blithe, Blith

Bo-bae (Korean) A treasured child

Bodgana (Polish) A gift of God
Bodganah, Bodganna, Bodgane, Bodgann, Bodganne, Bogna, Bohdana, Bohdanna

Bonamy (French) A very good friend
Bonamey, Bonami, Bonamie, Bonamee, Bonamei, Bonamea, Bonameah

Bonnie (English) Pretty face
Boni, Bona, Bonea, Boneah, Bonee

Borgny (Norwegian) One who offers help
Borgney, Borgni, Borgnie, Borgnee, Borgnea, Borgneah

Boudicca (Celtic) A victorious queen
Boudicea, Bodiccea, Bodicea, Bodicia

Bradana (Scottish) Resembling the salmon
Bradanah, Bradanna, Bradan, Bradane, Bradann, Bradanne, Braydan, Braydana

Brady (Irish) A large-chested woman
Bradey, Bradee, Bradi, Bradie, Bradea, Bradeah

Braima (African) Mother of multitudes
Braimah, Brayma, Braema, Braymah, Braemah

Brandy (English) A woman wielding a sword; an alcoholic drink
Brandey, Brandi, Brandie, Brandee, Branda, Brande, Brandelyn, Brandilyn

Braulia (Spanish) One who is glowing
Brauliah, Braulea, Brauleah, Brauliya, Brauliyah

Brazil (Spanish) Of the ancient tree
Brasil, Brazile, Brazille, Brasille, Bresil, Brezil, Bresille, Brezille

Brencis (Slavic) Crowned with laurel

Brenda (Irish) Feminine form of Brendan; a princess; wielding a sword
Brynda, Brinda, Breandan, Brendalynn, Brendolyn, Brend, Brienda

Brenna (Welsh) A raven-like woman
Brinna, Brenn, Bren, Brennah, Brina, Brena, Brenah

•**Brianna** (Irish) Feminine form of Brian; from the high hill; one who ascends
Breanna, Breanne, Breana, Breann, Breeana, Breeanna, Breona, Breonna

Brice (Welsh) One who is alert; ambitious
Bryce

Brie (French) Type of cheese
Bree

Bridget (Irish) A strong and protective woman; in mythology, goddess of fire, wisdom, and poetry
Bridgett, Bridgette, Briget, Brigette, Bridgit, Bridgitte, Birgit, Birgitte

^**Brielle** (French) Form of Brie, meaning "type of cheese"

Brilliant (American) A dazzling and sparkling woman

Brimlad (Anglo-Saxon)
From the seaway
Brymlad, Brimlod, Brymlod

Briseis (Greek) In mythology, the Trojan widow abducted by Achilles
Brisys, Brisa, Brisia, Brisha, Brissa, Briza, Bryssa, Brysa

Brittany (English) A woman from Great Britain
Britany, Brittanie, Brittaney, Brittani, Brittanee, Britney, Britnee, Britny

*Brook** (English) From the running stream
*Brooke, Brookie, **Brooklyn**, Brooklynn, Brooklynne*

*Brooklyn** (American) Borough of New York City
Brooklin, Brooklynn, Brooklynne

Brunhild (German) A dark and noble battle maiden; in Norse mythology, queen of the Valkyries
Brunhilde, Brunhilda

Brynn (Welsh) Hill
Brin, Brinn, Bryn, Brynlee, Brynly, Brinley, Brinli, Brynlie

Bryony (English) Of the healing place
Briony, Brionee, Bryonee, Bryoni, Brionie

C

Cable (American) Resembling a heavy rope; having great strength
Cabel

Cabrina (American) Form of Sabrina, meaning "a legendary princess"
Cabrinah, Cabrinna

Cabriole (French) An adorable girl
Cabriolle, Cabrioll, Cabriol, Cabryole, Cabryolle, Cabryoll, Cabryol, Cabriola

Cacalia (Latin) Resembling the flowering plant
Cacaliah, Cacalea, Cacaleah

Caden (English) A battle maiden
Cadan, Cadin, Cadon

Cadence (Latin) Rhythmic and melodious; a musical woman
Cadena, Cadenza, Cadian, Cadienne, Cadianne, Cadiene, Caydence, Cadencia, Kadence, Kaydence

Cadhla (Irish) A beautiful woman
Cadhlah

Caesaria (Greek)
Feminine form of Caesar;
an empress
Caesariah, Caesarea,
Caesareah, Caezaria,
Caezariah, Caezarea,
Caezareah, Cesaria

Caia (Latin) One who
rejoices
Cai, Cais

Cainwen (Welsh) A beauti-
ful treasure
Cainwenn, Cainwenne,
Cainwin, Cainwinn,
Cainwinne, Cainwyn,
Cainwynn, Cainwynne

Cairo (African) From the
city in Egypt

Caitlin (English) Form of
Catherine, meaning one
who is pure, virginal
Caitlyn, Catlin, Catline,
Catlyn, Caitlan, Caitlinn,
Caitlynn

Calais (French) From the
city in France

Cale (Latin) A respected
woman
Cayl, Cayle, Cael, Caele,
Cail, Caile

Caledonia (Latin) Woman
of Scotland
Caledoniah, Caledoniya,
Caledona, Caledonya,
Calydona

California (Spanish) From
paradise; from the state of
California
Califia

Calise (Greek) A gorgeous
woman
Calyse, Calice, Calyce

Calista (Greek) Most
beautiful; in mythology, a
nymph who changed into
a bear and then into the
Great Bear constellation
Calissa, Calisto, Callista,
Calyssa, Calysta, Calixte,
Colista, Collista

Calla (Greek) Resembling
a lily; a beautiful woman
Callah

Callie (Greek) A beautiful girl
Cali, Callee, Kali, Kallie

Calligenia (Greek) Daughter
born with beauty
Caligenia, Calligeniah,
Caligeniah, Callygenia,
Calygenia, Calligenea

Caltha (Latin) Resembling
a yellow flower
Calthah, Calthia, Calthiah,
Caltheah, Calthea

Calybe (Greek) In mythology, a nymph who was the
wife of Laomedon

Calypso (Greek) A woman
with secrets; in mythology,
a nymph who captivated
Odysseus for seven years

Camassia (American) One
who is aloof
*Camassiah, Camasia,
Camasiah, Camassea,
Camasseah, Camasea,
Camaseah*

Cambay (English) From
the town in India
Cambaye, Cambai, Cambae

Camdyn (English) Of the
enclosed valley
*Camden, Camdan,
Camdon, Camdin*

Cameron (Scottish)
Having a crooked nose
*Cameryn, Camryn, Camerin,
Camren, Camrin, Camron*

* ^ **Camila** (Italian)
Feminine form of
Camillus; a ceremonial
attendant; a noble virgin
*Camile, Camille, Camilla,
Camillia, Caimile,
Camillei, Cam, Camelai*

Campbell (Scottish)
Having a crooked mouth
*Campbel, Campbelle,
Campbele*

Candace (Ethiopian /
Greek) A queen / one who
is white and glowing
*Candice, Candiss, Candyce,
Candance, Candys,
Candyss, Candy*

Candida (Latin) White-
skinned
Candide, Candy

Candra (Latin) One who is
glowing

Candy (English) A sweet
girl; form of Candida,
meaning "white-skinned";
form of Candace, mean-
ing "a queen / one who is
white and glowing"
*Candey, Candi, Candie,
Candee, Candea, Candeah*

Caneadea (Native
American) From the hori-
zon
*Caneadeah, Caneadia,
Caneadiah*

Canika (American) A
woman shining with grace
*Canikah, Caneeka,
Canicka, Canyka, Canycka,
Caneekah, Canickah,
Canykah*

Canisa (Greek) One who is
very much loved
*Canisah, Canissa, Canysa,
Caneesa, Canyssa*

Cannes (French) A woman
from Cannes

Cantabria (Latin) From
the mountains
*Cantabriah, Cantebria,
Cantabrea, Cuntebrea*

Capeka (Slavic) Resembling
a young stork
*Capekah, Capecca,
Capeccah*

Caprina (Italian) Woman
of the island Capri
*Caprinah, Caprinna,
Capryna, Capreena,
Caprena, Capreenah,
Caprynah, Capriena*

^**Cara** (Italian / Gaelic)
One who is dearly loved /
a good friend
*Carah, Caralee, Caralie,
Caralyn, Caralynn, Carrah,
Carra, Chara*

Carissa (Greek) A woman
of grace
*Carisa, Carrisa, Carrissa,
Carissima*

Carla (Latin) Feminine
form of Carl; a free woman
*Carlah, Carlana, Carleen,
Carlena, Carlene, Carletta*

^**Carly** (American) Form
of Carla, meaning "a free
woman
*Carlee, Carleigh, Carli,
Carlie, Carley*

Carlessa (American) One
who is restless
*Carlessah, Carlesa,
Carlesah*

Carmel (Hebrew) Of the
fruitful orchid
Carmela, Carmella, Karmel

Carmen (Latin) A beauti-
ful song
*Carma, Carmelita,
Carmencita, Carmia,
Carmie, Carmina,
Carmine, Carmita*

Carna (Latin) In mythology, a goddess who ruled
the heart

Carni (Latin) One who is
vocal
*Carnie, Carny, Carney,
Carnee, Carnea, Carneah,
Carnia, Carniah*

Carol (English) Form of
Caroline, meaning "joyous
song"; feminine form of
Charles; a small, strong
woman
*Carola, Carole, Carolle,
Carolla, Caroly, Caroli,
Carolie, Carolee*

•**Caroline** (Latin) Joyous
song; feminine form of
Charles; a small, strong
woman
*Carol, Carolina, Carolyn,
Carolann, Carolanne,
Carolena, Carolene,
Carolena, Caroliana*

Carrington (English)
A beautiful woman; a
woman of Carrington
*Carington, Carryngton,
Caryngton*

Carson (Scottish) Son of the marshland
Carsan, Carsen, Carsin

Caryatis (Greek) In mythology, goddess of the walnut tree
Carya, Cariatis, Caryatiss, Cariatiss, Caryatys, Cariatys, Caryatyss, Cariatyss

Carys (Welsh) One who loves and is loved
Caryss, Carysse, Caris, Cariss, Carisse, Cerys, Ceryss, Cerysse

Cascadia (Latin) Woman of the waterfall
Cascadiya, Cascadea, Cascata

Casey (Greek, Irish) A vigilant woman
Casie, Casy, Caysie, Kasey

Cason (Greek) A seer
Cayson, Caison, Caeson

Cassandra (Greek) An unheeded prophetess; in mythology, King Priam's daughter who foretold the fall of Troy
Casandra, Cassandrea, Cassaundra, Cassondra, Cass, Cassy, Cassey, Cassi

Cassidy (Irish) Curly-haired girl
Cassady, Cassidey, Cassidi, Cassidie, Cassidee, Cassadi, Cassadie, Cassadee, Casidhe, Cassidea, Cassadea

Casta (Spanish) One who is pure; chaste
Castah, Castalina, Castaleena, Castaleina, Castaliena, Castaleana, Castalyna, Castara

Catherine (English) One who is pure; virginal
Catharine, Cathrine, Cathryn, Catherin, Catheryn, Catheryna, Cathi, Cathy, Katherine

Cathresha (American) One who is pure
Cathreshah, Cathreshia, Cathreshiah, Cathreshea, Cathresheah, Cathrisha

Catrice (Greek) A wholesome woman
Catrise, Catryce, Catryse, Catreece, Catreese, Catriece

Cavana (Irish) Feminine form of Cavan; from the hollow
Cavanna, Cavanah, Cavania, Cavaniya, Cavanea, Cavannah

Cayenne (French) Resembling the hot and spicy pepper

Cecilia (Latin) Feminine form of Cecil; one who is blind; patron saint of music
Cecelia, Cecile, Cecilee, Cicely, Cecily, Cecille, Cecilie, Cicilia, Sheila, Silka, Sissy

Celand (Latin) One who is
meant for heaven
*Celanda, Celande,
Celandia, Celandea*

Celandine (English)
Resembling a swallow
*Celandyne, Celandina,
Celandyna, Celandeena,
Celandena, Celandia*

Celeste (Latin) A heavenly
daughter
*Celesta, Celestia, Celisse,
Celestina, Celestyna,
Celestine*

Celia (Latin) Form of
Cecelia, meaning patron
saint of music

Celina (Latin) In mythology, one of the daughters of
Atlas who was turned into
a star of the Pleiades constellation; of the heavens;
form of Selena, meaning
"of the moon"
*Celena, Celinna, Celene,
Celenia, Celenne, Celicia*

Celka (Latin) A celestial
being
Celkah, Celki, Celkie

Celosia (Greek) A fiery
woman; burning; aflame
Celosiah, Celosea, Celoseah

Cera (French) A colorful
woman
Cerah, Cerrah, Cerra

Cerina (Latin) Form of
Serena, meaning "having
a peaceful disposition"
*Cerinah, Ceryna, Cerynah,
Cerena, Cerenah, Ceriena*

Cerise (French) Resembling
the cherry
Cerisa

Chadee (French) A divine
woman; a goddess
*Chadea, Chadeah, Chady,
Chadey, Chadi, Chadie*

Chai (Hebrew) One who
gives life
*Chae, Chaili, Chailie,
Chailee, Chaileigh, Chaily,
Chailey, Chailea*

Chailyn (American)
Resembling a waterfall
*Chailynn, Chailynne,
Chaelyn, Chaelynn,
Chaelynne, Chaylyn*

Chakra (Arabic) A center
of spiritual energy

Chalette (American)
Having good taste
*Chalett, Chalet, Chalete,
Chaletta, Chaleta*

Chalina (Spanish) Form
of Rosalina, meaning
"resembling a gentle
horse / resembling the
beautiful and meaningful
flower"
*Chalinah, Chalyna, Chaleena,
Chalena, Charo, Chaliena,
Chaleina, Chaleana*

Chameli (Hindi)
Resembling jasmine
*Chamelie, Chamely,
Chameley, Chamelee*

Chan (Sanskrit) A shining
woman

Chana (Hebrew) Form of
Hannah, meaning "having
favor and grace"
*Chanah, Channa, Chaanach,
Chaanah, Chanach, Channah*

Chance (American) One
who takes risks
*Chanci, Chancie, Chancee,
Chancea, Chanceah,
Chancy, Chancey*

Chanda (Sanskrit) An
enemy of evil
*Chandy, Chaand, Chand,
Chandey, Chandee, Chandi,
Chandie, Chandea*

Chandra (Hindi) Of the
moon; another name for
the goddess Devi
*Chandara, Chandria,
Chaundra, Chandrea,
Chandreah*

Chanel (French) From the
canal; a channel
*Chanell, Chanelle,
Channelle, Chenelle,
Chenel, Chenell*

Channary (Cambodian) Of
the full moon
*Channarie, Channari,
Channarey, Channaree,
Chantrea, Chantria*

Chantrice (French) A
singer
Chantryce, Chantrise, Chantryse

Chapawee (Native
American) Resembling a
beaver
*Chapawi, Chapawie,
Chapawy, Chapawea*

Charbonnet (French) A
giving and loving woman
*Charbonay, Charbonaye,
Charbonae, Charbonai,
Charbonnay, Charbonnae,
Charbonnai*

Charisma (Greek) Blessed
with charm
*Charismah, Charizma,
Charysma, Karisma*

Charlesia (American)
Feminine form of Charles;
small, strong woman
*Charlesiah, Charlesea,
Charleseah, Charlsie,
Charlsi*

·Charlotte (French) Form
of Charles, meaning "a
small, strong woman"
Charlize, Charlot, Charlotta

Charlshea (American)
Filled with happiness
*Charlsheah, Charlshia,
Charlshiah*

Charnee (American) Filled
with joy
*Charny, Charney, Charnea,
Charneah, Charni, Charnie*

Charnesa (American) One who gets attention
Charnessa, Charnessah

Charsetta (American) An emotional woman
Charsett, Charsette, Charset, Charsete, Charseta

Chartra (American) A classy lady
Chartrah

Charu (Hindi) One who is gorgeous
Charoo, Charou

Charumat (Hindi) An intelligent and beautiful woman
Charoomat, Charoumat

Chasia (Hebrew) One who is protected; sheltered
Chasiah, Chasea, Chaseah, Chasya, Chasyah

Chasidah (Hebrew) A religious woman; pious
Chasida, Chasyda, Chasydah

Chateria (Vietnamese) Born beneath the moonlight
Chateriah, Chaterea, Chatereah, Chateriya, Chateriyah

Chavi (Egyptian) A precious daughter
Chavie, Chavy, Chavey, Chavee, Chavea, Chaveah

Chavon (Hebrew) A giver of life
Chavonne, Chavonn, Chavona, Chavonna

Chazona (Hebrew) A prophetess
Chazonah, Chazonna, Chazonnah

Cheche (African) A small woman

Chedra (Hebrew) Filled with happiness
Chedrah

Cheer (American) Filled with joy
Cheere

Cheifa (Hebrew) From a safe harbor
Cheifah, Cheiffa, Cheiffah

Chekia (American) A saucy woman
Cheekie, Checki, Checkie, Checky, Checkey, Checkee, Checkea, Checkeah

Chelone (English) Resembling a flowering plant

Chelsea (English) From the landing place for chalk
Chelcie, Chelsa, Chelsee, Chelseigh, Chelsey, Chelsi, Chelsie, Chelsy

Chemarin (French) A dark
beauty
*Chemarine, Chemaryn,
Chemareen, Chemarein,
Chemarien*

Chemda (Hebrew) A charismatic woman
Chemdah

Chenille (American) A
soft-skinned woman
*Chenill, Chenil, Chenile,
Chenilla, Chenila*

Chephzibah (Hebrew)
Her father's delight

Cherika (French) One who
is dear
*Chericka, Cheryka,
Cherycka, Cherieka,
Cheriecka, Chereika,
Chereicka, Cheryka*

Cherry (English)
Resembling a fruit-bearing
tree
*Cherrie, Cherri, Cherrey,
Cherree, Cherrea, Cherreah*

Chesney (English) One
who promotes peace
*Chesny, Chesni, Chesnie,
Chesnea, Chesneah,
Chesnee*

Cheyenne (Native
American) Unintelligible
speaker
*Chayanne, Cheyane,
Cheyene, Shayan, Shyann*

Chiante (Italian)
Resembling the wine
*Chianti, Chiantie, Chiantee,
Chianty, Chiantey, Chiantea*

Chiara (Italian) Daughter
of the light
Chiarah, Chiarra, Chiarrah

Chiba (Hebrew) One who
loves and is loved
*Chibah, Cheeba, Cheebah,
Cheiba, Cheibah, Chieba,
Chiebah, Cheaba*

Chickoa (Native American)
Born at daybreak
Chickoah, Chikoa, Chikoah

Chidi (Spanish) One who
is cheerful
*Chidie, Chidy, Chidey,
Chidee, Chidea, Chideah*

Chidori (Japanese)
Resembling a shorebird
*Chidorie, Chidory,
Chidorey, Chidorea,
Chidoreah, Chidoree*

Chikira (Spanish) A tal-
ented dancer
*Chikirah, Chikiera,
Chikierah, Chikeira,
Chikeirah, Chikeera,
Chikeerah, Chikyra*

Chiku (African) A talkative
girl

Chinara (African) God
receives
*Chinarah, Chinarra,
Chinarrah*

Chinue (African) God's own blessing
Chinoo, Chynue, Chynoo

Chiriga (African) One who is triumphant
Chyrigu, Chyryga, Chiryga

Chislaine (French) A faithful woman
Chislain, Chislayn, Chislayne, Chislaen, Chislaene, Chyslaine, Chyslain, Chyslayn

Chitsa (Native American) One who is fair
Chitsah, Chytsa, Chytsah

Chizoba (African) One who is well-protected
Chizobah, Chyzoba, Chyzobah

*Chloe (Greek) A flourishing woman; blooming
Clo, Cloe, Cloey, Chloë

Cho (Japanese) Resembling a butterfly

Chofa (Polish) An able-bodied woman
Chofah, Choffa, Choffah

Christina (English) Follower of Christ
Christinah, Cairistiona, Christine, Christin, Christian, Christiana, Christiane, Christianna, Kristina

Chuki (African) Born during an unpleasant time
Chukie, Chuky, Chukey, Chukee, Chukea, Chukeah

Chula (Native American) Resembling a colorful flower
Chulah, Chulla, Chullah

Chulda (Hebrew) One who can tell fortunes
Chuldah

Chun (Chinese) Born during the spring

Chyou (Chinese) Born during autumn

Ciara (Irish) A dark beauty
Ceara, Ciaran, Ciarra, Ciera, Cierra, Ciere, Ciar, Ciarda

Cidrah (American) One who is unlike others
Cidra, Cydrah, Cydra

Cinnamon (American) Resembling the reddish-brown spice
Cinnia, Cinnie

Ciona (American) One who is steadfast
Cionah, Cyona, Cyonah

Claennis (Anglo-Saxon) One who is pure
Claenis, Claennys, Claenys, Claynnis, Claynnys, Claynys, Claynyss

•**Claire** (French) Form of Clara, meaning "famously bright"
Clare, Clair

Clancey (American) A light-hearted woman
Clancy, Clanci, Clancie, Clancee, Clancea, Clanceah

•**Clara** (Latin) One who is famously bright
*Clarie, Clarinda, Clarine, Clarita, Claritza, Clarrie, Clarry, Clarabelle, **Claire**, Clarice*

Clarice (French) A famous woman; also a form of Clara, meaning "one who is famously bright"
Claressa, Claris, Clarisa, Clarise, Clarisse, Claryce, Clerissa, Clerisse

Claudia (Latin / German / Italian) One who is lame
Claudelle, Gladys

Clelia (Latin) A glorious woman
Cloelia, Cleliah, Clelea, Cleleah, Cloeliah, Cloelea, Cloeleah

Clementine (French) Feminine form of Clement; one who is merciful
Clem, Clemence, Clemency, Clementia, Clementina, Clementya, Clementyna, Clementyn

Cleodal (Latin) A glorious woman
Cleodall, Cleodale, Cleodel, Cleodell, Cleodelle

Cleopatra (Greek) A father's glory; of the royal family
Clea, Cleo, Cleona, Cleone, Cleonie, Cleora, Cleta, Cleoni

Clever (American) One who is quick-witted and smart

Cloris (Greek) A flourishing woman; in mythology, the goddess of flowers
Clores, Clorys, Cloriss, Clorisse, Cloryss, Clorysse

Cloud (American) A light-hearted woman
Cloude, Cloudy, Cloudey, Cloudee, Cloudea, Cloudeah, Cloudi, Cloudie

Clydette (American) Feminine form of Clyde, meaning "from the river"
Clydett, Clydet, Clydete, Clydetta, Clydeta

Clymene (Greek) In mythology, the mother of Atlas and Prometheus
Clymena, Clymyne, Clymyn, Clymyna, Clymeena, Clymeina, Clymiena, Clymeana

Clytie (Greek) The lovely one; in mythology, a nymph who was changed into a sunflower
Clyti, Clytee, Clyty, Clytey, Clyte, Clytea, Clyteah

Co (American) A jovial woman
Coe

Coby (Hebrew) Feminine form of Jacob; the supplanter
Cobey, Cobi, Cobie, Cobee, Cobea, Cobeah

Cochava (Hebrew) Having a starlike quality
Cochavah, Cochavia, Cochavea, Cochaviah, Cochaveah

Coffey (American) A lovely woman
Coffy, Coffe, Coffee, Coffeu, Coffeah, Coffi, Coffie

Coira (Scottish) Of the churning waters
Coirah, Coyra, Coyrah

Colanda (American) Form of Yolanda, meaning "resembling the violet flower"
Colande, Coland, Colana, Colain, Colaine, Colane, Colanna, Corlanda

Cole (English) A swarthy woman; having coal-black hair
Col, Coal, Coale, Coli, Colie, Coly, Coley, Colee

Colemand (American) An adventurer
Colmand, Colemyan, Colemyand, Colmyan

Colette (French) Victory of the people
Collette, Kolette

Coligny (French) Woman from Cologne
Coligney, Colignie, Coligni, Colignee, Colignea, Coligneah

Colisa (English) A delightful young woman
Colisah, Colissa, Colissah, Colysa, Colysah, Colyssa, Colyssah

Colola (American) A victorious woman
Colo, Cola

Comfort (English) One who strengthens or soothes others
Comforte, Comfortyne, Comfortyna, Comforteene, Comforteena, Comfortene, Comfortena, Comfortiene

Conary (Gaelic) A wise woman
Conarey, Conarie, Conari, Conaree, Conarea, Conareah

Concordia (Latin) Peace and harmony; in mythology, goddess of peace
Concordiah, Concordea, Concord, Concorde, Concordeah

Coneisha (American) A giving woman
Coneishah, Coniesha, Conieshah, Conysha, Conyshah, Coneesha, Coneeshah, Coneasha

Constanza (American) One who is strong-willed
Constanzia, Constanzea

Consuela (Spanish) One who provides consolation
Consuelia, Consolata, Consolacion, Chela, Conswela, Conswelia, Conswelea, Consuella

Contessa (Italian) A titled woman; a countess
Countess, Contesse, Countessa, Countesa, Contesa

Cooper (English) One who makes barrels
Couper

Copper (American) A red-headed woman
Coper, Coppar, Copar

Cora (English) A young maiden,
Corah, Coraline, Corra

Coral (English) Resembling the semiprecious sea growth; from the reef
Coralee, Coralena, Coralie, Coraline, Corallina, Coralline, Coraly, Coralyn

Corazon (Spanish) Of the heart
Corazana, Corazone, Corazona

Cordelia (Latin) A good-hearted woman; a woman of honesty
Cordella, Cordelea, Cordilia, Cordilea, Cordy, Cordie, Cordi, Cordee

Corey (Irish) From the hollow; of the churning waters
Cory, Cori, Coriann, Corianne, Corie, Corri, Corrianna, Corrie

Corgie (American) A humorous woman
Corgy, Corgey, Corgi, Corgee, Corgea, Corgeah

Coriander (Greek) A romantic woman; resembling the spice
Coryander, Coriender, Coryender

Corinthia (Greek) A woman of Corinth
Corinthiah, Corinthe, Corinthea, Corintheah, Corynthia, Corynthea, Corynthe

Corky (American) An energetic young woman
Corki, Corkey, Corkie, Corkee, Corkea, Corkeah

Cornelia (Latin) Feminine
form of Cornelius; refer-
ring to a horn
*Cornalia, Corneelija,
Cornela, Cornelija,
Cornelya, Cornella,
Cornelle, Cornie*

Cota (Spanish) A lively
woman
Cotah, Cotta, Cottah

Coty (French) From the
riverbank
*Cotey, Coti, Cotie, Cotee,
Cotea, Coteah*

Courtney (English) A
courteous woman; courtly
*Cordney, Cordni, Cortenay,
Corteney, Cortland,
Cortnee, Cortneigh,
Cortney, Courteney*

Covin (American) An
unpredictable woman
Covan, Coven, Covyn, Covon

Coy (English) From the
woods, the quiet place
Coye, Coi

Cree (Native American) A
tribal name
Crei, Crey, Crea, Creigh

Creirwy (Welsh) One who
is lucky

Creola (American)
Daughter of American
birth but European heritage
*Creole, Creolla, Criole,
Criola, Criolla, Cryola,
Cryolla*

Cressida (Greek) The
golden girl; in mythology,
a woman of Troy
*Cressa, Criseyde, Cressyda,
Crissyda*

Criselda (American) Form
of Griselda, meaning "a
gray-haired battle maid; one
who fights the dark battle"
*Cricelda, Cricely, Crisel,
Criseldis, Crisella, Criselle,
Criselly, Crishelda*

Crishona (American) A
beautiful woman
*Crishonah, Cryshona,
Cryshonah, Crishonna,
Crishonnah, Cryshonna,
Cryshonnah*

Crisiant (Welsh) As clear
as a crystal
*Crisiante, Crisianta,
Crysiant, Crysyant,
Crysianta, Crysiante,
Crysyanta, Crysyante*

Cristos (Greek) A dedicated and faithful woman
Crystos, Christos, Chrystos

Cullodina (Scottish) From
the mossy ground
*Cullodena, Culodina,
Culodena, Cullodyna,
Culodyna*

Cushaun (American) An elegant lady
Cushawn, Cusean, Cushauna, Cushawna, Cuseana, Cooshaun, Cooshauna, Cooshawn

Cwen (English) A royal woman; queenly
Cwene, Cwenn, Cwenne, Cwyn, Cwynn, Cwynne, Cwin, Cwinn

Cylee (American) A darling daughter
Cyleigh, Cyli, Cylie, Cylea, Cyleah, Cyly, Cyley

Cyrene (Greek) In mythology, a maiden-huntress loved by Apollo
Cyrina, Cyrena, Cyrine, Cyreane, Cyreana, Cyreene, Cyreena

Czigany (Hungarian) A gypsy girl; one who moves from place to place
Cziganey, Czigani, Cziganie, Cziganee

d

Dacey (Irish) Woman from the south
Daicey, Dacee, Dacia, Dacie, Dacy, Daicee, Daicy, Daci

Daffodil (French) Resembling the yellow flower
Daffodill, Daffodille, Dafodil, Dafodill, Dafodille, Daff, Daffodyl, Dafodyl

Dagmar (Scandinavian) Born on a glorious day
Dagmara, Dagmaria, Dagmarie, Dagomar

Dahlia (Swedish) From the valley; resembling the flower
Dahlea, Dahl, Dahiana, Dayha, Daleia

Daira (Greek) One who is well-informed
Daeira, Danira, Dayeera

Daisy (English) Of the day's eye; resembling a flower
Daisee, Daisey, Daisi, Daisie, Dasie, Daizy, Daysi, Deysi

Dakota (Native American) A friend to all
Dakotah, Dakotta, Dakoda, Dakodah

Dalmace (Latin) Woman from Dalmatia, a region of Italy
Dalma, Dalmassa, Dalmatia, Dalmase, Dalmatea

Dalmar (African) A versatile woman
Dalmarr, Dalmare, Dalmarre

Damali (Arabic) A beautiful vision
Damalie, Damaly, Damaley, Damalee, Damaleigh, Damalea

Damani (American) Of a bright tomorrow
Damanie, Damany, Damaney, Damanee, Damanea, Damaneah

Damaris (Latin) A gentle woman
Damara, Damaress, Damariss, Damariz, Dameris, Damerys, Dameryss, Damiris

^**Dana** (English) Woman from Denmark
Danna, Daena, Daina, Danaca, Danah, Dane, Danet, Daney, Dania

Danica (Slavic) Of the morning star
Danika

Daniela (Spanish) Form of Danielle, meaning God is my judge
Daniella

•**Danielle** (Hebrew) Feminine form of Daniel; God is my judge
Daanelle, Danee, Danele, Danella, Danelle, Danelley, Danette, Daney

Daphne (Greek) Of the laurel tree; in mythology, a virtuous woman transformed into a laurel tree to protect her from Apollo
Daphna, Daphney, Daphni, Daphnie, Daffi, Daffie, Daffy, Dafna

Darby (English) Of the deer park
Darb, Darbee, Darbey, Darbie, Darrbey, Darrbie, Darrby, Derby, Larby

Daria (Greek) Feminine form of Darius; possessing good fortune; wealthy
Dari, Darian, Dariane, Darianna, Dariele, Darielle, Darien, Darienne

Daring (American) One who takes risks; a bold woman
Daryng, Derring, Dering, Deryng

Darlene (English) Our little darling
Dareen, Darla, Darleane, Darleen, Darleena, Darlena, Darlenny, Darlina

Darnell (English) A secretive woman
Darnelle, Darnella, Darnae, Darnetta, Darnisha, Darnel, Darnele, Darnela

Daryn (Greek) Feminine form of Darin; a gift of God
Darynn, Darynne, Darinne, Daren, Darenn, Darene

Daw (Thai) Of the stars
Dawe

Dawn (English) Born at daybreak; of the day's first light
Dawna, Dawne, Dawnelle, Dawnetta, Dawnette, Dawnielle, Dawnika, Dawnita

Day (American) A father's hope for tomorrow
Daye, Dai, Dae

^**Daya** (Hebrew) Resembling a bird of prey
*Dayah, **Dayana**, Dayanara, Dayania, Dayaniah, Dayanea, Dayaneah*

Dayton (English) From the sunny town
Dayten, Daytan

Dea (Greek) Resembling a goddess

Debonnaire (French) One who is suave; nonchalant
Debonair, Debonaire, Debonnayre, Debonayre, Debonaere, Debonnaere

Deborah (Hebrew) Resembling a bee; in the Bible, a prophetess
Debbera, Debbey, Debbi, Debbie, Debbra, Debby

Deidre (Gaelic) A brokenhearted or raging woman
Deadra, Dede, Dedra, Deedra, Deedre, Deidra, Deirdre, Deidrie

Deiondre (American) From the lush valley
Deiondra, Deiondria, Deiondrea, Deiondriya

Dekla (Latvian) In mythology, a trinity goddess
Decla, Deckla, Deklah, Decklah, Declah

Delaney (Irish / French) The dark challenger / from the elder-tree grove
Delaina, Delaine, Delainey, Delainy, Delane, Delanie, Delany, Delayna

Delaware (English) From the state of Delaware
Delawair, Delaweir, Delwayr, Delawayre, Delawaire, Delawaer, Delawaere

^**Delilah** (Hebrew) A seductive woman
Delila, Delyla, Delylah

Delta (Greek) From the mouth of the river; the fourth letter of the Greek alphabet
Dellta, Deltah, Delltah

Delu (African) The sole daughter
Delue, Deloo

Delyth (Welsh) A pretty young woman
Delythe, Delith, Delithe

Demeter (Greek) In mythology, the goddess of the harvest
Demetra, Demitra, Demitras, Dimetria, Demetre, Demetria, Dimitra, Dimitre

Denali (Indian) A superior woman
Denalie, Denaly, Denally, Denalli, Denaley, Denalee, Denallee, Denallie

Dendara (Egyptian) From the town on the river
Dendera, Dendaria, Denderia, Dendarra

Denver (English) From the green valley

Derora (Hebrew) As free as a bird
Derorah, Derorra, Derorit, Drora, Drorah, Drorit

Derry (Irish) From the oak grove
Derrey, Derri, Derrie, Derree, Derrea, Derreah

Deryn (Welsh) A birdlike woman
Derran, Deren, Derhyn, Deron, Derrin, Derrine, Derron, Derrynne

Desiree (French) One who is desired
Desaree, Desirae, Desarae, Desire, Desyre, Dezirae, Deziree, Desirat

•**Destiny** (English) Recognizing one's certain fortune; fate
Destanee, Destinee, Destiney, Destini, Destinie, Destine, Destina, Destyni

Deva (Hindi) A divine being
Devi, Daeva

Devera (Latin) In mythology, goddess of brooms
Deverah

Devon (English) From the beautiful farmland; of the divine
Devan, Deven, Devenne, Devin, Devona, Devondra, Devonna, Devonne

Dextra (Latin) Feminine form of Dexter; one who is skillful
Dex

Dharma (Hindi) The universal law of order
Darma

Dhisana (Hindi) In Hinduism, goddess of prosperity
Dhisanna, Disana, Disanna, Dhysana

Dhyana (Hindi) One who meditates

Diane (Latin) Form of Diana, meaning "of the divine"
Dayann, Dayanne, Deana, Deane, Deandra, Deann

Diana (Latin) Of the divine, in mythology, goddess of the moon and the hunt
Dianna, Dayanna

Diata (African) Resembling a lioness
Diatah, Dyata, Diatta, Dyatah, Dyatta, Diattah, Dyattah

Didina (French) One who is desired
Dideena, Dideina, Didiena, Dideana, Didyna

Dido (Latin) In mythology, the queen of Carthage who committed suicide
Dydo

Didrika (German) Feminine form of Dietrich; the ruler of the people
Diedericka, Diedricka, Diedrika, Dydrika, Didricka

Dielle (Latin) One who worships God
Diele, Diell, Diella, Diela, Diel

Dimity (English) Resembling a sheer cotton fabric
Dimitee, Dimitey, Dimitie, Dimitea, Dimiteah, Dimiti

Dimona (Hebrew) Woman from the south
Dimonah, Dymona, Demona, Demonah, Dymonah

Disa (English) Resembling an orchid

Discordia (Latin) In mythology, goddess of strife
Dyscordia, Diskordia, Dyskordia

Diti (Hindi) In Hinduism, an earth goddess
Dyti, Ditie, Dytie, Dity, Dyty, Ditey, Dytey, Ditee

Ditza (Hebrew) One who brings joy
Ditzah, Diza, Dizah, Dytza, Dytzah, Dyza, Dyzah

Dolores (Spanish) Woman of sorrow; refers to the Virgin Mary
Dalores, Delora, Delores, Deloria, Deloris, Dolorcita, Dolorcitas, Dolorita

Domela (Latin) The lady of the house
Domella, Domele, Domelle, Domell, Domhnulla, Domel

Domina (Latin) An elegant lady
Dominah, Domyna, Domynah

Dominique (French)
Feminine form of
Dominic; born on the
Lord's day
*Domaneke, Domanique,
Domenica, Domeniga,
Domenique, Dominee,
Domineek, Domineke*

Doreen (French / Gaelic)
The golden one / a brood-
ing woman
*Dorene, Doreyn, Dorine,
Dorreen, Doryne, Doreena,
Dore, Doirean*

Dorma (Latin) One who is
sleeping
Dorrma, Dorrmah, Dormah

Dorothy (Greek) A gift of
God
*Dasha, Dasya, Dodie,
Dody, Doe, Doll, Dolley,
Dolli*

Dove (American)
Resembling a bird of peace
Duv

Drisana (Indian) Daughter
of the sun
*Dhrisana, Drisanna, Drysana,
Drysanna, Dhrysana,
Dhrisanna, Dhrysanna*

Drury (French) One who is
greatly loved
*Drurey, Druri, Drurie,
Druree, Drurea, Drureah*

Duana (Irish) Feminine
form of Dwayne; little,
dark one
*Duane, Duayna, Duna,
Dwana, Dwayna, Dubhain,
Dubheasa*

Duena (Spanish) One who
acts as a chaperone

Dumia (Hebrew) One who
is silent
*Dumiya, Dumiah,
Dumiyah, Dumea, Dumeah*

Duvessa (Irish) A dark
beauty
*Duvessah, Duvesa,
Dubheasa, Duvesah*

Dylan (Welsh) Daughter of
the waves
*Dylana, Dylane, Dyllan,
Dyllana, Dillon, Dillan,
Dillen, Dillian*

Dympna (Irish) Fawn; the
patron saint of the insane
*Dymphna, Dimpna,
Dimphna*

Dyre (Scandinavian) One
who is dear to the heart

Dysis (Greek) Born at sun-
set
*Dysiss, Dysisse, Dysys,
Dysyss, Dysysse*

e

Eadlin (Anglo-Saxon) Born into royalty
Eadlinn, Eadlinne, Eadline, Eadlyn, Eadlynn, Eadlynne, Eadlina, Eadlyna

Eadrianne (American) One who stands out
Eadrian, Eadriann, Edriane, Edriana, Edrianna

Eara (Scottish) Woman from the east
Earah, Earra, Earrah, Earia, Earea, Earie, Eari, Earee

Earla (English) A great leader
Earlah

Earna (English) Resembling an eagle
Earnah, Earnia, Earnea, Earniah, Earneah

Easter (American) Born during the religious holiday
Eastere, Eastre, Eastir, Eastar, Eastor, Eastera, Easteria, Easterea

Easton (American) A wholesome woman
Eastan, Easten, Eastun, Eastyn

Eathelin (English) Noble woman of the waterfall
Eathelyn, Eathelinn, Eathelynn, Eathelina, Eathelyna, Ethelin, Ethelyn, Eathelen

Eathellreda (English) A noble young woman
Eathelreda, Eathellredia, Eathellredea, Eathelredia, Eathelredea, Ethelreda, Ethellreda

Eber (Hebrew) One who moves beyond

Ebere (African) One who shows mercy
Eberre, Ebera, Eberia, Eberea, Eberria, Eberrea, Ebiere, Ebierre

Ebony (Egyptian) A dark beauty
Eboni, Ebonee, Ebonie, Ebonique, Eboney, Ebonea, Eboneah

Ebrel (Cornish) Born during the month of April
Ebrell, Ebrele, Ebrelle, Ebriel, Ebriell, Ebriele, Ebrielle

Ebrill (Welsh) Born in April
Ebrille, Ebril, Evril, Evrill, Evrille

Edalene (Gaelic) A queenly woman; one who is noble
Edaleen, Edaleene, Edalena, Edaleena, Edalyne, Edalyna, Edaline, Edalina

Edana (Irish) Feminine form of Aidan; a fiery woman
Edanah, Edanna, Ena, Eideann, Eidana

Eden (Hebrew) Place of pleasure
Edan, Edin, Edon

Edna (Hebrew) One who brings pleasure; a delight
Ednah, Edena, Edenah

Edolia (Teutonic) A woman of good humor
Edoliah, Edolea, Edoleah, Edoli, Edolie, Edoly, Edoley, Edolee

Edra (English) A powerful and mighty woman
Edrah, Edrea, Edreah, Edria, Edriah

Eduarda (Portugese) Feminine form of Edward; a wealthy protector
Eduardia, Eduardea, Edwarda, Edwardia, Edwardea, Eduardina, Eduardyna, Edwardina

Edurne (Basque) Feminine form of Edur; woman of the snow
Edurna, Edurnia, Edurnea, Edurniya

Efterpi (Greek) A maiden with a pretty face
Efterpie, Efterpy, Efterpey, Efterpee, Efterpea, Efterpeah

Egan (American) A wholesome woman
Egann, Egen, Egun, Egon

Egberta (English) Feminine form of Egbert; wielding the shining sword
Egbertha, Egbertina, Egbertyna, Egberteena

Egeria (Latin) A wise counselor; in mythology, a water nymph
Egeriah, Egerea, Egereah, Egeriya, Egeriyah

Eglah (Hebrew) Resembling a heifer
Egla, Eglon, Eglona, Eglia, Egliah, Eglea, Egleah

Egzanth (American) A yellow-haired woman
Egzanthe, Egzantha, Egzanthia, Egzanthea, Egzanthiya, Egzanthya

Eileen (Gaelic) Form of Evelyn, meaning "a bird-like woman"
Eila, Eileene, Eilena, Eilene, Eilin, Eilleen, Eily, Eilean

Eiluned (Welsh) An idol worshipper
Luned

Eilwen (Welsh) One with a fair brow
Eilwenne, Eilwin, Eilwinne, Eilwyn, Eilwynne

Eirene (Greek) Form of Irene, meaning "a peaceful woman"
Eireen, Eireene, Eiren, Eir, Eireine, Eirein, Eirien, Eiriene

Eires (Greek) A peaceful woman
Eiress, Eiris, Eiriss, Eirys, Eiryss

Eirian (Welsh) One who is bright and beautiful
Eiriann, Eiriane, Eiriana, Eirianne, Eirianna

Ekron (Hebrew) One who is firmly rooted
Eckron, Ecron

Elaine (French) Form of Helen, meaning "the shining light"
Ellaine, Ellayne, Elaina, Elayna, Elayne, Elaene, Elaena, Ellaina

Elana (Hebrew) From the oak tree
Elanna, Elanah, Elanie, Elani, Elany, Elaney, Elanee, Elan

Elata (Latin) A high-spirited woman
Elatah, Elatta, Elattah, Elatia, Elatea, Elatiah, Elateah

Elath (Hebrew) From the grove of trees
Elathe, Elatha, Elathia, Elathea

Eldora (Greek) A gift of the sun
Eleadora, Eldorah, Eldorra, Eldoria, Eldorea

Eldoris (Greek) Woman of the sea
Eldorise, Eldoriss, Eldorisse, Eldorys, Eldoryss, Eldorysse

Eldreda (English) Feminine form of Eldred; one who provides wise counsel
Eldredah, Eldrida, Eldridah

Eleacie (American) One who is forthright
Eleaci, Eleacy, Eleacey, Eleacee, Eleacea

Eleanor (Greek) Form of Helen, meaning "the shining light"
Eleanora, Eleni, Eleonora, Eleonore, Elinor, Elnora, Eleanore, Elinora, Nora

Elena (Spanish) Form of Helen, meaning "the shining light"
Elenah, Eleena, Eleenah, Elyna, Elynah, Elina, Elinah, Eleni, Eliana

^**Eliana** (Hebrew) The Lord answers our prayers
Eleana, Elia, Eliane, Elianna, Elianne, Eliann, Elyana, Elyanna, Elyann, Elyan, Elyanne

Elica (German) One who is noble
Elicah, Elicka, Elika, Elyca, Elycka, Elyka, Elsha, Elsje

Elida (English) Resembling a winged creature
Elidah, Elyda, Eleeda, Eleda, Elieda, Eleida, Eleada

Elika (Hebrew) God will judge
Elikah, Elyka, Elicka, Elycka, Elica, Elyca

Eliphal (Hebrew) Delivered by God
Eliphala, Eliphall, Eliphalla, Eliphelet, Elipheleta

Elise (English) Form of Elizabeth, meaning "my God is bountiful"
Elisha, Elle, Elice, Elishia, Elissa, Elisa, Elisia, Elisse, Elysa, Elyse, Elysha, Elysia, Elyssa, Elysse, Ilyse

Elita (Latin) The chosen one
Elitah, Elyta, Elytah, Eleta, Eletah, Elitia, Elitea, Electa

•**Elizabeth** (Hebrew) My God is bountiful; God's promise
Liz, Elisabet, Elisabeth, Elisabetta, Elissa, Eliza, Elizabel, Elizabet, Elsa, Beth, Babette, Libby, Lisa, Tetty

•ᴛ**Ella** (German) From a foreign land
Elle, Ellee, Ellesse, Elli, Ellia, Ellie, Elly, Ela

Ellan (American) A coy woman
Ellane, Ellann

Ellen (English) Form of Helen, meaning "the shining light"
Elin, Elleen, Ellena, Ellene, Ellyn, Elynn, Elen, Ellin

Ellenweorc (Anglo-Saxon) A woman known for her courage

Ellery (English) Form of Hilary, meaning "a cheerful woman"
Ellerey, Elleri, Ellerie, Elleree, Ellerea, Ellereah

Ellie (English) Form of Eleanor, meaning "the shining light
Elli, Elly, Elley, Elleigh

Ellyanne (American) A shining and gracious woman
Ellianne, Ellyanna, Ellianna, Ellyann, Elliann, Ellyan, Ellian

Elma (German) Having God's protection
Elmah

Elpida (Greek) Feminine form of Elpidius; filled with hope
Elpidah, Elpyda, Elpeeda, Elpieda, Elpeida, Elpeada, Espe, Elpydah

Elrica (German) A great ruler
Elricah, Elrika, Elrikah, Elryca, Elrycah, Elryka, Elrykah, Elrick

Eltekeh (Hebrew) A God-fearing woman
Elteke, Elteckeh, Eltecke

Elton (American) A spontaneous woman
Elten, Eltan, Eltin, Eltyn, Eltun

Elvia (Irish) A friend of the elves
Elva, Elvie, Elvina, Elvinia, Elviah, Elvea, Elveah, Elvyna

Elvira (Latin) A truthful woman; one who can be trusted
Elvera, Elvita, Elvyra

Ema (Polynesian / German) One who is greatly loved / a serious woman

Emerson (German) offspring of Emery
Emmerson, Emyrson

^Emery (German) Industrious
Emeri, Emerie, Emori, Emorie, Emory

*ᵀEmily (Latin) An industrious and hardworking woman
Emilee, Emilie, Emilia, Emelia, Emileigh, Emeleigh, Emeli, Emelie, Emely

*ᵀEmma (German) One who is complete; a universal woman
Emmy, Emmajean, Emmalee, Emmi, Emmie, Emmaline, Emelina, Emeline

Emmylou (American) A universal ruler
Emmilou, Emmielou, Emylou, Emilou, Emielou

Ena (Irish) A fiery and passionate woman
Enah, Enat, Eny, Enya

Encarnacion (Spanish) Refers to the Incarnation festival

Engelbertha (German) A luminous angel
Engelberta, Engelberthe, Engelberte, Engelbertine, Engelbertina, Engelberteena, Engelberteen, Engelbertyna

Engracia (Spanish) A graceful woman
Engraciah, Engracea, Engraceah

Enslie (American) An emotional woman
Ensli, Ensley, Ensly, Enslee, Enslea, Ensleigh

Ephah (Hebrew) Woman of sorrow
Epha, Ephia, Ephea, Ephiah, Epheah

Ephesus (Hebrew) From the desired place

Eranthe (Greek) As delicate as a spring flower
Erantha, Eranth, Eranthia, Eranthea

Erasta (African) A peaceful woman

Ercilia (American) One who is frank
Erciliah, Ercilea, Ercileah, Ercilya, Ercilyah, Erciliya, Erciliyah

Erendira (Spanish) Daughter born into royalty
Erendirah, Erendiria, Erendirea, Erendyra, Erendyria, Erendyrea, Erendeera, Erendiera

Erica (Scandinavian / Latin) Feminine form of Eric; ever the ruler / resembling heather
Erika, Ericka, Erikka, Eryka, Erike, Ericca, Erics, Eiric, Rica

Erimentha (Greek) A devoted protector
Erimenthe, Erimenthia, Erimenthea

·Erin (Gaelic) Woman from Ireland
Erienne, Erina, Frinn, Erinna, Erinne, Eryn, Eryna, Erynn, Arin

Eriphyle (Greek) In mythology, the mother of Alcmaeon
Eriphile, Erifyle, Erifile

Ernestina (German) Feminine form of Ernest; one who is determined; serious
Ernesta, Ernestine, Ernesha, Erna, Ernestyne, Ernestyna, Ernesztina, Earnestyna

Esdey (American) A warm and caring woman
Essdey, Fsdee, Esdea, Esdy, Esdey, Esdi, Esdie, Esday

Eshah (African) An exuberant woman
Esha

Eshe (African) Giver of life
Eshey, Eshay, Esh, Eshae, Eshai

Esinam (African) God has heard
Esiname, Esynam, Esinama, Esynama, Esinamia, Esinamea

Esme (French) An esteemed woman
Esmai, Esmae, Esmay, Esmaye, Esmee

Esne (English) Filled with happiness
Esnee, Esney, Esnea, Esni, Esnie, Esny

Essence (American) A perfumed woman
Essince, Esense, Esince, Essynce, Esynce

Esthelia (Spanish) A shining woman
Estheliah, Esthelea, Estheleah, Esthelya, Esthelyah, Estheliya, Estheliyah

Esther (Persian) Resembling the myrtle leaf
Ester, Eszter, Eistir, Eszti

Estrid (Norse) Form of Astrid, meaning "one with divine strength"
Estread, Estreed, Estrad, Estri, Estrod, Estrud, Estryd, Estrida

Etana (Hebrew) A strong and dedicated woman
Etanah, Etanna, Etannah, Etania, Etanea, Ethana, Ethanah, Ethania

Etaney (Hebrew) One who is focused
Etany, Etanie, Etani, Etanee, Etanea

Etenia (Native American) One who is wealthy; prosperous
Eteniah, Etenea, Eteneah, Eteniya, Eteniyah

Eternity (American) Lasting forever
Eternitie, Eterniti, Eternitey, Eternitee, Eternyty, Eternyti, Eternytie, Eternytee

Ethna (Irish) A graceful woman
Ethnah, Eithne, Ethne, Eithna, Eithnah

Eudlina (Slavic) A generous woman
Eudlinah, Eudleena, Eudleenah, Eudleana, Eudleanah, Eudlyna, Eudlynah

Eudocia (Greek) One who is esteemed
Eudociah, Eudocea, Eudoceah, Eudokia, Eudokea, Eudosia, Eudosea, Eudoxia

Eugenia (Greek) A well-born woman
Eugenie, Gina, Zenechka

Eulanda (American) A fair woman
Eulande, Euland, Eulandia, Eulandea

Eunice (Greek) One who conquers
Eunise, Eunyce, Eunis, Euniss, Eunyss, Eunysse

Eurayle (Greek) In mythology, a Gorgon
Euryle, Euraile, Eurale, Eurael, Euraele

Eurybia (Greek) In mythology, a sea goddess and mother of Pallas, Perses, and Astraios
Eurybiah, Eurybea, Eurybeah, Euryba, Eurybah

Eurynome (Greek) In mythology, the mother of the Graces
Eurynomie, Eurynomi, Eurynomey, Eurynomee, Eurynomy, Eurynomea, Eurynomeah

Euvenia (American) A hardworking woman
Eveniah, Evenea, Eveneah, Eveniya, Eveniyah

Eva (Hebrew) Giver of life; a lively woman
Eve, Evetta, Evette, Evia, Eviana, Evie, Evita, Eeva

Evangeline (Greek) A bringer of good news
Evangelina, Evangelyn

•**Evelyn** (German) A birdlike woman
Evaleen, Evalina, Evaline, Evalyn, Evelin, Evelina, Eveline, Evelyne, Eileen

Everilde (American) A great huntress
Everild, Everilda, Everhilde, Everhild, Everhilda

Evline (French) One who loves nature
Evleen, Evleene, Evlean, Evleane, Evlene, Evlyn, Evlyne

f

Fadhiler (Arabic) A virtuous woman
Fadhyler, Fadheler, Fadheeler, Fadilah, Fadila, Fadillah, Fadyla, Fadylla

Faghira (Arabic) Resembling the jasmine flower
Faghirah, Fagira, Fagirah, Faghyra, Fagheera, Faaghira, Fagheara, Fagheira

Faida (Arabic) One who is bountiful
Faide, Fayda, Fayde, Faeda, Faede

Faillace (French) A delicate and beautiful woman
Faillase, Faillaise, Falace, Falase, Fallase, Fallace

Fairly (English) From the far meadow
Fairley, Fairlee, Fairleigh, Fairli, Fairlie, Faerly, Faerli, Faerlie

•**Faith** (English) Having a belief and trust in God
Faythe, Faithe, Faithful, Fayana, Fayanna, Fayanne, Fayane, Fayth

Fakhira (Arabic) A magnificent woman
Fakhirah, Fakhyra, Fakhyrah, Fakheera, Fakira, Fakirah, Fakeera, Fakyra

Fala (Native American) Resembling a crow
Falah, Falla, Fallah

Falesyia (Spanish) An exotic woman
Falesyiah, Falesiya, Falesiyah

Fallon (Irish) A commanding woman
Fallyn, Faline, Falinne, Faleen, Faleene, Falynne, Falyn, Falina

Falsette (American) A fanciful woman
Falsett, Falset, Falsete, Falsetta, Falseta

Fang (Chinese) Pleasantly fragrant

Fantasia (Latin) From the fantasy land
Fantasiah, Fantasea, Fantasiya, Fantazia, Fantazea, Fantaziya

Faqueza (Spanish) A weakness

Farley (English) From the fern clearing
Farly, Farli, Farlie, Farlee, Farleigh, Farlea, Farleah

Farrow (American) A narrow-minded woman
Farow, Farro, Faro

Fate (Greek) One's destiny
Fayte, Faite, Faete, Faet, Fait, Fayt

Fatima (Arabic) The perfect woman
Fatimah, Fahima, Fahimah

Fatinah (Arabic) A captivating woman
Fatina, Fateena, Fateenah, Fatyna, Fatynah, Fatin, Fatine, Faatinah

Fausta (Italian) A lucky lady; one who is fortunate
Fawsta, Faustina, Faustine, Faustyna, Faustyne, Fausteena, Fausteene, Fawstina

Fauve (French) An uninhibited and untamed woman

Favor (English) One who grants her approval
Faver, Favar, Favorre

Fay (English) From the fairy kingdom; a fairy or an elf
Faye, Fai, Faie, Fae, Fayette, Faylinn, Faylyn, Faylynn

Fayina (Russian) An independent woman
Fayinah, Fayena, Fayeena, Fayeana, Fayiena, Fayeina

February (American) Born in the month of February
Februari, Februarie, Februarey, Februaree, Februarea

Feechi (African) A woman who worships God
Feechie, Feechy, Feechey, Feechee, Fychi, Fychie, Fychey, Fychy

Felicity (Latin) Form of Felicia, meaning "happy"
Felicy, Felicie, Felisa

Femi (African) God loves me
Femmi, Femie, Femy, Femey, Femee, Femea, Femeah

Femise (American) One who desires love
Femeese, Femease, Femice, Femeece, Femeace, Femmis, Femmys

Fenia (Scandinavian) A gold worker
Feniah, Fenea, Feneah, Feniya, Feniyah, Fenya, Fenyah, Fenja

Fern (English) Resembling a green shade-loving plant
Ferne, Fyrn, Fyrne, Furn, Furne

Fernilia (American) A successful woman
Ferniliah, Fernilea, Fernileah, Fernilya, Fernilyah

Feryal (Arabic) Possessing the beauty of light
Feryall, Feryale, Feryalle

Fia (Portuguese / Italian / Scottish) A weaver / from the flickering fire / arising from the dark of peace
Fiah, Fea, Feah, Fya, Fiya, Fyah, Fiyah

Fianna (Irish) A warrior huntress
Fiannah, Fiana, Fianne, Fiane, Fiann, Fian

Fielda (English) From the field
Fieldah, Felda, Feldah

Fife (American) Having dancing eyes
Fyfe, Fifer, Fify, Fifey, Fifee, Fifea, Fifi, Fifie

Fifia (African) Born on a Friday
Fifiah, Fifea, Fifeah, Fifeea, Fifeeah

Filberta (English) Feminine form of Filibert; a very brilliant woman
Filiberta, Filbertha, Filibertha, Felabeorht, Felberta, Feliberta, Felbertha, Felibertha

Filipa (Spanish) Feminine form of Phillip; a friend of horses
Filipah, Filipina, Filipeena, Filipyna, Filippa, Fillipa, Fillippa

Filomena (Italian) Form of Philomena, meaning "a friend of strength"
Filomina, Filomeena, Filomyna, Filomenia

Fina (English) Feminine form of Joseph; God will add
Finah, Feena, Fyna, Fifine, Fifna, Fifne, Fini, Feana

Findabair (Celtic) Having fair eyebrows; in mythology, the daughter of Medb
Findabaire, Finnabair, Finnabaire, Findabhair, Findabhaire, Findabayr, Findabayre, Findabare

Finnea (Gaelic) From the stream of the wood
Finneah, Finnia, Fynnea, Finniah, Fynnia

Fiona (Gaelic) One who is fair; a white-shouldered woman
Fionna, Fione, Fionn, Finna, Fionavar, Fionnghuala, Fionnuala, Fynballa

Firdaus (Arabic) From the garden in paradise
Firdaws, Firdoos

Flair (English) An elegant woman of natural talent
Flaire, Flare, Flayr, Flayre, Flaer, Flaere

Flame (American) A passionate and fiery woman
Flaym, Flayme, Flaime, Flaim, Flaem, Flaeme

Flamina (Latin) A pious woman
Flaminah, Flamyna, Flamynah, Flamiena, Flamienah, Flameina, Flameinah, Flameena

Flannery (Gaelic) From the flatlands
Flanery, Flanneri, Flannerie, Flannerey, Flannaree, Flannerea

Fleming (English) Woman from Belgium
Flemyng, Flemming, Flemmyng

Fleta (English) One who is swift
Fletah, Flete, Fleda, Flita, Flyta

Flicky (American) A vivacious young woman
Flicki, Flickie, Flickea, Flickeah, Flickee, Flycki, Flyckie, Flyckee

Flirt (American) A playfully romantic woman
Flyrt, Flirti, Flirtie, Flirty, Flirtey, Flirtea, Flirteah, Flirtee

Florence (Latin) A flourishing woman; a blooming flower
Florencia, Florentina, Florenza, Florentine, Florentyna, Florenteena, Florenteene, Florentyne

Florizel (English) A young woman in bloom
Florizell, Florizelle, Florizele, Florizel, Florizella, Florizela, Florazel, Florazell

Fluffy (American) A fun-loving young woman
Fluffey, Fluffi, Fluffea, Fluffeah, Fluffee, Fluffie

Fola (African) Woman of honor
Folah, Folla, Follah

Fontenot (French) One who is special

Forest (English) A woodland dweller
Forrest

Forever (American) Everlasting

Francesca (Italian) Form of Frances, meaning one who is free
Francia, Francina, Francisca, Franchesca, Francie

Frederica (German) Peaceful ruler
Freda, Freida, Freddie, Rica

Freira (Spanish) A sister
Freirah, Freyira, Freyirah

Freydis (Norse) Woman born into the nobility
Freydiss, Freydisse, Freydys, Fredyss, Fraidis, Fradis, Fraydis, Fraedis

Frodina (Teutonic) A wise and beloved friend
Frodinah, Frodyna, Frodeena, Frodine, Frodyne, Frodeen, Frodeene, Frodeana

Fuchsia (Latin) Resembling the flower
Fusha, Fushia, Fushea, Fewsha, Fewshia, Fewshea

Fury (Greek) An enraged woman; in mythology, a winged goddess who punished wrongdoers
Furey, Furi, Furie, Furee

g

Gabbatha (Hebrew) From the temple mound
Gabbathah, Gabbathe, Gabatha, Gabbathia, Gabbathea, Gabathia, Gabathea

*ᵀ**Gabriella** (Italian /
Spanish) Feminine form
of Gabriel; heroine of God
*Gabriela, Gabriellia,
Gabrila, Gabryela,
Gabryella*

*ᵀ**Gabrielle** (Hebrew)
Feminine form of Gabriel;
heroine of God
*Gabriel, Gabriela, Gabriele,
Gabriell, **Gabriella**,
Gabriellen, Gabriellia,
Gabrila*

Gaira (Scottish) A petite
woman
*Gayra, Gara, Gairia,
Gairea, Gaera*

Galena (Greek) Feminine
form of Galen; one who is
calm and peaceful
*Galene, Galenah, Galenia,
Galenea*

Galiana (Arabic) The name
of a Moorish princess
*Galianah, Galianna,
Galianne, Galiane, Galian,
Galyana, Galyanna,
Galyann*

Galila (Hebrew) From the
rolling hills
*Galilah, Gelila, Gelilah,
Gelilia, Gelilya, Glila,
Glilah, Galyla*

Galilee (Hebrew) From the
sacred sea
*Galileigh, Galilea, Galiley,
Galily, Galili, Galilie*

Galina (Russian) Form
of Helen, meaning "the
shining light"
*Galinah, Galyna, Galynah,
Galeena, Galeenah, Galine,
Galyne, Galeene*

Gamma (Greek) The third
letter of the Greek alphabet
Gammah

Garbi (Basque) One who is
pure; clean
*Garbie, Garby, Garbey,
Garbee, Garbea, Garbeah*

Gardenia (English)
Resembling the sweet-
smelling flower
*Gardeniah, Gardenea,
Gardeneah, Gardeniya,
Gardynia, Gardynea,
Gardena, Gardyna*

Garima (Indian) A woman
of importance
*Garimah, Garyma,
Gareema, Garymah,
Gareemah, Gareama,
Gareamah, Gariema*

Garnet (English)
Resembling the dark-red
gem
*Garnette, Granata,
Grenata, Grenatta*

Gasha (Russian) One who
is well-behaved
*Gashah, Gashia, Gashea,
Gashiah, Gasheah*

Gath-rimmon (Hebrew)
Refers to the pomegranate
press

Gavina (Latin) Feminine
form of Gavin; resembling
the white falcom; woman
from Gabio
*Gavinah, Gaveena,
Gaveenah, Gavyna,
Gavynah, Gavenia,
Gavenea, Gaveana*

Gaza (Hebrew) Having
great strength
Gazah, Gazza, Gazzah

Gazit (Hebrew) Of the cut
stone
Giza, Gizah, Gisa, Gisah

Geila (Hebrew) One who
brings joy to others
*Geela, Geelah, Geelan,
Geilah, Geiliya, Geiliyah,
Gelisa, Gellah*

Gemma (Latin) As pre-
cious as a jewel
*Gemmalyn, Gemmalynn,
Gem, Gema, Gemmaline,
Jemma*

Genesis (Hebrew) Of the
beginning; the first book
of the Bible
*Genesies, Genesiss, Genessa,
Genisis*

Genevieve (French) White
wave; fair-skinned
*Genavieve, Geneve, Genevie,
Genivee, Genivieve,
Genoveva, Gennie, Genny*

Genista (Latin) Resembling
the broom plant
*Genistah, Geneesta,
Ginista, Genysta, Ginysta,
Gynysta, Geneasta,
Geneista*

Georgia (Greek) Feminine
form of George; one who
works the earth; a farmer;
from the state of Georgia
*Georgeann, Georgeanne,
Georgina, Georgena,
Georgene, Georgetta,
Georgette, Georgiana, Jeorjia*

Gerardine (English)
Feminine form of Gerard;
one who is mighty with a
spear
*Gerarda, Gerardina,
Gerardyne, Gererdina,
Gerardyna, Gerrardene,
Gerhardina, Gerhardine*

Gerizim (Hebrew) From
the mountains
*Gerizima, Gerizime,
Gerizimia, Gerizimea,
Gerizym, Gerizyme,
Gerizyma, Gerizymea*

Gertrude (German) Adored
warrior
*Geertruide, Geltruda,
Geltrudis, Gert, Gerta, Gerte,
Gertie, Gertina, Trudy*

Gethsemane (Hebrew)
Worker of the oil press
*Gethsemanie, Gethsemana,
Gethsemani, Gethsemaney,
Gethsemany, Gethsemanee,
Gethsemanea*

Gezana (Spanish) Refers to the doctrine of incarnation
Gezanah, Gezanna, Gezania, Gezanea, Gezane, Gizana, Gizane, Gizania

Gianna (Italian) Feminine form of John, meaning "God is gracious"
Gia, Giana, Giovana

Gibeah (Hebrew) From the hill town
Gibea, Gibia, Gibiah, Gibeon, Gibeona, Gibeonea, Gibeonia, Gibeoneah

Gillian (Latin) One who is youthful
Gilian, Giliana, Gillianne, Ghilian

Gimbya (African) Daughter born to royalty; a princess
Gimbyah, Gimbiya, Gimbeya, Gimbaya, Gimbiyah, Gimbayah, Gimbeyah

Gina (Japanese / English) A silvery woman / form of Eugenia, meaning "a well-born woman"; form of Jean, meaning "God is gracious"
Geana, Geanndra, Geena, Geina, Gena, Genalyn, Geneene, Genelle

Ginger (English) A lively woman; resembling the spice
Gingee, Gingie, Ginjer, Gingea, Gingy, Gingey, Gingi

Ginny (English) Form of Virginia, meaning "one who is chaste; virginal"
Ginnee, Ginnelle, Ginnette, Ginnie, Ginnilee, Ginna, Ginney, Ginni

Giona (Italian) Resembling the bird of peace
Gionah, Gionna, Gyona, Gyonna, Gionnah, Gyonah, Gyonnah

Giovanna (Italian) Feminine form of Giovanni; God is gracious
Geovana, Geovanna, Giavanna, Giovana, Giovani, Giovanni, Giovanie, Giovanee

Giselle (French) One who offers her pledge
Gisel, Gisela, Gisella, Jiselle

Gita (Hindi / Hebrew) A beautiful song / a good woman
Gitah, Geeta, Geetah, Gitika, Gatha, Gayatri, Gitel, Gittel

Gitana (Spanish) A gypsy woman
Gitanah, Gitanna, Gitannah, Gitane

Githa (Anglo-Saxon) A gift
from God
Githah

Giulia (Italian) form of Julia,
meaning one who is youth-
ful, daughter of the sky"
Giuliana, Giulie

Gladys (Welsh) Form of
Claudia, meaning "one
who is lame"
*Gladdis, Gladdys, Gladi,
Gladis, Gladyss, Gwladys,
Gwyladyss, Gleda*

Glenna (Gaelic) From the
valley between the hills
*Gleana, Gleneen, Glenene,
Glenine, Glen, Glenn,
Glenne, Glennene*

Glenys (Welsh) A holy
woman
*Glenice, Glenis, Glennice,
Glennis, Glennys, Glynis*

Godfreya (German)
Feminine form of
Godfrey; having the peace
of God
*Godfredya, Gotfreya,
Godafrid, Godafryd*

Godiva (English) Gift from
God
*Godivah, Godgifu, Godyva,
Godyvah*

Golda (English) Resembling
the precious metal
*Goldarina, Goldarine,
Goldee, Goldi, Goldie,
Goldina, Goldy, Goldia*

Gordana (Serbian /
Scottish) A proud woman /
one who is heroic
*Gordanah, Gordanna,
Gordania, Gordaniya,
Gordanea, Gordannah,
Gordaniah, Gordaniyah*

Gormghlaith (Irish)
Woman of sorrow
*Gormghlaithe, Gormley,
Gormly, Gormlie, Gormli,
Gormlee, Gormleigh*

*ᵀ**Grace** (Latin) Having
God's favor; in mythol-
ogy, the Graces were the
personification of beauty,
charm, and grace
*Gracee, Gracella,
Gracelynn, Gracelynne,
Gracey, Gracia, Graciana,
Gracie, Gracelyn*

*ᵀ**Gracie** (Latin) Form of
Grace, meaning "having
God's favor"
Gracee, Gracey, Graci

Granada (Spanish) From
the Moorish kingdom
*Granadda, Grenada,
Grenadda*

Greer (Scottish) Feminine
form of Gregory; one who
is alert and watchful
Grear, Grier, Gryer

Gregoria (Latin) Feminine form of Gregory; one who is alert and watchful
Gregoriana, Gregorijana, Gregorina, Gregorine, Gregorya, Gregoryna, Gregorea, Gregoriya

Greip (Norse) In mythology, a frost giantess

Greta (German) Resembling a pearl
Greeta, Gretal, Grete, Gretel, Gretha, Grethe, Grethel, Gretna, Gretchen

Grimhild (Norse) In mythology, a witch
Grimhilde, Grimhilda, Grimild, Grimilda, Grimilde

Griselda (German)A gray-haired battle maid; one who fights the dark battle
Grezelda, Grizelda, Criselda

Griswalda (German) Woman from the gray woodland
Griswalde, Grizwalda, Grizwalde, Griswald, Grizwald

Guadalupe (Spanish) From the valley of wolves
Guadelupe, Lupe, Lupita

Gudny (Swedish) One who is unspoiled
Gudney, Gudni, Gudnie, Gudne, Gudnee, Gudnea, Gudneah

Gudrun (Scandinavian) A battle maiden
Gudren, Gudrid, Gudrin, Gudrinn, Gudruna, Gudrunn, Gudrunne, Guthrun

Guinevere (Welsh) One who is fair; of the white wave; in mythology, King Arthur's queen
Guenever, Guenevere, Gueniver, Guenna, Guennola, Guinever, Guinna, Gwen

Guiseppina (Italian) Feminine form of Guiseppe; the Lord will add
Giuseppyna, Giuseppa, Giuseppia, Giuseppea, Guiseppie, Guiseppia, Guiseppa, Giuseppina

Gula (Babylonian) In mythology, a goddess
Gulah, Gulla, Gullah

Gulielma (German) Feminine form of Wilhelm; determined protector
Guglielma, Guillelmina, Guillielma, Gulielmina, Guillermina

Gulinar (Arabic) Resembling the pomegranate
Gulinare, Gulinear, Gulineir, Gulinara, Gulinaria, Gulinarea

Gullveig (Norse) In
mythology, a dark goddess
*Gullveiga, Gullveige,
Gulveig, Gulveiga, Gulveige*

Gwawr (Welsh) Born with
the morning light

Gwendolyn (Welsh) One
who is fair; of the white
ring
*Guendolen, Guendolin,
Guendolinn, Guendolynn,
Guenna, Gwen, Gwenda,
Gwendaline, Wendy*

Gwyneth (Welsh) One
who is blessed with hap-
piness
*Gweneth, Gwenith,
Gwenyth, Gwineth,
Gwinneth, Gwinyth,
Gwynith, Gwynna*

Gytha (English) One who
is treasured
Gythah

h

Habbai (Arabic) One who
is much loved
Habbae, Habbay, Habbaye

Habiba (Arabic) Feminine
form of Habib; one who is
dearly loved; sweetheart
*Habibah, Habeeba,
Habyba, Habieba,
Habeiba, Habika, Habyka,
Habicka*

Hachi (Native American /
Japanese) From the river /
having good fortune
*Hachie, Hachee, Hachiko,
Hachiyo, Hachy, Hachey,
Hachikka*

Hadara (Hebrew) A spec-
tacular ornament; adorned
with beauty
*Hadarah, Hadarit,
Haduraq, Hadarra,
Hadarrah*

Hadeel (Arabic)
Resembling a dove
*Hadil, Hadyl, Hadeil,
Hadiel, Hadeal*

Hadiya (Arabic) A gift from
God; a righteous woman
*Hadiyah, Hadiyyah,
Haadiyah, Haadiya,
Hadeeya, Hadeeyah,
Hadieya, Hadieyah*

Hadlai (Hebrew) In a rest-
ing state; one who hinders
Hadlae, Hadlay, Hadlaye

^**Hadley** (English) From
the field of heather
*Hadlea, Hadleigh, Hadly,
Hedlea, Hedleigh, Hedley,
Hedlie, Hadlee*

Hadria (Latin) From the town in northern Italy
Hadrea, Hadriana, Hadriane, Hadrianna, Hadrien, Hadrienne, Hadriah, Hadreah

Hafthah (Arabic) One who is protected by God
Haftha

Hagab (Hebrew) Resembling a grasshopper
Hagabah, Hagaba, Hagabe

Hagai (Hebrew) One who has been abandoned
Hagae, Hagay, Hagaye, Haggai, Haggae, Hagie, Haggie, Hagi

Hagen (Irish) A youthful woman
Hagan, Haggen, Haggan

Haggith (Hebrew) One who rejoices; the dancer
Haggithe, Haggyth, Haggythe, Hagith, Hagithe, Hagyth, Hagythe

Haidee (Greek) A modest woman; one who is well-behaved
Hadee, Haydee, Haydy, Haidi, Haidie, Haydi, Haydie, Haidy

•Hailey (English) from the field of hay
Haley, Hayle, Hailee, Haylee, Haylie, Haleigh, Hayley, Haeleigh

Haimati (Indian) A queen of the snow-covered mountains
Haimatie, Haimaty, Haimatey, Haimatee, Haymati, Haymatie, Haymatee, Haimatea

Haimi (Hawaiian) One who searches for the truth
Haimie, Haimy, Haimey, Haimee, Haymi, Haymie, Haymee, Haimea

Hakana (Turkish) Feminine form of Hakan; ruler of the people; an empress
Hakanah, Hakanna, Hakane, Hakann, Hakanne

Hakkoz (Hebrew) One who has the qualities of a thorn
Hakoz, Hakkoze, Hakoze, Hakkoza, Hakoza

Halak (Hebrew) One who is bald; smooth

Haleigha (Hawaiian) Born with the rising sun
Haleea, Haleya, Halya

Hall (American) One who is distinguished
Haul

Hallie (Scandinavian, Greek, English) From the hall; woman of the sea; from the field of hay
Halley, Hallie, Halle, Hallee, Hally, Halleigh, Hallea, Halleah

Halo (Latin) Having a blessed aura
Haylo, Haelo, Hailo

Halsey (American) A playful woman
Halsy, Halsee, Halsea, Halsi, Halsie, Halcie, Halcy, Halcey

Halyn (American) A unique young woman
Halynn, Halynne, Halin, Halinn, Halinne

Hamida (Arabic) One who gives thanks
Hamidah, Hamyda, Hameeda, Hameida, Hamieda, Hameada, Hamydah, Hameedah

Hammon (Hebrew) Of the warm springs

Hamula (Hebrew) Feminine form of Hamul; spared by God
Hamulah, Hamulla, Hamullah

Hana (Japanese / Arabic) Resembling a flower blossom / a blissful woman
Hanah, Hanako

Hanan (Arabic) One who shows mercy and compassion

Hang (Vietnamese) Of the moon

Hanika (Hebrew) A graceful woman
Hanikah, Haneeka, Haneekah, Hanyka, Hanykah, Haneika, Haneikah, Hanieka

Hanita (Indian) Favored with divine grace
Hanitah, Hanyta, Haneeta, Hanytah, Haneetah, Haneita, Haneitah, Hanieta

Haniyah (Arabic) One who is pleased; happy
Haniya, Haniyyah, Haniyya, Hani, Hanie, Hanee, Hany, Haney

*T**Hannah** (Hebrew) Having favor and grace; in the Bible, mother of Samuel
Hanalee, Hanalise, Hanna, Hanne, Hannele, Hannelore, Hannie, Hanny, Chana

Hanya (Aboriginal) As solid as a stone

Happy (American) A joyful woman
Happey, Happi, Happie, Happee, Happea

Hara (Hebrew) From the mountainous land
Harah, Harra, Harrah

Haradah (Hebrew) One who is filled with fear
Harada

Harika (Turkish) A superior woman
Harikah, Haryka, Hareeka, Harykah, Hareekah, Hareaka, Hareakah

Harimanti (Indian) Born during the spring
Harimantie, Harymanti, Harimanty, Harymanty, Harymantie, Harimantea, Harymantea

Hariti (Indian) In mythology, the goddess for the protection of children
Haritie, Haryti, Harytie, Haritee, Harytee, Haritea, Harytea

Harla (English) From the fields
Harlah

^**Harley** (English) From the meadow of the hares
Harlea, Harlee, Harleen, Harleigh, Harlene, Harlie, Harli, Harly

Harlow (American) An impetuous woman

^**Harper** (English) One who plays or makes harps

Harriet (German) Feminine form of Henry; ruler of the house
Harriett, Hanriette, Hanrietta, Harriette, Harrietta, Harrette

Harva (English) A warrior of the army

Hasibah (Arabic) Feminine form of Hasib; one who is noble and respected
Hasiba, Hasyba, Hasybah, Haseeba, Haseebah

Hasina (African) One who is good and beautiful
Hasinah, Hasyna, Hasynah, Haseena, Haseenah, Hasiena, Hasienah, Haseina

Hatsu (Japanese) The firstborn daughter

Haukea (Hawaiian) Of the white snow
Haukia, Haukeah, Haukiah, Haukiya, Haukiyah

Haurana (Hebrew) Feminine form of Hauran; woman from the caves
Hauranna, Hauranah, Haurann, Hauranne

Havva (Turkish) A giver of the breath of life
Havvah, Havvia, Havviah

^**Hayden** (English) From the hedged valley
Haden, Haydan, Haydn, Haydon, Haeden, Haedyn, Hadyn

Hayud (Arabic) From the mountain
Hayuda, Hayudah, Hayood, Hayooda

Heartha (Teutonic) A gift from Mother Earth

Heather (English) Resembling the evergreen flowering plant
Hether, Heatha, Heath, Heathe

Heaven (American) From paradise; from the sky
Heavely, Heavenly, Hevean, Hevan, Heavynne, Heavenli, Heavenlie, Heavenleigh, Heavenlee, heavenley, Heavenlea, Heavyn

Hecate (Greek) In mythology, a goddess of fertility and witchcraft
Hekate

Heirnine (Greek) Form of Helen, meaning "the shining light"
Heirnyne, Heirneine, Heirniene, Heirneene, Heirneane

Helen (Greek) The shining light; in mythology, Helen was the most beautiful woman in the world
Helene, Halina, Helaine, Helana, Heleena, Helena, Helenna, Hellen, Aleen, Elaine, Eleanor, Elena, Ellen, Galina, Heirnine, Helice, Leanna, Yalena

Helga (German) A holy woman; one who is successful

Helia (Greek) Daughter of the sun
Heliah, Helea, Heleah, Heliya, Heliyah, Heller, Hellar

Helice (Greek) Form of Helen, meaning "the shining light"
Helyce, Heleece, Heliece, Heleace

Helike (Greek) In mythology, a willow nymph who nurtured Zeus
Helica, Helyke, Helika, Helyka, Helyca

Helle (Greek) In mythology, the daughter of Athamas who escaped sacrifice on the back of a golden ram

Helma (German) Form of Wilhelmina, meaning "determined protector"
Helmah, Helmia, Helmea, Helmina, Helmyna, Helmeena, Helmine, Helmyne

Heloise (French) One who is famous in battle
Helois, Heloisa, Helewidis

Hemanti (Indian) Born during the early winter
Hemantie, Hemanty, Hemantey, Hemantee, Hemantea

Hen (English) Resembling the mothering bird

Henrietta (German)
Feminine form of Henry;
ruler of the house
*Henretta, Henrieta, Henriette,
Henrika, Henryetta, Hetta,
Hette, Hettie*

Hephzibah (Hebrew) She
is my delight
*Hepsiba, Hepzibeth,
Hepsey, Hepsie, Hepsy,
Hepzibah, Hepsee, Hepsea*

Herdis (Scandinavian) A
battle maiden
*Herdiss, Herdisse, Herdys,
Herdyss, Herdysse*

Hermelinda (Spanish)
Bearing a powerful shield
*Hermelynda, Hermalinda,
Hermalynda, Hermelenda,
Hermalenda*

Hermia (Greek) Feminine
form of Hermes; a mes-
senger of the gods
*Hermiah, Hermea, Hermila,
Hermilla, Hermilda,
Herminia, Hermenia, Herma*

Hermona (Hebrew) From
the mountain peak
*Hermonah, Hermonna,
Hermonnah*

Hernanda (Spanish) One
who is daring
*Hernandia, Hernandea,
Hernandiya*

Herra (Greek) Daughter of
the earth
Herrah

Hersala (Spanish) A lovely
woman
*Hersalah, Hersalla,
Hersallah, Hersalia,
Hersaliah, Hersalea,
Hersaleah*

Hesiena (African) The
firstborn of twins
*Hesienna, Hesienah,
Heseina, Hasana, Hasanah,
Hasanna, Hasane*

Hesione (Greek) In
mythology, a Trojan prin-
cess saved by Hercules
from a sea monster

Hester (Greek) A starlike
woman
*Hestere, Hesther, Hesta,
Hestar*

Heven (American) A pret-
ty young woman
*Hevin, Hevon, Hevun,
Hevven, Hevvin, Hevvon,
Hevvun*

Hezer (Hebrew) A woman
of great strength
*Hezir, Hezyr, Hezire,
Hezyre, Hezere*

Hiah (Korean) A bright
woman
Heija, Heijah, Hia

Hiawatha (Native
American) She who
makes rivers
*Hiawathah, Hyawatha,
Hiwatha, Hywatha*

Hibiscus (Latin)
Resembling the showy
flower
*Hibiskus, Hibyscus,
Hibyskus, Hybiscus,
Hybiskus, Hybyscus,
Hybyskus*

Hicks (American) A saucy
woman
*Hiks, Hycks, Hyks, Hicksi,
Hicksie, Hicksee, Hicksy,
Hicksey*

Hide (Japanese) A superior
woman
Hideyo

Hikmah (Arabic) Having
great wisdom
Hikmat, Hikma

Hilan (Greek) Filled with
happines
*Hylan, Hilane, Hilann,
Hilanne, Hylane, Hylann,
Hylanne*

Hilary (Latin) A cheerful
woman
Hillary, Hillery, Ellery

Hina (Polynesian) In
mythology, a dual goddess
symbolizing day and night
*Hinna, Henna, Hinaa,
Hinah, Heena, Hena*

Hind (Arabic) Owning a
group of camels; a wife of
Muhammed
Hynd, Hinde, Hynde

Hinda (Hebrew)
Resembling a doe
*Hindah, Hindy, Hindey,
Hindee, Hindi, Hindie,
Hynda, Hyndy*

Hiriwa (Polynesian) A silvery woman

Hitomi (Japanese) One
who has beautiful eyes
*Hitomie, Hitomee,
Hitomea, Hitomy, Hitomey*

Holda (German) A secretive woman; one who is
hidden
Holde

Hollander (Dutch) A
woman from Holland
*Hollynder, Hollender,
Holander, Holynder,
Holender, Hollande,
Hollanda*

Holly (English) Of the
holly tree
*Holli, Hollie, Hollee,
Holley, Hollye, Hollyanne,
Holle, Hollea*

Holton (American) One
who is whimsical
*Holten, Holtan, Holtin,
Holtyn, Holtun*

Holy (American) One who
is pious or sacred
*Holey, Holee, Holeigh,
Holi, Holie, Holye, Holea,
Holeah*

Hope (English) One who has high expectations through faith

Horem (Hebrew) One who is dedicated to God
Horema, Horemah, Horym, Horyma

Horonaim (Hebrew) Of the two caverns
Horonaima, Horonama, Horonayma, Horonayme, Horonaem, Horonaema

Hortensia (Latin) Woman of the garden
Hartencia, Hartinsia, Hortencia, Hortense, Hortenspa, Hortenxia, Hortinzia, Hortendana

Hoshi (Japanese) One who shines as brightly as a star
Hoshiko, Hoshie, Hoshee, Hoshy, Hoshey, Hoshiyo, Hoshea

Hourig (Slavic) A small, fiery woman

Hova (African) Born into the middle class

Hoyden (American) A spirited woman
Hoiden, Hoydan, Hoidan, Hoydyn, Hoidyn, Hoydin, Hoidin

Hudel (Scandinavian) One who is lovable
Hudell, Hudele, Hudelle, Hudela, Hudella

Hudes (Hebrew) Form of Judith, meaning " woman from Judea"

Hudson (English) One who is adventurous; an explorer
Hudsen, Hudsan, Hudsun, Hudsyn, Hudsin

Hueline (German) An intelligent woman
Huelene, Huelyne, Hueleine, Hueliene, Hueleene, Huleane

Huhana (Maori) Form of Susannah, meaning "white lily"
Huhanah, Huhanna, Huhanne, Huhann, Huhane

Humita (Native American) One who shells corn
Humitah, Humyta, Humeeta, Humieta, Humeita, Humeata, Humytah, Humeetah

Hutena (Hurrian) In mythology, the goddess of fate
Hutenah, Hutenna, Hutyna, Hutina

Huwaidah (Arabic) One who is gentle
Huwaydah, Huwaida, Huwayda, Huwaeda, Huwaedah

Huyen (Vietnamese) A woman with jet-black hair

Hvergelmir (Norse) In
mythology, the wellspring
of cold waters
*Hvergelmire, Hvergelmira,
Hvergelmeer, Hvergelmeera*

Hydeira (Greek) Woman
of the water
*Hydira, Hydyra, Hydeyra,
Hydeera, Hydeara, Hydiera*

Hygeia (Greek) In mythology, the goddess of health
Hygia, Hygeiah, Hygea

Hypatia (Greek) An intel-
lectually superior woman
Hypasia, Hypacia, Hypate

Hypermnestra (Greek) In
mythology, the mother of
Amphiareos

I

Ianeke (Hawaiian) God is
gracious
*Ianeki, Ianekie, Ianeky,
Ianekey, Ianekea, Ianekee*

Ianthe (Greek) Resembling
the violet flower; in
mythology, a sea nymph, a
daughter of Oceanus
*Iantha, Ianthia, Ianthina,
Ianthyna, Ianthea,
Ianthiya, Ianthya*

Ibtesam (Arabic) One who
smiles often
Ibtisam, Ibtysam

Ibtihaj (Arabic) A delight;
bringer of joy
Ibtehaj, Ibtyhaj

Ida (Greek) One who is
diligent; hardworking; in
mythology, the nymph
who cared for Zeus on
Mount Ida
*Idania, Idaea, Idalee, Idaia,
Idania, Idalia, Idalie, Idana*

Idil (Latin) A pleasant
woman
Idyl, Idill, Idyll

Idoia (Spanish) Refers to
the Virgin Mary
*Idoea, Idurre, Iratze,
Izazkun*

Idona (Scandinavian) A
fresh-faced woman
*Idonah, Idonna, Idonnah,
Idonia, Idoniah, Idonea,
Idoneah, Idonya*

Idowu (African) Daughter
born after twins

Ife (African) One who
loves and is loved
Ifeh, Iffe

Ignatia (Latin) A fiery
woman; burning brightly
*Igantiah, Ignacia, Ignazia,
Iniga*

Iheoma (Hawaiian) Lifted up by God

Ikeida (American) A spontaneous woman
Ikeidah, Ikeyda, Ikeydah, Ikeda, Ikedah, Ikieda, Ikiedah, Ikeeda

Ilamay (French) From the island
Ilamaye, Ilamai, Ilamae

Ilandere (American) Moon woman
Ilander, Ilanderre, Ilandera, Ilanderra

Ilia (Greek) From the ancient city
Iliah, Ilea, Ileah, Iliya, Iliyah, Ilya, Ilyah

Ilisapesi (Tonga) The blessed child
Ilisapesie, Ilysapesi, Ilysapesy, Ilisapesy, Ilisapesea, Ilysapesie, Ilysapesea

Ilithyia (Greek) In mythology, goddess of childbirth
Ilithya, Ilithiya, Ilithyiah

Ilma (German) Form of Wilhelmina, meaning "determined protector"
Ilmah, Illma, Illmah

Ilori (African) A special child; one who is treasured
Illori, Ilorie, Illorie, Ilory, Illory, Ilorey, Illorey, Iloree

Ilta (Finnish) Born at night
Iltah, Illta

Ilyse (German / Greek) Born into the nobility / form of Elyse, meaning "blissful"
Ilysea, Ilysia, Ilysse, Ilysea

Imala (Native American) One who disciplines others
Imalah, Imalla, Imallah, Immala, Immalla

Imanuela (Spanish) A faithful woman
Imanuella, Imanuel, Imanuele, Imanuell

Imari (Japanese) Daughter of today
Imarie, Imaree, Imarea, Imary, Imarey

Imelda (Italian) Warrior in the universal battle
Imeldah, Imalda, Imaldah

Imperia (Latin) A majestic woman
Imperiah, Imperea, Impereah, Imperial, Imperiel, Imperielle, Imperialle

Ina (Polynesian) In mythology, a moon goddess
Inah, Inna, Innah

Inaki (Asian) Having a generous nature
Inakie, Inaky, Inakey, Inakea, Inakee

Inanna (Sumerian) A lady
of the sky; in mythology,
goddess of love, fertility,
war, and the earth
*Inannah, Inana, Inanah,
Inann, Inanne, Inane*

Inara (Arabic) A heaven-
sent daughter; one who
shines with light
Inarah, Innara, Inarra, Innarra

Inari (Finnish / Japanese)
Woman from the lake /
one who is successful
*Inarie, Inaree, Inary,
Inarey, Inarea, Inareah*

Inaya (Arabic) One who
cares for the well-being of
others
Inayah, Inayat

Inca (Indian) An adventurer
*Incah, Inka, Inkah, Incka,
Inckah*

India (English) From the
river; woman from India
*Indea, Indiah, Indeah,
Indya, Indiya, Indee, Inda,
Indy*

Indiana (English) From
the land of the Indians;
from the state of Indiana
*Indianna, Indyana,
Indyanna*

Indiece (American) A
capable woman
*Indeice, Indeace, Indeece,
Indiese, Indeise, Indeese,
Indease*

Indigo (English)
Resembling the plant; a
purplish-blue dye
Indygo, Indeego

Indre (Hindi) Woman of
splendor

Ineesha (American) A
sparkling woman
*Ineeshah, Ineisha, Ineishah,
Iniesha, Inieshah, Ineasha,
Ineashah, Ineysha*

Ingalls (American) A
peaceful woman

Ingegard (Scandinavian)
Of the god Ing's kingdom
*Ingagard, Ingegerd,
Ingagerd, Ingigard, Ingigerd*

Ingelise (Danish) Having
the grace of the god Ing
*Ingelisse, Ingeliss, Ingelyse,
Ingelisa, Ingelissa, Ingelysa,
Ingelyssa*

Inghean (Scottish) Her
father's daughter
*Ingheane, Inghinn,
Ingheene, Ingheen, Inghynn*

Inis (Irish) Woman from
Ennis
*Iniss, Inisse, Innis, Inys,
Innys, Inyss, Inysse*

Intisar (Arabic) One who
is victorious; triumphant
*Intisara, Intisarah, Intizar,
Intizara, Intizarah,
Intisarr, Intysarr, Intysar*

Iolanthe (Greek)
Resembling a violet flower
*Iolanda, Iolanta, Iolantha,
Iolante, Iolande, Iolanthia,
Iolanthea*

Iona (Greek) Woman from
the island
Ionna, Ioane, Ioann, Ioanne

Ionanna (Hebrew) Filled
with grace
*Ionannah, Ionana, Ionann,
Ionane, Ionanne*

Ionia (Greek) Of the sea
and islands
*Ionya, Ionija, Ioniah, Ionea,
Ionessa, Ioneah, Ioniya*

Iosepine (Hawaiian) Form
of Josephine, meaning
"God will add"
*Iosephine, Iosefa, Iosefena,
Iosefene, Iosefina, Iosefine,
Iosepha, Iosephe*

Iowa (Native American) Of
the Iowa tribe; from the
state of Iowa

Iphedeiah (Hebrew) One
who is saved by the Lord
*Iphedeia, Iphedia, Iphedea,
Iphidea, Iphidia, Iphideia*

Iphigenia (Greek) One
who is born strong; in
mythology, daughter of
Agamemnon
*Iphigeneia, Iphigenie,
Iphagenia, Iphegenia,
Iphegenie, Iphegeneia,
Ifigenia, Ifegenia*

Ipsa (Indian) One who is
desired
*Ipsita, Ipsyta, Ipseeta,
Ipseata, Ipsah*

Iratze (Basque) Refers to
the Virgin Mary
*Iratza, Iratzia, Iratzea,
Iratzi, Iratzie, Iratzy,
Iratzey, Iratzee*

Irem (Turkish) From the
heavenly gardens
Irema, Ireme, Iremia, Iremea

Irene (Greek) A peaceful
woman; in mythology, the
goddess of peace
*Ira, Irayna, Ireen, Iren, Irena,
Irenea, Irenee, Irenka, Eirene*

Ireta (Greek) One who is
serene
*Iretah, Iretta, Irettah, Irete,
Iret, Irett, Ireta*

Irma (German) A universal
woman
*Irmina, Irmine, Irmgard,
Irmgarde, Irmagard,
Irmagarde, Irmeena, Irmyna*

Irodell (American) A
peaceful woman
*Irodelle, Irodel, Irodele,
Irodella, Irodela*

Irta (Greek) Resembling
a pearl
Irtah

Irune (Basque) Refers to
the Holy Trinity
Iroon, Iroone, Iroun, Iroune

*ᵀIsabel (Spanish) Form of
Elizabeth, meaning "my
God is bountiful; God's
promise"
*Isabeau, Isabela, Isabele,
Isabelita, Isabell, **Isabelle**,
Ishbel, Ysabel*

*ᵀIsabella (Italian /
Spanish) Form of Isabel,
meaning consecrated to
God
*Isabela, Isabelita, Isobella,
Izabella, Isibella, Isibela,
Isahella*

Isadore (Greek) A gift
from the goddess Isis
*Isadora, Isador, Isadoria,
Isidor, Isidoro, Isidorus,
Isidro, Isidora*

Isana (German) A strong-
willed woman
*Isunah, Isanna, Isane,
Isann, Isanne, Isan*

Isela (American) A giving
woman
Iselah, Isella, Isellah

Isla (Gaelic) From the
island
Islae, Islai, Isleta

Isleen (Gaelic) Form of
Aisling, meaning "a dream
or vision; an inspiration"
*Isleene, Islyne, Islyn, Isline,
Isleine, Isliene, Islene,
Isleyne*

Isolde (Celtic) A woman
known for her beauty; in
mythology, the lover of
Tristan
*Iseult, Iseut, Isold, Isolda,
Isolt, Isolte, Isota, Isotta*

Isra (Arabic) One who travels in the evening
Israh, Isria, Isrea, Israt

Itiah (Hebrew) One who is
comforted by God
*Itia, Iteah, Itea, Itiyah,
Itiya, Ityah, Itya*

Itidal (Arabic) One who is
cautious
Itidalle, Itidall, Itidale

Itsaso (Basque) Woman of
the ocean
Itasasso, Itassaso, Itassasso

Iudita (Hawaiian) An
affectionate woman
*Iuditah, Iudyta, Iudytah,
Iudeta, Iudetah*

Iuginia (Hawaiian) A high-
born woman
*Iuginiah, Iuginea,
Iugineah, Iugynia*

Ivory (English) Having a
creamy-white complexion;
as precious as elephant
tusks
*Ivorie, Ivorine, Ivoreen,
Ivorey, Ivoree, Ivori,
Ivoryne, Ivorea*

Ivy (English) Resembling the evergreen vining plant
Ivie, Ivi, Ivea

Iwilla (American) She shall rise
Iwillah, Iwilah, Iwila, Iwylla, Iwyllah, Iwyla, Iwylah

Ixchel (Mayan) The rainbow lady; in mythology, the goddess of the earth, moon, and healing
Ixchell, Ixchelle, Ixchela, Ixchella, Ixchal, Ixchall, Ixchalle, Ixchala

Iyabo (African) The mother is home

Izanne (American) One who calms others
Izann, Izane, Izana, Izan, Izanna

Izefia (African) A childless woman
Izefiah, Izefya, Izefiya, Izephia, Izefa, Izepha, Izefea, Izephea

Izolde (Greek) One who is philosophical
Izold, Izolda

J

Jaakkina (Finnish) Feminine form of Jukka; God is gracious
Jakkina, Jaakkinah, Jaakina, Jakina, Jakyna

Jacey (American) Form of Jacinda, meaning "resembling the hyacinth"
Jacee, Jacelyn, Jaci, Jacine, Jacy, Jaicee, Jaycee, Jacie

Jacinda (Spanish) Resembling the hyacinth
Jacenda, Jacenia, Jacenta, Jacindia, Jacinna, Jacinta, Jacinth, Jacintha, Jacey

Jacqueline (French) Feminine form of Jacques; the supplanter
Jackie, Xaquelina, Jacalin, Jacalyn, Jacalynn, Jackalin, Jackalinne, Jackelyn, Jacquelyn

Jade (Spanish) Resembling the green gemstone
Jadeana, Jadee, Jadine, Jadira, Jadrian, Jadrienne, Jady

Jaden (Hebrew / English) One who is thankful to God / form of Jade, meaning "resembling the green gemstone"
Jadine, Jadyn, Jadon, Jayden, Jadyne, Jaydyn, Jaydon, Jaydine

Jadwige (Polish) One who is protected in battle
Jadwyge, Jadwig, Jadwyg, Jadwiga, Jadwyga, Jadriga, Jadryga, Jadreega

Jadzia (Polish) A princess; born into royalty
Jadziah, Jadzea, Jadzeah, Jadziya, Jadziyah, Jadzya

Jae (English) Feminine form of Jay; resembling a jaybird
Jai, Jaelana, Jaeleah, Jaelyn, Jaenelle, Jaya

Jael (Hebrew) Resembling a mountain goat
Jaella, Jaelle, Jayel, Jaele, Jayil

Jaen (Hebrew) Resembling an ostrich
Jaena, Jaenia, Jaenea, Jaenne

Jaffa (Hebrew) A beautiful woman
Jaffah, Jafit, Jafita

Jalila (Arabic) An important woman; one who is exalted
Jalilah, Jalyla, Jalylah, Jaleela, Jaleelah, Jalil

Jamaica (American) From the island of springs
Jamaeca, Jamaika, Jemaica, Jamika, Jamieka

Jamie (Hebrew) Feminine form of James; she who supplants
Jaima, Jaime, Jaimee, Jaimelynn, Jaimey, Jaimi, Jaimie, Jaimy

Janan (Arabic) Of the heart and soul

Jane (Hebrew) Feminine form of John; God is gracious
Jaina, Jaine, Jainee, Janey, Jana, Janae, Janaye, Jandy, Sine, Janel, Janelle

^Janiyah (American) Form of Jana, meaning gracious, merciful
Janiya, Janiah

Janis (English) Feminine form of John; God is gracious
Janice, Janeece, Janess, Janessa, Janesse, Janessia, Janicia, Janiece

Jarah (Hebrew) A sweet and kind woman

Jasher (Hebrew) One who is righteous; upright
Jashiere, Jasheria, Jasherea

^Jaslene (American) Form of Jocelyn, meaning joy
*Jaslin, Jaslyn, **Jazlyn**, Jazlynn*

*Jasmine (Persian)
Resembling the climbing
plant with fragrant flowers
Jaslyn, Jaslynn, Jasmin,
Jasmyn, Jazmin, Jazmine,
Jazmyn

Javiera (Spanish)
Feminine form of Xavier;
one who is bright; the
owner of a new home
Javierah, Javyera, Javyerah,
Javeira, Javeirah

ᵀJayda (Resembling the
green gemstone)
Jada, Jaydah

Jayla (Arabic) One who is
charitable
Jaela, Jaila, Jaylah, Jaylee,
Jaylen, Jaylene, Jayleen,
Jaylin, Jaylyn, Jaylynn

Jean (Hebrew) Feminine
form of John; God is gra-
cious
Jeanae, Jeanay, Jeane,
Jeanee, Jeanelle, Jeanetta,
Jeanette, Jeanice, Gina

Jehaleleel (Hebrew) One
who praises God
Jehalelel, Jahaleleil, Jehaleliel,
Jehalelyl, Jehaleleal

Jehonadab (Hebrew) The
Lord gives liberally
Jonadab

Jemima (Hebrew) Dovelike
Jamima, Mima

Jemma (English) Form of
Gemma, meaning "as pre-
cious as a jewel"
Jemmah, Jema, Jemah,
Jemmalyn, Jemalyn,
Jemmalynn, Jemalynn

Jena (Arabic) Our little bird
Jenna, Jenah

Jendayi (Egyptian) One
who is thankful
Jendayie, Jendayey,
Jendayee, Jendaya,
Jendayia, Jendayea

*ᵀJennifer (Welsh) One
who is fair; a beautiful girl
Jenefer, Jeni, Jenifer,
Jeniffer, Jenn, Jennee, Jenni,
Jen, **Jenna,** *Jenny*

Jeorjia (American) Form
of Georgia, meaning "one
who works the earth; a
farmer"
Jeorgia, Jeorja, Jorja,
Jorjette, Jorgette, Jorjeta,
Jorjetta, Jorgete

Jereni (Slavic) One who is
peaceful
Jerenie, Jereny, Jereney,
Jerenee

Jermaine (French) Woman
from Germany
Jermainaa, Jermane,
Jermayne, Jermina,
Jermana, Jermayna,
Jermaen, Jermaena

---

*ᵀ**Jessica** (Hebrew) The Lord sees all
Jess, Jessa, Jessaca, Jessaka, Jessalin, Jessalyn, Jesse, Jesseca, Yessica

Jethetha (Hebrew) Feminine form of Jetheth; a princess
Jethethia, Jethethea, Jethethiya

Jethra (Hebrew) Feminine form of Jethro; the Lord's excellence; one who has plenty; abudance
Jethrah, Jethria, Jethrea, Jethriya, Jeth, Jethe

Jetta (Danish) Resembling the jet-black lustrous gem-stone
Jette, Jett, Jeta, Jete, Jettie, Jetty, Jetti, Jettey

Jewel (French) One who is playful; resembling a precious gem
Jewell, Jewelle, Jewelyn, Jewelene, Jewelisa, Jule, Jewella, Juelline

Jezebel (Hebrew) One who is not exalted; in the Bible, the queen of Israel punished by God
Jessabell, Jetzabel, Jezabel, Jezabella, Jezebelle, Jezibel, Jezibelle, Jezybell

Jie (Chinese) One who is pure; chaste

Jiera (Lithuanian) A lively woman
Jierah, Jyera, Jyerah, Jierra, Jyerra

Jillian (English) Form of Gillian, meaning "one who is youthful"
Jilian, Jiliana, Jilllaine, Jillan, Jillana, Jillane, Jillanne, Jillayne, Jillene, Jillesa, Jilliana, Jilliane, Jilliann, Jillianna, Jill

^**Jimena** (Spanish) One who is heard

Jinelle (Welsh) Form of Genevieve, meaning "white wave; fair-skinned"
Jinell, Jinele, Jinel, Jynelle, Jynell, Jynele, Jynel

Jinx (Latin) One who performs charms or spells
Jynx, Jinxx, Jynxx

Jiselle (American) Form of Giselle, meaning "one who offers her pledge"
Jisell, Jisele, Jisela, Jizelle, Joselle, Jisella, Jizella, Jozelle

Jo (English) Feminine form of Joseph; God will add
Jobelle, Jobeth, Jodean, Jodelle, Joetta, Joette, Jolinda, Jolisa

Joakima (Hebrew) Feminine form of Joachim; God will judge
Joachima, Joaquina, Joaquine, Joaquima

Jocasta (Greek) In mythology, the queen of Thebes who married her son
Jocastah, Jokasta, Jokastah, Jockasta, Joccasta

•**Jocelyn** (German / Latin) From the tribe of Gauts / one who is cheerful, happy
Jocelin, Jocelina, Jocelinda, Joceline, Jocelyne, Jocelynn, Jocelynne, Josalind, Joslyn, Joslynn, Joselyn

Joda (Hebrew) An ancestor of Christ

Jokim (Hebrew) Blessed by God
Jokima, Jokym, Jokyme, Jokeem, Jokimia, Jokimea, Joka, Jokeam

Jolan (Greek) Resembling a violet flower
Jola, Jolaine, Jolande, Jolanne, Jolanta, Jolantha, Jolandi, Jolanka

Jolene (English) Feminine form of Joseph; God will add
Joeline, Joeleen, Joeline, Jolaine, Jolean, Joleen, Jolena, Jolina

Jonina (Israeli) Resembling a little dove
Joninah, Jonyna, Jonynah, Joneena, Joneenah, Jonine, Jonyne, Joneene

Jorah (Hebrew) Resembling an autumn rose
Jora

Jord (Norse) In mythology, goddess of the earth
Jorde

⊤**Jordan** (Hebrew) Of the down-flowing river; in the Bible, the river where Jesus was baptized
Jardena, Johrdan, Jordain, Jordaine, Jordana, Jordane, Jordanka, Jordyn

Josephine (French) Feminine form of Joseph; God will add
Josefina, Josephene, Jo, Josie, Iosepine

Jovana (Spanish) Feminine form of Jovian; daughter of the sky
Jeovana, Jeovanna, Jovanna, Jovena, Jovianne, Jovina, Jovita, Joviana

Joy (Latin) A delight; one who brings pleasure to others
Jioia, Jioya, Joi, Joia, Joie, Joya, Joyann, Joyanna

Joyce (English) One who brings joy to others
Joice, Joyceanne, Joycelyn, Joycelynn, Joyse, Joyceta

Jozachar (Hebrew) God has remembered
Jozachare, Jozachara, Jozacharia, Jozacharea

Judith (Hebrew) Woman from Judea
Judithe, Juditha, Judeena, Judeana, Judyth, Judit, Judytha, Judita, Hudes

•**Julia** (Latin) One who is youthful; daughter of the sky
Jiulia, Joleta, Joletta, Jolette, Julaine, Julayna, Julee, Juleen, Julie, Julianne

Juliana (Spanish) form of Julia, meaning "one who is youthful"
Julianna

ʌ**Juliet** (French) Form of Julia, meaning one who is youthful
Juliette, Julitta, Julissa

July (Latin) Form of Julia, meaning "one who is youthful; daughter of the sky"; born during the month of July
Julye

June (Latin) One who is youthful; born during the month of June
Junae, Junel, Junelle, Junette, Junita, Junia

Justice (English) One who upholds moral rightness and fairness
Justyce, Justiss, Justyss, Justis, Justus, Justise

Juturna (Latin) In mythology, goddess of fountains and springs
Jutorna, Jutourna

Jwahir (African) The golden woman
Jwahyr, Jwaheer, Jwahear

Jyotsna (Indian) Woman of the moonlight

k

Kachina (Native American) A spiritual dancer
Kachine, Kachinah, Kachineh, Kachyna, Kacheena, Kachynah, Kacheenah, Kacheana

Kacondra (American) One who is bold
Kacondrah, Kacondria, Kacondriah, Kacondrea, Kacondreah, Kaecondra, Kaycondra, Kakondra

Kadin (Arabic) A beloved companion
Kadyn, Kadan, Kaden, Kadon, Kadun, Kaedin, Kaeden, Kaydin

Kaelyn (English) A beautiful girl from the meadow
Kaelynn, Kaelynne, Kaelin, Kailyn, Kaylyn, Kaelinn, Kaelinne

Kagami (Japanese) Displaying one's true image
Kagamie, Kagamy, Kagamey, Kagamee, Kagamea

Kailasa (Indian) From the silver mountain
Kailasah, Kailassa, Kaylasa, Kaelasa, Kailas, Kailase

•Kaitlyn (Greek) Form of Katherine, meaning one who is pure, virginal
*Kaitlin, Kaitlan, Kaitleen, Kaitlynn, Katalin, Katalina, Katalyn, Katelin, Kateline, Katelinn, **Katelyn**, Katelynn, Katilyn, Katlin*

Kakra (Egyptian) The younger of twins
Kakrah

Kala (Arabic / Hawaiian) A moment in time / form of Sarah, meaning "a princess; lady"
Kalah, Kalla, Kallah

Kalifa (Somali) A chaste and holy woman
Kalifah, Kalyfa, Kalyfah, Kaleefa, Kaleefah, Kalipha, Kalypha, Kaleepha

Kalinda (Indian) Of the sun
Kalindah, Kalynda, Kalinde, Kalindeh, Kalindi, Kalindie, Kalyndi, Kalyndie

Kallie (English) Form of Callie, meaning "a beautiful girl"
Kalli, Kallita, Kally, Kalley, Kallee, Kalleigh, Kallea, Kalleah

Kalma (Finnish) In mythology, goddess of the dead

Kalpana (Indian) Having a great imagination
Kalpanah, Kalpanna, Kalpannah

Kalwa (Finnish) A heroine

Kalyan (Indian) A beautiful and auspicious woman
Kalyane, Kalyanne, Kalyann, Kaylana, Kaylanna, Kalliyan, Kaliyan, Kaliyane

Kama (Indian) One who loves and is loved
Kamah, Kamma, Kammah

Kamala (Arabic) A woman of perfection
Kamalah, Kammala, Kamalla

Kamaria (African) Of the moon
Kamariah, Kamarea, Kamareah, Kamariya, Kamariyah

Kambiri (African) Newest addition to the family
Kambirie, Kambiry, Kambyry, Kambiree, Kambirea, Kambyree, Kambyrea, Kambyri

Kamea (Hawaiian) The one and only; precious one
Kameo

Kamyra (American) Surrounded by light
Kamira, Kamera, Kamiera, Kameira, Kameera, Kameara

Kanan (Indian) From the garden

Kanda (Native American) A magical woman
Kandah

Kanika (African) A dark, beautiful woman
Kanikah, Kanyka, Kanicka, Kanycka, Kaneeka, Kaneecka, Kaneaka, Kaneacka

Kantha (Indian) A delicate woman
Kanthah, Kanthe, Kantheh, Kanthia, Kanthia, Kanthea, Kantheah, Kanthiya

Kanya (Thai) A young girl; a virgin

Kaoru (Japanese) A fragrant girl
Kaori

Kara (Greek / Italian / Gaelic) One who is pure / dearly loved / a good friend
Karah, Karalee, Karalie, Karalyn, Karalynn, Karrah, Karra, Khara

Karcsi (French) A joyful singer
Karcsie, Karcsy, Karcsey, Karcsee, Karcsea

Karen (Greek) Form of Katherine, meaning "one who is pure; virginal"
Karan, Karena, Kariana, Kariann, Karianna, Karianne, Karin, Karina

Karina (Scandinavian / Russian) One who is dear and pure
Karinah, Kareena, Karyna

Karisma (English) Form of Charisma, meaning "blessed with charm"
Kharisma, Karizma, Kharizma

Karissa (Greek) Filled with grace and kindess; very dear
Karisa, Karyssa, Karysa, Karessa, Karesa, Karis, Karise

Karmel (Latin) Form of Carmel, meaning "of the fruitful orchard"
Karmelle, Karmell, Karmele, Karmela, Karmella

Karla (German) Feminine form of Karl; a small strong woman
Karly, Karli, Karlie, Karleigh, Karlee, Karley, Karlin, Karlyn, Karlina, Karleen

Karoline (English) A small and strong woman
Karolina, Karolinah, Karolyne, Karrie, Karie, Karri, Kari, Karry

Karsten (Greek) The anointed one
Karstin, Karstine, Karstyn, Karston, Karstan, Kiersten, Keirsten

Kasey (Irish) Form of Casey, meaning "a vigilant woman"
Kacie, Kaci, Kacy, KC, Kacee, Kacey, Kasie, Kasi

Kashawna (American) One who enjoys debate
Kashawn, Kaseana, Kasean, Kashaun, Kashauna, Kashona, Kashonna

Kashonda (American) A dramatic woman
Kashondah, Kashaunda, Kashaundah, Kashawnda, Kashawndah, Kashanda, Kashandah

Kasi (Indian) From the holy city; shining

Kasmira (Slavice) A peacemaker
Kasmirah, Kasmeera, Kasmeerah, Kasmyra, Kasmyrah, Kazmira, Kazmirah, Kazmyrah

Kate (English) Form of Katherine, meaning "one who is pure, virginal"
Katie, Katey, Kati

•**Katherine** (Greek) Form of Catherine, meaning "one who is pure; virginal"
Katharine, Katharyn, Kathy, Kathleen, Katheryn, Kathie, Kathrine, Kathryn, Karen, Kay

Katriel (Hebrew) Crowned by God
Katriele, Katrielle, Katriell

Kaveri (Indian) From the sacred river
Kaverie, Kauveri, Kauverie, Kavery, Kaverey, Kaveree, Kaverea, Kauvery

Kavinli (American) One who is eager
Kavinlie, Kavinly, Kavinley, Kavinlee, Kavinlea, Kavinleigh

Kawthar (Arabic) From the river in paradise
Kawthare, Kawthara, Kawtharr

Kay (English / Greek) The keeper of the keys / form of Katherine, meaning "one who is pure; virginal"
Kaye, Kae, Kai, Kaie, Kaya, Kayana, Kayane, Kayanna

^**Kayden** (American) Form of Kaden, meaning "a beloved companion"

***Kayla** (Arabic / Hebrew) Crowned with laurel
Kaylah, Kalan, Kalen, Kalin, Kalyn, Kalynn, Kaylan, Kaylana, Kaylin, Kaylen, Kaylynn, Kaylyn, Kayle

***Kaylee** (American) Form of Kayla, meaning crowned with laurel
Kaleigh, Kaley, Kaelee, Kaeley, Kaeli, Kailee, Kailey, Kalee, Kayleigh, Kayley, Kayli, Kaylie

Kearney (Irish) The winner
Kearny, Kearni, Kearnie, Kearnee, Kearnea

Keaton (English) From a shed town
Keatan, Keatyn, Keatin, Keatun

Keavy (Irish) A lovely and graceful girl
Keavey, Keavi, Keavie, Keavee, Keavea

Keeya (African) Resembling a flower
Keeyah, Kieya, Keiya, Keyya

Kefira (Hebrew) Resembling a young lioness
Kefirah, Kefiera, Kefeira, Kefeera, Kefyra, Kephira

Keira (Irish) Form of Kiera, meaning little dark-haired one
Kierra, Kyera, Kyerra, Keiranne, Kyra, Kyrie, Kira, Kiran

Keisha (American) The favorite child; form of Kezia, meaning "of the spice tree"
Keishla, Keishah, Kecia, Kesha, Keysha, Keesha, Kiesha, Keshia

Kelly (Irish) A lively and bright-headed woman
Kelley, Kelli, Kellie, Kellee, Kelliegh, Kellye, Keely, Keelie, Keeley, Keelyn

Kelsey (English) From the island of ships
Kelsie, Kelcey, Kelcie, Kelcy, Kellsie, Kelsa, Kelsea, Kelsee, Kelsi, Kelsy, Kellsey

Kendall (Welsh) From the royal valley
Kendal, Kendyl, Kendahl, Kindall, Kyndal, Kenley

Kendra (English) Feminine form of Kendrick; having royal power; from the high hill
Kendrah, Kendria, Kendrea, Kindra, Kindria

Kennedy (Gaelic) A
helmeted chief
*Kennedi, Kennedie,
Kennedey, Kennedee,
Kenadia, Kenadie, Kenadi,
Kenady, Kenadey*

Kensington (English) A
brash lady
*Kensyngton, Kensingtyn,
Kinsington, Kinsyngton,
Kinsingtyn*

Kenwei (Arabic)
Resembling a water lily

Kenyangi (Ugandan)
Resembling the white
egret
*Kenyangie, Kenyangy,
Kenyangey, Kenyangee*

Kerensa (Cornish) One
who loves and is loved
*Kerinsa, Keransa, Kerensia,
Kerensea, Kerensya, Kerenz,
Kerenza, Keranz*

Kerr (Scottish) From the
marshland

Keshon (American) Filled
with happiness
*Keyshon, Keshawn,
Keyshawn, Kesean, Keysean,
Keshaun, Keyshaun,
Keshonna*

Kevina (Gaelic) Feminine
form of Kevin; a beautiful
and beloved child
*Kevinah, Keva, Kevia,
Kevinne, Kevyn, Kevynn*

Keyla (English) A wise
daughter

Kezia (Hebrew) Of the
spice tree
*Keziah, Kesia, Kesiah, Kesi,
Kessie, Ketzia, Keisha*

Khai (American) Unlike
the others; unusual
Khae, Khay, Khaye

Khalida (Arabic) Feminine
form of Khalid; an immor-
tal woman
*Khalidah, Khaleeda,
Khalyda, Khaalida, Khulud,
Khulood, Khaleada*

Khaliqa (Arabic) Feminine
form of Khaliq; a creator;
one who is well-behaved
*Khaliqah, Khalyqa,
Khaleeqa, Kaliqua,
Kaleequa, Kalyqua,
Khaleaqa, Kaleaqua*

Khanh (Vietnamese)
Resembling a precious
stone
Khann, Khan

Khatiba (Arabic) Feminine
form of Khatib; one who
leads the prayers; an orator
*Khateeba, Khatyba, Khateba,
Khatibah, Khateaba*

Khatun (Arabic) A daugh-
ter born to nobility; a lady
*Khatune, Khatoon,
Khaatoon, Khanom,
Kanom, Khanam,
Khaanam, Khatoun*

Khayriyyah (Arabic) A charitable woman
Khayriyah, Khariyyah, Khariya, Khareeya

Khepri (Egyptian) Born of the morning sun
Kheprie, Kepri, Keprie, Khepry, Kepry, Khepree, Kepree, Kheprea

Khiana (American) One who is different
Khianna, Khiane, Khianne, Khian, Khyana, Khyanna, Kheana, Kheanna

^**Khloe** (Greek) Form of Chloe, meaning "a flourishing woman, blooming"

Kiara (American) Form of Chiara, meaning "daughter of the light"

Kichi (Japanese) The fortunate one
Kichie, Kichy, Kichey, Kichee, Kichea

Kidre (American) A loyal woman
Kidrea, Kidreah, Kidria, Kidriah, Kidri, Kidrie, Kidry, Kidrey

Kiele (Hawaiian) Resembling the gardenia
Kielle, Kiel, Kiell, Kiela, Kiella

Kikka (German) The mistress of all
Kika, Kykka, Kyka

^**Kiley** (American) Form of Kylie, meaning "a boomerang"

Kimana (American) Girl from the meadow
Kimanah, Kimanna, Kimannah, Kymana, Kymanah, Kymanna, Kymannah

Kimball (English) Chief of the warriors; possessing royal boldness
Kimbal, Kimbell, Kimbel, Kymball, Kymbal

*****Kimberly** (English) Of the royal fortress
Kimberley, Kimberli, Kimberlee, Kimberleigh, Kimberlin, Kimberlyn, Kymberlie, Kymberly

Kimeo (American) Filled with happiness
Kimeyo

Kimetha (American) Filled with joy
Kimethah, Kymetha, Kymethah, Kimethia, Kymethia, Kimethea, Kymethea

Kimiko (Japanese) A noble child; without equal

^**Kimora** (American) Form of Kimberly, meaning "royal"

Kina (Hawaiian) Woman of China

Kineks (Native American) Resembling a rosebud

Kineta (Greek) One who is active; full of energy
Kinetikos

Kinipela (Hawaiian) One who is fair; white wave

Kinsey (English) The king's victory
Kinnsee, Kinnsey, Kinnsie, Kinsee, Kinsie, Kinzee, Kinzie, Kinzey

Kintra (American) A joyous woman
Kintrah, Kentra, Kentrah, Kintria, Kentria, Kintrea, Kentrea, Kintrey

Kioko (Japanese) A daughter born with happiness

Kirima (Eskimo) From the hill
Kirimah, Kiryma, Kirymah, Kirema, Kiremah, Kireema, Kireemah, Kireama

Kismet (English) One's destiny; fate

Kiss (American) A caring and compassionate woman
Kyss, Kissi, Kyssi, Kissie, Kyssie, Kissy, Kyssy, Kissey

Kissa (African) Daughter born after twins
Kissah, Kyssa, Kyssah

Kita (Japanese) Woman from the north

Kobi (American) Woman from California
Kobie, Koby, Kobee, Kobey, Kobea

Koko (Japanese) The stork has come

Kolette (English) Form of Colette, meaning "victory of the people"
Kolete, Kolett, Koleta, Koletta, Kolet

Kolinka (Danish) Born to the victors
Kolinka, Koleenka, Kolynka, Kolenka

Komala (Indian) A delicate and tender woman
Komalah, Komalla, Komal, Komali, Komalie, Komalee, Komaleigh, Komalea

Kona (Hawaiian) A girly woman
Konah, Konia, Koniah, Konea, Koneah, Koni, Konie, Koney

Konane (Hawaiian) Daughter of the moonlight

Kreeli (American) A charming and kind girl
Kreelie, Krieli, Krielie, Kryli, Krylie, Kreely, Kriely, Kryly

Krenie (American) A capable woman
Kreni, Kreny, Kreney, Krenee, Krenea

Kristina (English) Form of Christina, meaning "follower of Christ"
Kristena, Kristine, Kristyne, Kristyna, Krystina, Krystine

Kumi (Japanese) An everlasting beauty
Kumie, Kumy, Kumey, Kumee, Kumea

Kunti (Hindi) In Hinduism, the mother of the Pandavas
Kuntie, Kunty, Kuntey, Kuntea, Koonti, Koontie, Koonty, Koontey

•Kyla (English) Feminine form of Kyle; from the narrow channel
Kylah, Kylar, Kyle

•Kylie (Australian) A boomerang
Kylee, Kyleigh, Kyley, Kyli, Kyleen, Kyleen, Kyler, Kily, Kileigh, Kilee, Kilie, Kili, Kilea, Kylea

Kyra Kyra (Greek) Form of Cyrus, meaning "noble"
Kyrah, Kyria, Kyriah, Kyrra, Kyrrah

Labana (Hebrew) Feminine form of Labon; white; fair-skinned
Labanah, Labanna, Labania, Labanea, Labaniya, Labannah, Labaniah, Labaneah

Labiba (Arabic) Having great wisdom; one who is intelligent
Labibah, Labeeba, Labeebah, Labyba, Labybah, Labieba, Labiebah, Labeiba

Lacey (French) Woman from Normandy; as delicate as lace
Lace, Lacee, Lacene, Laci, Laciann, Lacie, Lacina, Lacy

Lachesis (Greek) In mythology, one of the three Fates
Lachesiss, Lachesisse, Lachesys, Lacheses

Lacole (American) A sly woman
Lakole, Lucole, Lukole

Lady (English) One who kneads bread; the head of the house
Lady, Ladee, Ladi, Ladie, Laidy, Laydy, Laydi, Laydie

Lael (Hebrew) One who belongs to God
Laele, Laelle

Laila (Arabic) A beauty of the night, born at nightfall
Layla, Laylah

Lainil (American) A soft-hearted woman
Lainill, Lainyl, Lainyll, Laenil, Laenill, Laenyl, Laenyll, Laynil

Lais (Greek) A legendary courtesan
Laise, Lays, Layse, Laisa, Laes, Laese

Lajita (Indian) A truthful woman
Lajyta, Lajeeta, Lajeata

Lake (American) From the still waters
Laken, Laiken, Layken, Layk, Layke, Laik, Laike, Laeken

Lala (Slavic) Resembling a tulip
Lalah, Lalla, Lallah, Laleh

Lalaine (American) A hardworking woman
Lalain, Lalaina, Lalayn, Lalayne, Lalayna, Lalaen, Lalaene, Lalaena

Lalia (Greek) One who is well-spoken
Lali, Lallia, Lalya, Lalea, Lalie, Lalee, Laly, Laley

Lalita (Indian) A playful and charming woman
Lalitah, Laleeta, Laleetah, Lalyta, Lalytah, Laleita, Laleitah, Lalieta

Lamarian (American) One who is conflicted
Lamariane, Lamarean, Lamareane

Lamia (Greek) In mythology, a female vampire
Lamiah, Lamiya, Lamiyah, Lamea, Lameah

Lamya (Arabic) Having lovely dark lips
Lamyah, Lamyia, Lama

Lanassa (Russian) A light-hearted woman; cheerful
Lanasa, Lanassia, Lanasia, Lanassiya, Lanasiya

Lang (Scandinavian) Woman of great height

Lani (Hawaiian) From the sky; one who is heavenly
Lanikai

Lansing (English) Filled with hope
Lanseng, Lansyng

Lanza (Italian) One who is noble and willing
Lanzah, Lanzia, Lanziah, Lanzea, Lanzeah

Lapis (Egyptian)
Resembling the dark-blue
gemstone
*Lapiss, Lapisse, Lapys,
Lapyss, Lapysse*

Laquinta (American) The
fifth-born child

Laramie (French)
Shedding tears of love
*Larami, Laramy, Laramey,
Laramee, Laramea*

Larby (American) Form of
Darby, meaning "of the
deer park"
*Larbey, Larbi, Larbie,
Larbee, Larbea*

Larch (American) One
who is full of life
Larche

Lark (English) Resembling
the songbird
Larke

Larue (American) Form of
Rue, meaning "a medici-
nal herb"
LaRue, Laroo, Larou

Lashawna (American)
Filled with happiness
*Lashauna, Laseana,
Lashona, Lashawn, Lasean,
Lashone, Lashaun*

Lata (Indian) Of the lovely
vine
Latah

Latanya (American)
Daughter of the fairy
queen
*Latanyah, Latonya,
Latania, Latanja, Latonia,
Latanea*

LaTeasa (Spanish) A flirtatious woman
Lateasa, Lateaza

Latona (Latin) In mythol-
ogy, the Roman equivalent
of Leto, the mother of
Artemis and Apollo
*Latonah, Latonia, Latonea,
Lantoniah, Latoneah*

Latrelle (American) One
who laughs a lot
*Latrell, Latrel, Latrele,
Latrella, Latrela*

Laudonia (Italian) Praises
the house
*Laudonea, Laudoniya,
Laudomia, Laudomea,
Laudomiya*

Laura (Latin) Crowned
with laurel; from the lau-
rel tree
*Lauraine, Lauralee, Laralyn,
Laranca, Larea, Lari,
Lauralee, Lauren, Loretta*

•**Lauren** (French) Form of
Laura, meaning "crowned
with laurel; from the lau-
rel tree"
*Laren, Larentia, Larentina,
Larenzina, Larren, Laryn,
Larryn, Larrynn*

•**Leah** (Hebrew) One who is weary; in the Bible, Jacob's first wife
Leia, Leigha, Lia, Liah, Leeya

Leanna (Gaelic) Form of Helen, meaning "the shining light"
Leana, Leann, Leanne, Lee-Ann, Leeann, Leeanne, Leianne, Leyanne

Lecia (English) Form of Alice, meaning "woman of the nobility; truthful; having high moral character"
Licia, Lecea, Licea, Lisha, Lysha, Lesha

Ledell (Greek) One who is queenly
Ledelle, Ledele, Ledella, Ledela, Ledel

Legend (American) One who is memorable
Legende, Legund, Legunde

Legia (Spanish) A bright woman
Legiah, Legea, Legeah, Legiya, Legiyah, Legya, Legyah

Leila (Persian) Night, dark beauty
Leela, Lela

Lenis (Latin) One who has soft and silky skin
Lene, Leneta, Lenice, Lenita, Lennice, Lenos, Lenys, Lenisse

Leona (Latin) Feminine form of Leon; having the strength of a lion
Leeona, Leeowna, Leoine, Leola, Leone, Leonelle, Leonia, Leonie

Lequoia (Native American) Form of Sequoia, meaning "of the giant redwood tree"
Lequoya, Lequoiya, Lekoya

Lerola (Latin) Resembling a blackbird
Lerolla, Lerolah, Lerolia, Lerolea

Leslie (Gaelic) From the holly garden; of the gray fortress
Leslea, Leslee, Lesleigh, Lesley, Lesli, Lesly, Lezlee, Lezley

Leucippe (Greek) In mythology, a nymph
Lucippe, Leucipe, Lucipe

Leucothea (Greek) In mythology, a sea nymph
Leucothia, Leucothiah, Leucotheah

Levora (American) A homebody
Levorah, Levorra, Levorrah, Levoria, Levoriah, Levorea, Levoreah, Levorya

Lewa (African) A very beautiful woman
Lewah

Lewana (Hebrew) Of the white moon
Lewanah, Lewanna, Lewannah

^**Lia** (Italian) Form of Leah, meaning "one who is weary

Libby (English) Form of Elizabeth, meaning "my God is bountiful; God's promise"
Libba, Libbee, Libbey, Libbie, Libet, Liby, Lilibet, Lilibeth

Liberty (English) An independent woman; having freedom
Libertey, Libertee, Libertea, Liberti, Libertie, Libertas, Libera, Liber

Libra (Latin) One who is balanced; the seventh sign of the zodiac
Leebra, Leibra, Liebra, Leabra, Leighbra, Lybra

Librada (Spanish) One who is free
Libradah, Lybrada, Lybradah

Lieu (Vietnamese) Of the willow tree

Ligia (Greek) One who is musically talented
Ligiah, Ligya, Ligiya, Lygia, Ligea, Lygea, Lygya, Lygiya

^**Lila** (Arabic / Greek) Born at night / resembling a lily
Lilah, Lyla, Lylah

Lilac (Latin) Resembling the bluish-purple flower
Lilack, Lilak, Lylac, Lylack, Lylak, Lilach

Lilette (Latin) Resembling a budding lily
Lilett, Lilete, Lilet, Lileta, Liletta, Lylette, Lylett, Lylete

Liliana (Italian, Spanish) Form of Lillian, meaning "resembling the lily"
Lilliana, Lillianna, Liliannia, Lilyana, Lilia

Lilith (Babylonian) Woman of the night
Lilyth, Lillith, Lillyth, Lylith, Lyllith, Lylyth, Lyllyth, Lilithe

*·**Lillian** (Latin) Resembling the lily
Lilian, Liliane, Lilianne, Lilias, Lilas, Lillas, Lillias

Lilo (Hawaiian) One who is generous
Lylo, Leelo, Lealo, Leylo, Lielo, Leilo

*·τ**Lily** (English) Resembling the flower; one who is innocent and beautiful
Leelee, Lil, Lili, Lilie, Lilla, Lilley, Lilli, Lillie, Lilly

Limor (Hebrew) Refers to myrrh
Limora, Limoria, Limorea, Leemor, Leemora, Leemoria, Leemorea

Lin (Chinese) Resembling jade; from the woodland

Linda (Spanish) One who is soft and beautiful
Lindalee, Lindee, Lindey, Lindi, Lindie, Lindira, Lindka, Lindy, Lynn

Linden (English) From the hill of lime trees
Lindenn, Lindon, Lindynn, Lynden, Lyndon, Lyndyn, Lyndin, Lindin

Lindley (English) From the pastureland
Lindly, Lindlee, Lindleigh, Lindli, Lindlie, Leland, Lindlea

Lindsay (English) From the island of linden trees; from Lincoln's wetland
Lind, Lindsea, Lindsee, Lindseigh, Lindsey, Lindsy, Linsay, Linsey

Lisa (English) Form of Elizabeth, meaning "my God is bountiful; God's promise"
Leesa, Liesa, Lisebet, Lise, Liseta, Lisette, Liszka, Lisebeth

Lishan (African) One who is awarded a medal
Lishana, Lishanna, Lyshan, Lyshana, Lyshanna

Lissie (American) Resembling a flower
Lissi, Lissy, Lissey, Lissee, Lissea

Liv (Scandinavian / Latin) One who protects others / from the olive tree
Livia, Livea, Liviya, Livija, Livvy, Livy, Livya, Lyvia

Liya (Hebrew) The Lord's daughter
Liyah, Leeya, Leeyah, Leaya, Leayah

Lo (American) A fiesty woman
Loe, Low, Lowe

Loicy (American) A delightful woman
Loicey, Loicee, Loicea, Loici, Loicie, Loyce, Loice, Loyci

Lokelani (Hawaiian) Resembling a small red rose
Lokelanie, Lokelany, Lokelaney, Lokelanee, Lokelanea

Loki (Norse) In mythology, a trickster god
Lokie, Lokee, Lokey, Loky, Lokea, Lokeah, Lokia, Lokiah

Lola (Spanish) Form of Dolores, meaning "woman of sorrow"
Lolah, Loe

^**London** (English) From the capital of England
Londyn

Lorelei (German) From the rocky cliff; in mythology, a siren who lured sailors to their deaths
Laurelei, Laurelie, Loralee, Loralei, Loralie, Loralyn

Loretta (Italian) Form of Laura, meaning "crowned with laurel; from the laurel tree"
Laretta, Larretta, Lauretta, Laurette, Leretta, Loreta, Lorette, Lorretta

Lorraine (French) From the kingdom of Lothair
Laraine, Larayne, Laurraine, Leraine, Lerayne, Lorain, Loraina, Loraine

Lo-ruhamah (Hebrew) One who does not receive mercy

Louvain (English) From the city in Belgium
Leuven, Loovain

Love (English) One who is full of affection
Lovey, Loveday, Lovette, Lovi, Lovie, Lov, Luv, Luvey

Lovella (Native American) Having a soft spirit
Lovell, Lovela, Lovele, Lovelle, Lovel

Lovely (American) An attractive and pleasant woman
Loveli, Loveley, Lovelie, Lovelee, Loveleigh, Lovelea

Luana (Hawaiian) One who is content and enjoys life
Lewanna, Lou-Ann, Louann, Louanna, Louanne, Luanda, Luane, Luann

Lucretia (Latin) A bringer of light; a successful woman; in mythology, a maiden who was raped by the prince of Rome
Lacretia, Loucrecia, Loucresha, Loucretia, Loucrezia, Lucrece, Lucrecia, Lucreecia

Lucy (Latin) Feminine form of Lucius; one who is illuminated
Luce, Lucetta, Lucette, Luci, Lucia, Luciana, Lucianna, Lucida, Lucille

Lucylynn (American) A light-hearted woman
Lucylyn, Lucylynne, Lucilynn, Lucilyn, Lucilynne

Ludmila (Slavic) Having the favor of the people
Ludmilah, Ludmilla, Ludmillah, Ludmyla, Ludmylla, Lyubochka

Luenetter (American) A self-centered woman
Luenette, Luenett, Luenete, Luenet, Luenetta, Lueneta

^**Luna** (Latin) Of the moon
Lunah

Lunet (English) Of the crescent moon
Lunett, Lunette, Luneta, Lunete, Lunetta

Lupita (Spanish) Form of Guadalupe, meaning "from the valley of wolves"
Lupe, Lupyta, Lupelina, Lupeeta, Lupieta, Lupeita, Lupeata

Lurissa (American) A beguiling woman
Lurisa, Luryssa, Lurysa, Luressa, Luresa

Luvina (English) Little one who is dearly loved
Luvinah, Luvena, Luvyna, Luveena, Luveina, Luviena, Luveana

Luyu (Native American) Resembling the dove

Lydia (Greek) A beautiful woman from Lydia
Lidia, Lidie, Lidija, Lyda, Lydie, Lydea, Liddy, Lidiy

^**Lyla** (Arabic) Form of Lila, meaning "born at night, resembling a lily"
Lylah

✷**Lynn** (English) Woman of the lake; form of Linda, meaning "one who is soft and beautiful"
Linell, Linnell, Lyn, Lynae, Lyndel, Lyndell, Lynell, Lynelle

^**Lyric** (French) Of the lyre; the words of a song
Lyrica, Lyricia, Lyrik, Lyrick, Lyrika, Lyricka

Lytanisha (American) A scintillating woman
Lytanesha, Lytaniesha, Lytaneisha, Lytanysha, Lytaneesha, Lytaneasha

m

Maachah (Hebrew) One who has been oppressed; in the Bible, one of David's wives
Maacha

Macanta (Gaelic) A kind and gentle woman
Macan, Macantia, Macantea, Macantah

Machi (Taiwanese) A good friend
Machie, Machy, Machey, Machee, Machea

Mackenna (Gaelic) Daughter of the handsome man
Mackendra, Mackennah, McKenna, McKendra, Makenna, Makennah

*ᵀMackenzie (Gaelic)
Daughter of a wise leader;
a fiery woman; one who
is fair
Mackenzey, Makensie,
Makenzie, *M'Kenzie,*
McKenzie, Meckenzie,
Mackenzee, Mackenzy

Macy (French) One who
wields a weapon
Macee, Macey, Maci,
Macie, Maicey, Maicy,
Macea, Maicea

Mada (Arabic) One who has
reached the end of the path
Madah

Madana (Ethiopian) One
who heals others
Madayna, Madaina,
Madania, Madaynia,
Madainia

Maddox (English) Born
into wealth and prosperity
Madox, Madoxx, Maddoxx

*^Madeline (Hebrew)
Woman from Magdala
Mada, Madalaina,
Madaleine, Madalena,
Madalene, **Madelyn,**
Madalyn, **Madelynn,**
Madilyn

Madhavi (Indian)
Feminine form of Madhav;
born in the springtime
Madhavie, Madhavee,
Madhavey, Madhavy,
Madhavea

Madhu (Indian) As sweet
as honey
Madhul, Madhula, Madhulika,
Madhulia, Madhulea

Madini (Swahili) As pre-
cious as a gemstone
Madinie, Madiny, Madiney,
Madinee, Madyny, Madyni,
Madinea, Madynie

*ᵀ^Madison (English)
Daughter of a mighty
warrior
Maddison, Madisen,
Madisson, *Madisyn, Madyson*

Madoline (English) One
who is accomplished with
the stringed instrument
Mandalin, Mandalyn,
Mandalynn, Mandelin,
Mandellin, Mandellyn,
Mandolin, Mandolyn

Madonna (Italian) My lady;
refers to the Virgin Mary
Madonnah, Madona, Madonah

Maeve (Irish) An intoxicat-
ing woman
Mave, Meave, Medb, Meabh

Maggie (English) Form
of Margaret, meaning
"resembling a pearl"
Maggi

Magnolia (French)
Resembling the flower
Magnoliya, Magnoliah,
Magnolea, Magnoleah,
Magnoliyah, Magnolya,
Magnolyah

Mahal (Native American) A tender and loving woman
Mahall, Mahale, Mahalle

Mahari (African) One who offers forgiveness
Maharie, Mahary, Maharey, Maharee, Maharai, Maharae, Maharea

Maheona (Native American) A medicine woman
Maheo, Maheonia, Maheonea

Mahesa (Indian) A powerful and great lady
Maheshvari

Mahira (Arabic) A clever and adroit woman
Mahirah, Mahir, Mahire, Mahiria, Mahirea, Maheera, Mahyra, Mahiera

Maia (Latin / Maori) The great one; in mythology, the goddess of spring / a brave warrior
Maiah, Mya, Maja

Maida (English) A maiden; a virgin
Maidel, Maidie, Mayda, Maydena, Maydey, Mady, Maegth, Magd

Maiki (Japanese) Resembling the dancing flower
Maikie, Maikei, Maikki, Maikee

Maimun (Arabic) One who is lucky; fortunate
Maimoon, Maimoun

Maimuna (Arabic) One who is trustworthy
Maimoona, Maimouna

Maine (French) From the mainland; from the state of Maine

Maiolaine (French) As delicate as a flower
Maiolainie, Maiolani, Maiolaney, Maiolany, Maiolanee, Maiolayne, Maiolanea

Maisara (Arabic) One who lives an effortless life
Maisarah, Maisarra, Maisarrah

Maisha (African) Giver of life
Maysha, Maishah, Mayshah, Maesha, Maeshah

Maisie (Scottish) Form of Margaret, meaning "resembling a pearl"
Maisee, Maisey, Maisy, Maizie, Mazey, Mazie, Maisi, Maizi

Maitreya (Sanskrit) One who offers love to all
Maitreyah, Maetreya, Maitraya, Maetraya

Majaya (Indian) A victorious woman
Majayah

Makala (Hawaiian)
Resembling myrtle
Makalah, Makalla, Makallah

*T**Makayla** (Celtic / Hebrew /
English) Form of
Michaela, meaning "who
is like God?"
*Macaela, MacKayla,
Mak,Mechaela, Meeskaela,
Mekea, Mekelle*

Makani (Hawaiian) Of the
wind
*Makanie, Makaney,
Makany, Makanee*

Makareta (Maori) Form
of Margaret, meaning
"resembling a pearl / the
child of light"
Makaretah, Makarita

Makea (Finnish) One who
is sweet
Makeah, Makia, Makiah

Makeda (African) A
queenly woman; greatness
Makedah

Makelina (Hawaiian)
Form of Madeline,
meaning "woman from
Magdala"
*Makelinah, Makeleena,
Makelyna, Makeleana*

Makenna (Irish) Form of
McKenna, meaning "of
the Irish one"
Makennah

Makena (African) One who
is filled with happiness
*Makenah, Makeena,
Makeenah, Makeana,
Makeanah, Makyna,
Makynah, Mackena*

Malak (Arabic) A heavenly
messenger; an angel
*Malaka, Malaika, Malayka,
Malaeka, Malake, Malayk,
Malaek, Malakia*

Malati (Indian) Resembling
a fragrant flower
*Malatie, Malaty, Malatey,
Malatee, Malatea*

Malcomina (Scottish)
Feminine form of
Malcolm; devotee of St.
Columba
*Malcomeena, Malcomyna,
Malcominia, Malcominea,
Malcomena, Malcomeina,
Malcomiena, Malcomeana*

Malcsi (Hungarian) An
industrious woman
*Malcsie, Malcsee, Malcsey,
Malcsy, Malksi, Malksie,
Malksy, Malksee*

Maleda (Ethiopian) Born
with the rising sun
Maledah

Mali (Thai / Welsh)
Resembling a flower /
form of Molly, meaning
"star of the sea / from the
sea of bitterness"
*Malie, Malee, Maleigh,
Maly, Maley*

^**Malia** (Hawaiian) Form of Mary, meaning "star of the sea / from the sea of bitterness
Maliah, Malea, Maleah

Malika (Arabic) Destined to be queen
Malikah, Malyka, Maleeka, Maleika, Malieka, Maliika, Maleaka

Malina (Hawaiian) A peaceful woman
Malinah, Maleena, Maleenah, Malyna, Malynah, Maleina, Maliena, Maleana

Malinka (Russian) As sweet as a little berry
Malinkah, Malynka, Maleenka, Malienka, Maleinka, Maleanka

Maluna (Hawaiian) One who rises above
Maloona, Malunia, Malunai, Maloonia, Maloonai, Malouna, Malounia, Malounai

Malva (Greek) One who is soft and slender
Malvah, Malvia, Malvea

Mana (Polynesian) A charismatic and prestigious woman
Manah

Manal (Arabic) An accomplished woman
Manala, Manall, Manalle, Manalla, Manali

Manami (Japanese) Having a love of the ocean
Manamie, Manamy, Manamey, Manamee, Manamea

Mangena (Hebrew) As sweet as a melody
Mangenah, Mangenna, Mangennah

Manyara (African) A humble woman
Manyarah

Maola (Irish) A handmaiden
Maoli, Maole, Maolie, Maolia, Maoly, Maoley, Maolee, Maolea

Mapenzi (African) One who is dearly loved
Mpenzi, Mapenzie, Mapenze, Mapenzy, Mapenzee, Mapenzea

Maram (Arabic) One who is wished for
Marame, Marama, Marami, Maramie, Maramee, Maramy, Maramey, Maramea

Marcella (Latin) Dedicated to Mars, the God of war
Marcela, Marsela, Marsella, Maricela, Maricel

Marcia (Latin) Feminine form of Marcus; dedicated to Mars, the god of war
Marcena, Marcene, Marchita, Marciana, Marciane, Marcianne, Marcilyn, Marcilynn

Marde (Latin) A woman warrior
Mardane, Mardayne

Mardea (African) The last-born child
Mardeah

^**Marely** (American) form of Marley, meaning of the marshy meadow

Margaret (Greek / Persian) Resembling a pearl / the child of light
Maighread, Mairead, Mag, Maggi, Maggie, Maggy, Maiga, Malgorzata, Megan, Marwarid, Marjorie, Marged, Makareta

Marged (Welsh) Form of Margaret, meaning "resembling a pearl / the child of light"
Margred, Margeda, Margreda

*****Maria** (Spanish) Form of Mary, meaning "star of the sea / from the sea of bitterness"
Mariah, Marialena, Marialinda, Marialisa, Maaria, Mayria, Maeria, Mariabella

*****Mariah** (Latin) Form of Mary, meaning star of the sea

Mariamne (Hebrew) A rebellious woman
Mamre, Meria

Mariana (Spanish / Italian) Form of Mary, meaning "star of the sea"
Marianna

Mariane (French) Blend of Mary, meaning "star of the sea / from the sea of bitterness," and Ann, meaning "a woman graced with God's favor"
Mariam, Mariana, Marian, Marion, Maryann, Maryanne, Maryanna, Maryane

Marietta (French) Form of Mary, meaning "star of the sea / from the sea of bitterness"
Mariette, Maretta, Mariet, Maryetta, Maryette, Murieta

Marika (Danish) Form of Mary, meaning "star of the sea / from the sea of bitterness"
Marieke, Marijke, Marike, Maryk, Maryka

Mariko (Japanese) Daughter of Mari; a ball or sphere
Maryko, Mareeko, Marieko, Mareiko

Marilyn (English) Form of Mary, meaning "star of the sea / from the sea of bitterness"
Maralin, Maralyn, Maralynn, Marelyn, Marilee, Marilin, Marillyn, Marilynn

Marissa (Latin) Woman of the sea
Maressa, Maricia, Marisabel, Marisha, Marisse, Maritza, Mariza, Marrissa

Marjam (Slavic) One who is merry
Marjama, Marjamah, Marjami, Marjamie, Marjamy, Marjamey, Marjamee, Marjamea

Marjani (African) Of the coral reef
Marjanie, Marjany, Marjaney, Marjanee, Marjean, Marjeani, Marjeanie, Marijani

Marjorie (English) Form of Margaret, meaning "resembling a pearl / the child of light"
Marcharie, Marge, Margeree, Margery, Margerie, Margery, Margey, Margi

Marley (English) Of the marshy meadow
Marlee, Marleigh, Marli, Marlie, Marly

Marlene (German) Blend of Mary, meaning "star of the sea / from the sea of bitterness," and Magdalene, meaning "woman from Magdala"
Marlaina, Marlana, Marlane, Marlayna

Marlis (German) Form of Mary, meaning "star of the sea / from the sea of bitterness"
Marlisa, Marliss, Marlise, Marlisse, Marlissa, Marlys, Marlyss, Marlysa

Marlo (English) One who resembles driftwood
Marloe, Marlow, Marlowe, Marlon

Marmara (Greek) From the sparkling sea
Marmarra, Marmarah, Marmarrah

Marsala (Italian) From the place of sweet wine
Marsalah, Marsalla, Marsallah

Martha (Aramaic) Mistress of the house; in the Bible, the sister of Lazarus and Mary
Maarva, Marfa, Marhta, Mariet, Marit, Mart, Marta, Marte

Marvina (English) Feminine form of Marvin; friend of the sea
Marvinah, Marveena, Marveene, Marvyna, Marvyne, Marvadene, Marvene, Marvena

Marwarid (Arabic) Form of Margaret, meaning "resembling a pearl / the child of light"
Marwaareed, Marwareed, Marwaryd, Marwaryde, Marwaride

•**Mary** (Latin / Hebrew) Star of the sea / from the sea of bitterness
Mair, Mal, Mallie, Manette, Manon, Manya, Mare, Maren, Maria, Marietta, Marika, Marilyn, Marlis, Maureen, May, Mindel, Miriam, Molly, Mia

Maryweld (English) Mary of the woods
Marywelde, Marywelda, Mariweld, Mariwelde, Mariwelda

Masami (African / Japanese) A commanding woman / one who is truthful
Masamie, Masamee, Masamy, Masamey, Masamea

Mashaka (African) A troublemaker; a mischievous woman
Mashakah, Mashakia, Mashake, Mashaki, Mashakie, Mashaky, Mashakey, Mashakee

Ma'sma (Arabic) One who is innocent
Maa'sma

Massachusetts (Native American) From the big hill; from the state of Massachusetts
Massachusets, Massachusette, Massachusetta, Massa, Massachute, Massachusta

Mastura (Arabic) One who is pure; chaste
Mastoora, Masturah, Masturia, Masturiya, Mastooria, Mastoura, Mastrouria

Matana (Hebrew) A gift from God
Matanah, Matanna, Matannah, Matai

Matangi (Hindi) In Hinduism, the patron of inner thought
Matangy, Matangie, Matangee, Matangey, Matangea

Matsuko (Japanese) Child of the pine tree

Maureen (Irish) Form of Mary, meaning "star of the sea / from the sea of bitterness"
Maura, Maurene, Maurianne, Maurine, Maurya, Mavra, Maure, Mo

Mauve (French) Of the mallow plant
Mawve

Maven (English) Having great knowledge
Mavin, Mavyn

Maverick (American) One who is wild and free
Maverik, Maveryck, Maveryk, Mavarick, Mavarik

Mavis (French) Resembling a songbird
Mavise, Maviss, Mavisse, Mavys, Mavyss, Mavysse

Mawunyaga (African) God is great

May (Latin) Born during the month of May; form of Mary, meaning "star of the sea / from the sea of bitterness"
Mae, Mai, Maelynn, Maelee, Maj, Mala, Mayana, Maye

•**Maya** (Indian / Hebrew) An illusion, a dream / woman of the water
Mya

Mayumi (Japanese) One who embodies truth, wisdom, and beauty
Mayumie, Mayumee, Mayumy, Mayumey, Mayumea

Mazarine (French) Having deep-blue eyes
Mazareen, Mazareene, Mazaryn, Mazaryne, Mazine, Mazyne, Mazeene

Mazhira (Hebrew) A shining woman
Mazhirah, Mazheera, Mazhyra, Mazheira, Mazhiera, Mazheara

McKayla (Gaelic) A fiery woman
McKale, McKaylee, McKaleigh, McKay, McKaye, McKaela

Meara (Gaelic) One who is filled with happiness
Mearah

Medea (Greek) A cunning ruler; in mythology, a sorceress
Madora, Medeia, Media, Medeah, Mediah, Mediya, Mediyah

Medini (Indian) Daughter of the earth
Medinie, Mediny, Mediney, Medinee, Medinea

Meditrina (Latin) The healer; in mythology, goddess of health and wine
Meditreena, Meditryna, Meditriena

Medora (Greek) A wise ruler
Medoria, Medorah, Medorra, Medorea

Medusa (Greek) In mythology, a Gorgon with snakes for hair
Medoosa, Medusah, Medoosah, Medousa, Medousah

Meenakshi (Indian)
Having beautiful eyes

Megan (Welsh) Form
of Margaret, meaning
"resembling a pearl / the
child of light"
*Maegan, Meg, Magan,
Magen, Megin, Maygan,
Meagan, Meaghan, Meghan*

Mehalia (Hebrew) An
affectionate woman
*Mehaliah, Mehalea,
Mehaleah, Mehaliya,
Mehaliyah*

Meishan (Chinese)
One who is virtuous
and beautiful
*Meishana, Meishawn,
Meishaun, Meishon*

Meiwei (Chinese) One
who is forever enchanting

Melangell (Welsh) A sweet
messenger from heaven
*Melangelle, Melangela,
Melangella, Melangele,
Melangel*

Melanie (Greek) A dark-
skinned beauty
*Malaney, Malanie, Mel,
Mela, Melaina, Melaine,
Melainey, Melany*

Meli (Native American)
One who is bitter
*Melie, Melee, Melea,
Meleigh, Mely, Meley*

Melia (Hawaiian / Greek)
Resembling the plumeria /
of the ash tree; in mythol-
ogy, a nymph
*Melidice, Melitine, Meliah,
Meelia, Melya*

Melika (Turkish) A great
beauty
*Melikah, Melicka, Melicca,
Melyka, Melycka, Meleeka,
Meleaka*

Melinda (Latin) One who
is sweet and gentle
*Melynda, Malinda, Malinde,
Mallie, Mally, Malynda,
Melinde, Mellinda, Mindy*

Melisande (French) Having
the strength of an animal
*Mulisande, Malissande,
Malyssandre, Melesande,
Melisandra, Melisandre,
Melissande, Melissandre*

Melissa (Greek)
Resembling a honeybee;
in mythology, a nymph
*Malissa, Mallissa, Mel,
Melesa, Melessa, Melisa,
Melise, Melisse*

Melita (Greek) As sweet as
honey
*Malita, Malitta, Melida,
Melitta, Melyta, Malyta,
Meleeta, Meleata*

Melka (Polish) A dark-
skinned beauty
Melkah

Melody (Greek) A beautiful song
Melodee, Melodey, Melodi, Melodia, Melodie, Melodea

Menula (Lithuanian) Born beneath the moon
Menulah, Menoola, Menoolah, Menoula, Menoulah

Mephaath (Hebrew) A lustrous woman
Mephath, Mephatha, Mephaatha

Merana (American) Woman of the waters
Meranah, Meranna, Merannah

Mercer (English) A prosperous merchant

Meredith (Welsh) A great ruler; protector of the sea
Maredud, Meridel, Meredithe, Meredyth, Meridith, Merridie, Meradith, Meredydd

Meribah (Hebrew) A quarrelsome woman
Meriba

Merope (Greek) In mythology, one of the Pleiades
Meropi, Meropie, Meropy, Meropey, Meropee, Meropea

Meroz (Hebrew) From the cursed plains
Meroza, Merozia, Meroze

Merry (English) One who is lighthearted and joyful
Merree, Merri, Merrie, Merrielle, Merrile, Merrilee, Merrili, Merrily

Mertice (English) A well-known lady
Mertise, Mertyce, Mertyse, Mertysa, Mertisa, Mertiece, Merteace

Merton (English) From the village near the pond
Mertan, Mertin, Mertun

Mesopotamia (Hebrew) From the land between two rivers
Mesopotama, Mesopotamea

Metea (Greek) A gentle woman
Meteah, Metia, Metiah

Metin (Greek) A wise counselor
Metine, Metyn, Metyne

Metis (Greek) One who is industrious
Metiss, Metisse, Metys, Metyss, Metysse

Mettalise (Danish) As graceful as a pearl
Metalise, Mettalisse, Mettalisa, Mettalissa

Mhina (African) A delightful lady
Mhinah, Mhinna, Mhena, Mhenah

⁺ᵀ**Mia** (Israeli / Latin) Who is like God? / form of Mary, meaning "star of the sea / from the sea of bitterness"
Miah, Mea, Meah, Meya

⁺ᵀ**Michaela** (Celtic, Gaelic, Hebrew, English, Irish) Feminine form of Michael; who is like God?
*Macaela, MacKayla, **Makayla**, Mak, Mechaela, Meeskaela, Mekea, Micaela*

Michelle (French) Feminine form of Michael; who is like God?
Machelle, Mashelle, M'chelle, Mechelle, Meechelle, Me'Shell, Meshella, Mischa

Michewa (Tibetan) Sent from heaven
Michewah

Michima (Japanese) Possessing beautiful wisdom

Michri (Hebrew) Gift from God
Michrie, Michry, Michrey, Michree, Michrea

Mide (Irish) One who is thirsty
Meeda, Mida

Midori (Japanese) Having green eyes
Midorie, Midory, Midorey, Midoree, Midorea

Mignon (French) One who is cute and petite
Mignonette, Mignonne, Mingnon, Minyonne, Minyonette

Mikayla (English) Feminine form of Michael, meaning "who is like God?"

Mila (Slavic) One who is industrious and hardworking
Milaia, Milaka, Milla, Milia

Milan (Latin) From the city in Italy; one who is gracious
Milaana

Milena (Slavic) The favored one
Mileena, Milana, Miladena, Milanka, Mlada, Mladena

^**Miley** (American) Form of Mili, meaning "a virtuous woman"
*Milee, **Mylee**, Mareli*

Miliana (Latin) Feminine of Emeliano; one who is eager and willing
Milianah, Milianna, Miliane, Miliann, Milianne

Milima (Swahili) Woman from the mountains
Milimah, Mileema, Milyma

Millo (Hebrew) Defender of the sacred city
Milloh, Millowe, Milloe

Miloslava (Russian) Feminine form of Miloslav; having the favor and glory of the people
Miloslavah, Miloslavia, Miloslavea

Mima (Hebrew) Form of Jemima, meaning "our little dove"
Mimah, Mymah, Myma

Minda (Native American, Hindi) Having great knowledge
Mindah, Mynda, Myndah, Menda, Mendah

Mindel (Hebrew) Form of Mary, meaning "star of the sea / from the sea of bitterness"
Mindell, Mindelle, Mindele, Mindela, Mindella

Mindy (English) Form of Melinda, meaning "one who is sweet and gentle"
Minda, Mindee, Mindi, Mindie, Mindey, Mindea

Ming Yue (Chinese) Born beneath the brigh moon

Mingmei (Chinese) A bright and beautiful girl

Minjonet (French) Resembling the small blue flower
Minjonett, Minjonete, Minjonette, Minjoneta, Minjonetta

Minka (Teutonic) One who is resolute; having great strength
Minkah, Mynka, Mynkah, Minna, Minne

Minowa (Native American) One who has a moving voice
Minowah, Mynowa, Mynowah

Minuit (French) Born at midnight
Minueet

Miracle (American) An act of God's hand
Mirakle, Mirakel, Myracle, Myrakle

Miranda (Latin) Worthy of admiration
Maranda, Myranda, Randi

Mirai (Basque / Japanese) A miracle child / future
Miraya, Mirari, Mirarie, Miraree, Mirae

Miremba (Ugandan) A promoter of peace
Mirembe, Mirem, Mirembah, Mirembeh, Mirema

Miriam (Hebrew) Form of Mary, meaning "star of the sea / from the sea of bitterness"
Mariam, Maryam, Meriam, Meryam, Mirham, Mirjam, Mirjana, Mirriam

Mirinesse (English) Filled with joy
Miriness, Mirinese, Mirines, Mirinessa, Mirinesa

Mirit (Hebrew) One who is strong-willed

Miroslava (Slavic) Feminine form of Miroslav; one who basks in peaceful glory
Miroslavia, Miroslavea, Myroslava, Myroslavia, Myroslavea

Mischa (Russian) Form of Michelle, meaning "who is like God?"
Misha

Mistico (Italian) A mystical woman
Mistica, Mystico, Mystica, Mistiko, Mystiko

Misumi (Japanese) A pure, beautiful woman
Misumie, Misumee, Misumy, Misumey, Misumea

Mitali (Indian) A friendly and sweet woman
Mitalie, Mitalee, Mitaleigh, Mitaly, Mitaley, Meeta, Mitalea

Mitexi (Native American) Born beneath the sacred moon
Mitexie, Mitexee, Mitexy, Mitexey, Mitexa, Mitexea

Miya (Japenese) From the sacred temple
Miyah

Miyo (Japanese) A beautiful daughter
Miyoko

Mizar (Hebrew) A little woman; petite
Mizarr, Mizarre, Mizare, Mizara, Mizaria, Mizarra

Mliss (Cambodian) Resembling a flower
Mlissu, Mlisse, Mlyss, Mlysse, Mlyssa

Mocha (Arabic) As sweet as chocolate
Mochah

Modesty (Latin) One who is without conceit
Modesti, Modestie, Modestee, Modestus, Modestey, Modesta, Modestia, Modestina

Moesha (American) Drawn from the water
Moisha, Moysha, Moeesha, Moeasha, Moeysha

Mohini (Indian) The most beautiful
Mohinie, Mohinee, Mohiny, Mohiney, Mohinea

Moladah (Hebrew) A giver
of life
Molada

Molly (Irish) Form of
Mary, meaning "star of
the sea / from the sea of
bitterness"
*Moll, Mollee, Molley, Molli,
Mollie, Molle, Mollea, Mali*

Mona (Gaelic) One who is
born into the nobility
*Moina, Monah, Monalisa,
Monalissa, Monna, Moyna,
Monalysa, Monalyssa*

Monahana (Gaelic) A reli-
gious woman
*Monahanah, Monahanna,
Monahannah*

Moncha (Irish) A solitary
woman
Monchah

Monica (Greek / Latin) A
solitary woman / one who
advises others
*Monnica, Monca, Monicka,
Monika, Monike*

Monique (French) One
who provides wise counsel
*Moniqua, Moneeque,
Moneequa, Moneeke,
Moeneek, Moneaque,
Moneaqua, Moneake*

Monisha (Hindi) Having
great intelligence
*Monishah, Monesha,
Moneisha, Moniesha,
Moneysha, Moneasha*

Monroe (Gaelic) Woman
from the river
Monrow, Monrowe, Monro

Monserrat (Latin) From
the jagged mountain
Montserrat

Montana (Latin) Woman
of the mountains; from
the state of Montana
*Montanna, Montina,
Monteene, Montese*

Morcan (Welsh) Of the
bright sea
*Morcane, Morcana,
Morcania, Morcanea*

Moreh (Hebrew) A great
archer; a teacher

*T**Morgan** (Welsh) Circling
the bright sea; a sea
dweller
*Morgaine, Morgana,
Morgance, Morgane,
Morganica, Morgann,
Morganne, Morgayne*

Morguase (English) In
Arthurian legend, the
mother of Gawain
*Marguase, Margawse,
Morgawse, Morgause,
Margause*

Morina (Japanese) From
the woodland town
*Morinah, Moreena,
Moryna, Moriena, Moreina,
Moreana*

Mubarika (Arabic) One who is blessed
Mubaarika, Mubaricka, Mubaryka, Mubaricca, Mubarycca

Mubina (Arabic) One who displays her true image
Mubeena, Mubinah, Mubyna, Mubeana, Mubiena

Mudan (Mandarin) Daughter of a harmonious family
Mudane, Mudana, Mudann, Mudaen, Mudaena

Mufidah (Arabic) One who is helpful to others
Mufeeda, Mufeyda, Mufyda, Mufeida, Mufieda, Mufeada

Mugain (Irish) In mythology, the wife of the king of Ulster
Mugayne, Mugaine, Mugane, Mugayn, Mugaen, Mugaene, Mugaina, Mugayna

Muirne (Irish) One who is dearly loved
Muirna

Mukantagara (Egyptian) Born during a time of war

Mukarramma (Egyptian) One who is honored and respected
Mukarama, Mukaramma, Mukkarama

Munay (African) One who loves and is loved
Manay, Munaye, Munae, Munai

Munazza (Arabic) An independent woman; one who is free
Munazzah, Munaza, Munazah

Muriel (Irish) Of the shining sea
Merial, Meriel, Merrill, Miureall, Murial, Muriella, Murielle, Merill

Murphy (Celtic) Daughter of a great sea warrior
Murphi, Murphie, Murphey, Murphee, Murfi, Murfy, Murfie, Murphea

Musoke (African) Having the beauty of a rainbow

Mutehhara (Arabic) One who is pure; chaste
Mutehara, Mutehharah, Muteharra, Muteharah

Mya (American) Form of Maya, meaning an illusion, woman of the water
Myah

Myisha (Arabic) Form of Aisha, meaning "lively; womanly"
Myesha, Myeisha, Myeshia, Myiesha, Myeasha

Myka (Hebrew) Feminine of Micah, meaning "who is like God?"
Micah

Myrina (Latin) In mythology, an Amazon
Myrinah, Myreena, Myreina, Myriena, Myreana

Myrrh (Egyptian) Resembling the fragrant oil

n

Naama (Hebrew) Feminine form of Noam; an attractive woman; good-looking
Naamah

Naava (Hebrew) A lovely and pleasant woman
Naavah, Nava, Navah, Navit

Nabila (Arabic) Daughter born into nobility; a high-born daughter
Nabilah, Nabeela, Nabyla, Nabeelah, Nabylah, Nabeala, Nabealah

Nachine (Spanish) A fiery young woman
Nacheene, Nachyne, Nachina, Nachinah, Nachyna, Nacheena

Nadda (Arabic) A very generous woman
Naddah, Nada, Nadah

Nadia (Slavic) One who is full of hope
Nadja, Nadya, Naadiya, Nadine, Nadie, Nadiyah, Nadea, Nadija

Nadirah (Arabic) One who is precious; rare
Nadira, Nadyra, Nadyrah, Nadeera, Nadeerah, Nadra, Nadrah

Naeemah (Egyptian) A kind and benevolent woman
Nayma, Nayima, Nayema

Naeva (French) Born in the evening
Naevah, Naevia, Naevea, Nayva, Nayvah, Nayvia, Nayvea

Nafuna (African) A child who is delivered feetfirst
Nafunah, Nafunna, Nafoona, Nafoonah, Naphuna, Naphunah, Naphoona, Naphoonah

Nagesa (African) Born during the time of harvest
Nagesah, Nagessa, Nagessah

Nagge (Hebrew) A radiant woman

Nagina (Arabic) As precious as a pearl
Nageena, Naginah, Nageenah, Nagyna, Nagynah, Nageana, Nageanah

Nailah (Arabic) Feminine form of Nail; a successful woman; the acquirer
Na'ila, Na'ilah, Naa'ilah, Naila, Nayla, Naylah, Naela, Naelah

Najia (Arabic) An independent woman; one who is free
Naajia

Najja (African) The second-born child
Najjah

Namid (Native American) A star dancer
Namide, Namyd, Namyde

Namita (Papuan) In mythology, a mother goddess
Namitah, Nameeta, Namyta, Nameetah, Namytah, Nameata, Nameatah

Nana (Hawaiian / English) Born during the spring; a star / a grandmother or one who watches over children

Nancy (English) Form of Anna, meaning "a woman graced with God's favor"
Nainsey, Nainsi, Nance, Nancee, Nancey, Nanci, Nancie, Nancsi

Nandalia (Australian) A fiery woman
Nandaliah, Nandalea, Nandaleah, Nandali, Nandalie, Nandalei, Nandalee, Nandaleigh

Nandita (Indian) A delightful daughter
Nanditah, Nanditia, Nanditea

Naomi (Hebrew / Japanese) One who is pleasant / a beauty above all others
Namoie, Nayomi, Naomee

Narella (Greek) A bright woman; intelligent
Narellah, Narela, Narelah, Narelle, Narell, Narele

Nascio (Latin) In mythology, goddess of childbirth

Nashita (Arabic) A lively woman; one who is energetic
Nashitah, Nashyta, Nasheeta, Nasheata, Nashieta, Nasheita

Nasiha (Arabic) One who gives good advice
Naasiha, Nasihah, Naseeha, Naseehah, Nasyha, Nasyhah, Naseaha, Naseahah

Natalia (Spanish / Latin) form of Natalie, born on Christmas day
Natalya, Natalja

*ᴛ**Natalie** (Latin) Refers to Christ's birthday; born on Christmas Day
Natala, Natalee, Natalene, Nataline, Nataly, Natasha

Natane (Native American) Her father's daughter
Natanne

Natasha (Russian) Form of Natalie, meaning "born on Christmas Day"
Nastaliya, Nastalya, Natacha, Natascha, Natashenka, Natashia, Natasia, Natosha, Tosha

Natividad (Spanish) Refers to the Nativity
Natividade, Natividada, Natyvydad, Nativydad, Natyvidad

Natsuko (Japanese) Child born during the summer
Natsu, Natsumi

Navida (Iranian) Feminine form of Navid; bringer of good news
Navyda, Navidah, Navyda, Naveeda, Naveedah, Naveada, Naveadah

Navya (Indian) One who is youthful
Navyah, Naviya, Naviyah

Nawal (Arabic) A gift of God
Nawall, Nawalle, Nawala, Nawalla

Nawar (Arabic) Resembling a flower
Nawaar

Nazahah (Arabic) One who is pure and honest
Nazaha, Nazihah, Naziha

Nechama (Hebrew) One who provides comfort
Nehama, Nehamah, Nachmanit, Nachuma, Nechamah, Nechamit

Neda (Slavic) Born on a Sunday
Nedda, Nedah, Nedi, Nedie, Neddi, Neddie, Nedaa

Neeharika (Indian) Of the morning dew
Neharika, Neeharyka, Neharyka

Neena (Hindi) A woman who has beautiful eyes
Neenah, Neanah, Neana, Neyna, Neynah

Nefertiti (Egyptian) A queenly woman
Nefertari, Nefertyty, Nefertity, Nefertitie, Nefertitee, Nefertytie, Nefertitea

Neith (Egyptian) In mythology, goddess of war and hunting
Neitha, Neytha, Neyth, Neit, Neita, Neitia, Neitea, Neithe

Nekana (Spanish) Woman of sorrow
Nekane, Nekania, Nekanea

Neneca (Spanish) Form of Amelia, meaning "one who is industrious and hardworking"
Nenecah, Nenica, Nenneca, Nennica

Neo (African) A gift from God

Nephthys (Egyptian) In mythology, one of the nine most important deities; the lady of the house
Nebt-het, Nebet-het

Nerissa (Italian / Greek) A black-haired beauty / sea nymph
Narissa, Naryssa, Nericcia, Neryssa, Narice, Nerice, Neris

Nessa (Hebrew / Greek) A miracle child / form of Agnes, meaning "one who is pure; chaste"
Nesha, Nessah, Nessia, Nessya, Nesta, Neta, Netia, Nessie

Netis (Native American) One who is trustworthy
Netiss, Netisse, Netys, Netyss, Netysse

*Nevaeh** (American) Child from heaven

Nevina (Scottish) Feminine form of Nevin; daughter of a saint
Nevinah, Neveena, Nevyna, Nevinne, Nevynne, Neveene, Neveana, Neveane

Newlyn (Gaelic) Born during the spring
Newlynn, Newlynne, Newlin, Newlinn, Newlinne, Newlen, Newlenn, Newlenne

Neziah (Hebrew) One who is pure; a victorious woman
Nezia, Nezea, Nezeah, Neza, Nezah, Neziya, Neziyah

Niabi (Native American) Resembling a fawn
Niabie, Niabee, Niabey, Niaby, Nyabi, Nyabie, Niabea, Nyabea

Niagara (English) From the famous waterfall
Niagarah, Niagarra, Niagarrah, Nyagara, Nyagarra

Nicole (Greek) Feminine form of Nicholas; of the victorious people
Necole, Niccole, Nichol, Nichole, Nicholle, Nickol, Nickole, Nicol

Nicosia (English) Woman from the capital of Cyprus
Nicosiah, Nicosea, Nicoseah, Nicotia, Nicotea

Nidia (Spanish) One who is gracious
Nydia, Nidiah, Nydiah, Nidea, Nideah, Nibia, Nibiah, Nibea

Nighean (Scottish) A
young woman; a maiden
Nighinn, Nigheen

Nike (Greek) One who
brings victory; in mythology, goddess of victory
Nikee, Nikey, Nykee, Nyke

Nilam (Arabic) Resembling
a precious blue stone
*Neelam, Nylam, Nilima,
Nilyma, Nylyma, Nylima,
Nealam, Nealama*

Nilsine (Scandinavian)
Feminine form of Neil; a
champion
*Nilsina, Nilsyne, Nilsyna,
Nylsine, Nylsyna, Nylsina,
Nylsyne, Nilsa*

Nimeesha (African) A
princess; daughter born to
royalty
*Nimeeshah, Nimiesha,
Nimisha, Nimysha,
Nymeesha, Nymisha,
Nymysha, Nimeasha*

Nini (African) As solid as
a stone
*Ninie, Niny, Niney, Ninee,
Ninea*

Nishan (African) One who
wins awards
*Nishann, Nishanne,
Nishana, Nishanna,
Nyshan, Nyshana*

Nitya (Indian) An eternal
beauty
Nithya, Nithyah, Nityah

Nixie (German) A beauti-
ful water sprite
*Nixi, Nixy, Nixey, Nixee,
Nixea*

Nizhoni (Native American)
A beautiful woman
*Nizhonie, Nyzhoni,
Nyzhonie, Nizhony,
Nizhoney, Nizhonea,
Nyzhony, Nyzhoney*

ˆ**Noel** (French) Born at
Christmastime
Noelle, Noela, Noele, Noe

Nokomis (Native
American) A daughter of
the moon
*Nokomiss, Nokomisse,
Nokomys, Nokomyss,
Nokomysse*

Nolcha (Native American)
Of the sun
Nolchia, Nolchea

Nomusa (African) One
who is merciful
*Nomusah, Nomusha,
Nomusia, Nomusea,
Nomushia, Nomushea*

Nora (English) Form of
Eleanor, meaning "the
shining light"
*Norah, Noora, Norella,
Norelle, Norissa, Norri,
Norrie, Norry*

Nordica (German) Woman from the north
Nordika, Nordicka, Nordyca, Nordyka, Nordycka, Norda, Norell, Norelle

Nosiwe (African) Mother of the homeland

Noura (Arabic) Having an inner light
Nureh, Nourah, Nure

Nsia (African) The sixth-born child

Nsonowa (African) The seventh-born child

Nuo (Chinese) A graceful woman

Nyala (African) Resembling an antelope
Nyalah, Nyalla, Nyallah

Nyneve (English) In Arthurian legend, another name for the lady of the lake
Nineve, Niniane, Ninyane, Nyniane, Ninieve, Niniveve

Nyura (Ukrainian) A graceful woman
Nyrurah, Nyrurra, Niura, Neura

Oaisara (Arabic) A great ruler; an empress
Oaisarah, Oaisarra, Oaisarrah

Oamra (Arabic) Daughter of the moon
Oamrah, Oamira, Oamyra, Oameera

Oba (African) In mythology, the goddess of rivers
Obah, Obba, Obbah

Obioma (African) A kind and caring woman
Obiomah, Obeoma, Obeomah, Obyoma, Obyomah

Octavia (Latin) Feminine form of Octavius; the eighth-born child
Octaviana, Octavianne, Octavie, Octiana, Octoviana, Ottavia, Octavi, Octavy

Odahingum (Native American) Of the rippling waters

Oddrun (Scandinavian) Our secret love

Oddveig (Scandinavian) One who wields a spear

Ode (Egyptian / Greek)
Traveler of the road / a
lyric poem
Odea

Odessa (Greek) Feminine
form of Odysseus; one who
wanders; an angry woman
*Odissa, Odyssa, Odessia,
Odissia, Odyssia, Odysseia*

Odina (Latin /
Scandinavian) From the
mountain / feminine
form of Odin, the highest
of the gods
*Odinah, Odeena, Odeene,
Odeen, Odyna, Odyne,
Odynn, Odeana*

Ogenya (Hebrew) God
provides assistance
*Ogenyah, Ogeniya,
Ogeniyah*

Ogin (Native American)
Resembling the wild rose

Oheo (Native American) A
beautiful woman

Oira (Latin) One who
prays to God
Oyra, Oirah, Oyrah

Okalani (Hawaiian) From
the heavens
*Okalanie, Okalany,
Okalaney, Okalanee,
Okaloni, Okalonie,
Okalonee, Okalony*

Okei (Japanese) Woman of
the ocean

Oksana (Russian)
Hospitality
Oksanah, Oksie, Aksana

Ola (Nigerian / Hawaiian
/ Norse) One who is pre-
cious / giver of life; well-
being / a relic of one's
ancestors
Olah, Olla, Ollah

Olaide (American) A
thoughtful woman
*Olaid, Olaida, Olayd,
Olayde, Olayda, Olaed,
Olaede, Olaeda*

Olathe (Native American)
A lovely young woman

Olaug (Scandinavian) A
loyal woman

Olayinka (Yoruban)
Surrounded by wealth and
honor
Olayenka, Olayanka

Oldriska (Czech) A noble
ruler
*Oldryska, Oldri, Oldrie,
Oldry, Oldrey, Oldree,
Oldrea*

Oleda (English) Resembling
a winged creature
*Oldedah, Oleta, Olita,
Olida, Oletah, Olitah,
Olidah*

Olethea (Latin) Form of
Alethea, meaning "one
who is truthful"
*Oletheia, Olethia, Oletha,
Oletea, Olthaia, Olithea,
Olathea, Oletia*

Olina (Hawaiian) One who
is joyous
*Oline, Oleen, Oleene,
Olyne, Oleena, Olyna, Olin*

*ˈ***Olivia** (Latin) Feminine
form of Oliver; of the olive
tree; one who is peaceful
*Oliviah, Oliva, Olive,
Oliveea, Olivet, Olivetta,
Olivette, Olivija*

Olwen (Welsh) One who
leaves a white footprint
Olwynn, Olvyen, Olvyin

Olympia (Greek) From
Mount Olympus; a god-
dess
*Olympiah, Olimpe,
Olimpia, Olimpiada,
Olimpiana, Olypme,
Olympie, Olympi*

Omri (Arabic) A red-haired
woman
*Omrie, Omree, Omrea,
Omry, Omrey*

Omusa (African) One who
is adored
Omusah, Omousa, Omousah

Ona (Hebrew) Filled with
grace
Onit, Onat, Onah

Ondine (Latin) Resembling
a small wave
*Ondina, Ondyne, Ondinia,
Ondyna*

Ondrea (Slavic) Form of
Andrea, meaning "coura-
geous and strong / wom-
anly"
*Ondria, Ondrianna,
Ondreia, Ondreina,
Ondreya, Ondriana,
Ondreana, Ondera*

Oneida (Native American)
Our long-awaited daughter
*Onieda, Oneyda, Onida,
Onyda*

Onida (Native American)
The one who has been
expected
Onidah, Onyda, Onydah

Ontibile (African)
Protected by God
*Ontibyle, Ontybile,
Ontybyle*

Ontina (American) An
open-minded woman
*Ontinah, Onteena,
Onteenah, Onteana,
Onteanah, Ontiena,
Ontienah, Onteina*

Oona (Gaelic) Form of
Agnes, meaning "one who
is pure; chaste"
*Oonaugh, Oonagh, Oonah,
Ouna, Ounah, Ounagh,
Ounaugh*

Opal (Sanskrit) A treasured jewel; resembling the iridescent gemstone
Opall, Opalle, Opale, Opalla, Opala, Opalina, Opaline, Opaleena

Ophelia (Greek) One who offers help to others
Ofelia, Ofilia, OphÈlie, Ophelya, Ophilia, Ovalia, Ovelia, Opheliah

Ophrah (Hebrew) Resembling a fawn; from the place of dust
Ofra, Ofrit, Ophra, Oprah, Orpa, Orpah, Ofrat, Ofrah

Oraleyda (Spanish) Born with the light of dawn
Oraleydah, Oraleida, Oraleidah, Oralida, Oralidah, Oralyda, Oralydah, Oraleda

Orange (Latin) Resembling the sweet fruit
Orangetta, Orangia, Orangina, Orangea

Orbelina (American) One who brings excitement
Orbelinah, Orbeleena, Orbeleenah, Orbeleana, Orbeleanah, Orbelyna, Orbelynah, Orbie

Orea (Greek) From the mountains
Oreah

Orenda (Iroquois Indian) A woman with magical powers

Oriana (Latin) Born at sunrise
Oreana, Orianna, Oriane, Oriann, Orianne

Oribel (Latin) A beautiful golden child
Orabel, Orabelle, Orabell, Orabela, Orabella, Oribell, Oribelle, Oribele

Orin (Irish) A dark-haired beauty
Orine, Orina, Oryna, Oryn, Oryne

Orinthia (Hebrew / Gaelic) Of the pine tree / a fair lady
Orrinthia, Orenthia, Orna, Ornina, Orinthea, Orenthea, Orynthia, Orynthea

Oriole (Latin) Resembling the gold-speckled bird
Oreolle, Oriolle, Oreole, Oriola, Oriolla, Oriol, Oreola, Oreolla

Orion (Greek) The huntress; a constellation

Orithna (Greek) One who is natural
Orithne, Orythna, Orythne, Orithnia, Orythnia, Orithnea, Orythnea

Orla (Gaelic) The golden queen
Orlah, Orrla, Orrlah, Orlagh, Orlaith, Orlaithe, Orghlaith, Orghlaithe

Orna (Irish / Hebrew) One who is pale-skinned / of the cedar tree
Ornah, Ornette, Ornetta, Ornete, Orneta, Obharnait, Ornat

Ornella (Italian) Of the flowering ash tree

Ornice (Irish) A pale-skinned woman
Ornyce, Ornise, Orynse, Orneice, Orneise, Orniece, Orniese, Orneece

Ortygia (Greek) In mythology, an island where Artemis and Apollo were born
Ortegia, Ortigia

Orva (Anglo-Saxon / French) A courageous friend / as precious as gold

Orynko (Ukrainian) A peaceful woman
Orinko, Orynka, Orinka

Osaka (Japanese) From the city of industry
Osaki, Osakie, Osakee, Osaky, Osakey, Osakea

Osma (English) Feminine form of Osmond; protected by God
Osmah, Ozma, Ozmah

Otina (American) A fortunate woman
Otinah, Otyna, Otynah, Oteena, Oteenah, Oteana, Oteanah, Otiena

Ourania (Greek) A heavenly woman
Ouraniah, Ouranea, Ouraneah, Ouraniya, Ouraniyah

Overton (English) From the upper side of town
Overtown

Owena (Welsh) A high-born woman
Owenah, Owenna, Owennah, Owenia, Owenea

Ozora (Hebrew) One who is wealthy
Ozorah, Ozorra, Ozorrah

p

Paavna (Hindi) One who is pure; chaste
Pavna, Paavnah, Pavnah, Paavani, Pavani, Pavany, Pavaney, Pavanie

Pace (American) A charismatic young woman
Paice, Payce, Paeece, Pase, Paise, Payse, Paese

Pacifica (Spanish) A peaceful woman
Pacifika, Pacyfyca, Pacyfyka, Pacifyca, Pacifyka, Pacyfica, Pacyfika

Pageant (American) A dramatic woman
Pagent, Padgeant, Padgent

*Paige** (English) A young assistant
Page, Payge, Paege

^**Paisley** (English) Woman of the church

Paki (African) A witness of God
Pakki, Packi, Pacci, Pakie, Pakkie, Paky, Pakky, Pakey

Palakika (Hawaiian) One who is dearly loved
Palakyka, Palakeka, Palakeeka, Palakieka, Palakeika, Palakeaka

Palba (Spanish) A fair-haired woman

Palemon (Spanish) A kindhearted woman
Palemond, Palemona, Palemonda

Palesa (African) Resembling a flower
Palessa, Palesah, Palysa, Palisa, Paleesa

Paloma (Spanish) Dove-like
Palloma, Palomita, Palometa, Peloma, Aloma

Pamela (English) A woman who is as sweet as honey
Pamelah, Pamella, Pammeli, Pammelie, Pameli, Pamelie, Pamelia, Pamelea

Panagiota (Greek) Feminine form of Panagiotis; a holy woman

Panchali (Indian) A princess; a high-born woman
Panchalie, Panchaly, Panchalli, Panchaley, Panchalee, Panchalea, Panchaleigh

Panda (English) Resembling the bamboo-eating animal
Pandah

Pandara (Indian) A good wife
Pandarah, Pandarra, Pandaria, Pandarea

Pandora (Greek) A gifted, talented woman; in mythology, the first mortal woman, who unleashed evil upon the world
Pandorah, Pandorra, Pandoria, Pandorea, Pandoriya

Pantxike (Latin) A woman who is free
Pantxikey, Pantxikye, Pantxeke, Pantxyke

Paras (Indian) A woman against whom others are measured

Parcae (Latin) In mythology, a name that refers to the Fates
Parca, Parcia, Parcee, Parsae, Parsee, Parsia, Parcea

Paris (English) Woman of the city in France
Pariss, Parisse, Parys, Paryss, Parysse

Parry (Welsh) Daughter of Harry
Parri, Parrie, Parrey, Parree, Parrea

Parvani (Indian) Born during a full moon
Parvanie, Parvany, Parvaney, Parvanee, Parvanea

Parvati (Hindi) Daughter of the mountain; in Hinduism, a name for the wife of Shiva
Parvatie, Parvaty, Parvatey, Parvatee, Pauravi, Parvatea, Pauravie, Pauravy

Paterekia (Hawaiian) An upper-class woman
Paterekea, Pakelekia, Pakelekea

Patience (English) One who is patient; an enduring woman
Patiencia, Paciencia, Pacencia, Pacyncia, Pacincia, Pacienca

Patricia (English) Feminine form of Patrick; of noble descent
Patrisha, Patrycia, Patrisia, Patsy, Patti, Patty, Patrizia, Pattie, Trisha

Patrina (American) Born into the nobility
Patreena, Patriena, Patreina, Patryna, Patreana

Paula (English) Feminine form of Paul; a petite woman
Paulina, Pauline, Paulette, Paola, Pauleta, Pauletta, Pauli, Paulete

Pausha (Hindi) Resembling the moon
Paushah

Pax (Latin) One who is peaceful; in mythology, the goddess of peace
Paxi, Paxie, Paxton, Paxten, Paxtan, Paxy, Paxey, Paxee

^**Payton** (English) From the warrior's village
Paton, Paeton, Paiton, Payten, Paiten

Pearl (Latin) A precious gem of the sea
Pearla, Pearle, Pearlie, Pearly, Pearline, Pearlina, Pearli, Pearley

Pelopia (Greek) In mythology, the wife of Thyestes and mother of Aegisthus
Pelopiah, Pelopea, Pelopeah, Pelopiya

Pembroke (English) From the broken hill
Pembrook, Pembrok, Pembrooke

Pendant (French) A decorated woman
Pendent, Pendante, Pendente

^**Penelope** (Greek) Resembling a duck; in mythology, the faithful wife of Odysseus
Peneloppe, Penelopy, Penelopey, Penelopi, Penelopie, Penelopee, Penella, Penelia

Penia (Greek) In mythology, the personification of poverty
Peniah, Penea, Peniya, Peneah, Peniyah

Penthesilea (Greek) In mythology, a queen of the Amazons

Peony (Greek) Resembling the flower
Peoney, Peoni, Peonie, Peonee, Peonea

Pepin (French) An awe-inspiring woman
Peppin, Pepine, Peppine, Pipin, Pippin, Pepen, Pepan, Peppen

Pepita (Spanish) Feminine form of Joseph; God will add
Pepitah, Pepitta, Pepitia, Pepitina

Perdita (Latin) A lost woman
Perditah, Perditta, Perdy, Perdie, Perdi, Perdee, Perdea, Perdeeta

Perdix (Latin) Resembling a partridge
Perdixx, Perdyx, Perdyxx

Peri (Persian / English) In mythology, a fairy / from the pear tree
Perry, Perri, Perie, Perrie, Pery, Perrey, Perey, Peree

Perpetua (Latin) One who is constant; steadfast

Persephone (Greek) In mythology, the daughter of Demeter and Zeus who was abducted to the underworld
Persephoni, Persephonie, Persephony, Persephoney, Persephonee, Persefone, Persefoni, Persefonie

Persis (Greek) Woman of Persia
Persiss, Persisse, Persys, Persyss, Persysse

Pesha (Hebrew) A flourishing woman
Peshah, Peshia, Peshiah, Peshea, Pesheah, Peshe

Petronela (Latin) Feminine form of Peter, as solid and strong as a rock
Petronella, Petronelle, Petronia, Petronilla, Petronille, Petrona, Petronia, Petronel

Petunia (English) Resembling the flower
Petuniah, Petuniya, Petunea, Petoonia, Petounia

*^**Peyton** (English) From the warrior's village
Peyten

Phaedra (Greek) A bright woman; in mythology, the wife of Theseus
Phadra, Phaidra, Phedra, Phaydra, Phedre, Phaedre

Phailin (Thai) Resembling a sapphire
Phaylin, Phaelin, Phalin

Phashestha (American) One who is decorated
Phashesthea, Phashesthia, Phashesthiya

Pheakkley (Vietnamese) A faithful woman
Pheakkly, Pheakkli, Pheakklie, Pheakklee, Pheakkleigh, Pheakklea

Pheodora (Greek) A supreme gift
Pheodorah, Phedora, Phedorah

Phernita (American) A well-spoken woman
Pherneeta, Phernyta, Phernieta, Pherneita, Pherneata

Phia (Italian) A saintly woman
Phiah, Phea, Pheah

Philippa (English) Feminine form of Phillip; a friend of horses
Phillippa, Philipa, Phillipa, Philipinna, Philippine, Phillipina, Phillipine, Pilis

Philomena (Greek) A friend of strength
Filomena, Philomina, Mena

Phoebe (Greek) A bright, shining woman; in mythology, another name for the goddess of the moon
Phebe, Phoebi, Phebi, Phoebie, Phebie, Pheobe, Phoebee, Phoebea

Phoena (Greek) Resembling a mystical bird
Phoenah, Phoenna, Phena, Phenna

Phoenix (Greek) A dark-red color; in mythology, an immortal bird
Phuong, Phoenyx

Phyllis (Greek) Of the foliage; in mythology, a girl who was turned into an almond tree
Phylis, Phillis, Philis, Phylys, Phyllida, Phylida, Phillida, Philida

Pili (Egyptian) The second-born child
Pilie, Pily, Piley, Pilee, Pilea, Pileigh

Pililani (Hawaiian) Having great strength
Pililanie, Pililany, Pililaney, Pililanee, Pililanea

Piluki (Hawaiian) Resembling a small leaf
Pilukie, Piluky, Pilukey, Pilukee, Pilukea

Pineki (Hawaiian) Resembling a peanut
Pinekie, Pineky, Pinekey, Pinekee, Pinekea

Ping (Chinese) One who is peaceful
Pyng

Pinga (Inuit) In mythology, goddess of the hunt, fertility, and healing
Pingah, Pyngah, Pyngah

Pinquana (Native American) Having a pleasant fragrance
Pinquan, Pinquann, Pinquanne, Pinquanna, Pinquane

Piper (English) One who plays the flute
Pipere, Piperel, Piperell, Piperele, Piperelle, Piperela, Piperella, Pyper

Pippi (French / English) A friend of horses / a blushing young woman
Pippie, Pippy, Pippey, Pippee, Pippea

Pirouette (French) A ballet dancer
Piroette, Pirouett, Piroett, Piroueta, Piroeta, Pirouetta, Piroetta, Pirouet

Pisces (Latin) The twelfth sign of the zodiac; the fishes
Pysces, Piscees, Pyscees, Piscez, Pisceez

Pithasthana (Hindi) In Hinduism, a name for the wife of Shiva

Platinum (English) As precious as the metal
Platynum, Platnum, Platie, Plati, Platee, Platy, Platey, Platea

Platt (French) From the plains
Platte

Pleshette (American) An extravagent woman
Pleshett, Pleshet, Pleshete, Plesheta, Pleshetta

Pleun (American) One who is good with words
Pleune

Po (Italian) A lively woman

Podarge (Greek) In mythology, one of the Harpies

Poetry (American) A romantic woman
Poetrey, Poetri, Poetrie, Poetree, Poetrea

Polete (Hawaiian) A kind young woman
Polet, Polett, Polette, Poleta, Poletta

Polina (Russian) A small woman
Polinah, Poleena, Poleenah, Poleana, Poleunah, Poliena, Polienah, Poleina

Polyxena (Greek) In mythology, a daughter of Priam and loved by Achilles
Polyxenah, Polyxenia, Polyxenna, Polyxene, Polyxenea

Pomona (Latin) In mythology, goddess of fruit trees
Pomonah, Pomonia, Pomonea, Pamona, Pamonia, Pamonea

Poni (African) The second-born daughter
Ponni, Ponie, Ponnie, Pony, Ponny, Poney, Ponney, Ponee

Poodle (American) Resembling the dog; one with curly hair
Poudle, Poodel, Poudel

Poonam (Hindi) A kind and caring woman
Pounam

Porter (Latin) The doorkeeper

Posala (Native American) Born at the end of spring
Posalah, Posalla, Posallah

Posh (American) A fancy young woman
Poshe, Posha

Potina (Latin) In mythology, goddess of children's food and drink
Potinah, Potyna, Potena, Poteena, Potiena, Poteina, Poteana

Powder (American) A light-hearted woman
Powdar, Powdir, Powdur, Powdor, Powdi, Powdie, Powdy, Powdey

Praise (Latin) One who expresses admiration
Prayse, Praize, Prayze, Praze, Praese, Praeze

Pramada (Indian) One who is indifferent

Pramlocha (Hindi) In Hinduism, a celestial nymph

Precious (American) One who is treasured
Preshis, Preshys

Prima (Latin) The firstborn child
Primalia, Primma, Pryma, Primia, Primea, Preema, Preama

Primola (Latin) Resembling a primrose
Primolah, Primolia, Primoliah, Primolea, Primoleah

Princess (English) A high-born daughter; born to royalty
Princessa, Princesa, Princie, Princi, Princy, Princee, Princey, Princea

Prisca (Latin) From an ancient family
Priscilla, Priscella, Precilla, Presilla, Prescilla, Prisilla, Prisella, Prissy, Prissi

Promise (American) A faithful woman
Promice, Promyse, Promyce, Promis, Promiss, Promys, Promyss

Prudence (English) One who is cautious and exercises good judgment
Prudencia, Prudensa, Prudensia, Prudentia, Predencia, Predentia, Prue, Pru

Pryce (American / Welsh) One who is very dear / an enthusiastic child
Price, Prise, Pryse

Pulcheria (Italian) A chubby baby
Pulcheriah, Pulcherea, Pulchereah, Pulcherya, Pulcheryah, Pulcheriya

Pulika (African) An obedient and well-behaved girl
Pulikah, Pulicca, Pulicka, Pulyka, Puleeka, Puleaka

Pyrena (Greek) A fiery woman
Pyrenah, Pyrina, Pyrinah, Pyryna, Pyrynah, Pyreena, Pyreenah, Pyriena

Pyria (American) One who is cherished
Pyriah, Pyrea, Pyreah, Pyriya, Pyriyah, Pyra

q

Qadesh (Syrian) In mythology, goddess of love and sensuality
Quedesh, Qadesha, Quedesha, Qadeshia, Quedeshia, Quedeshiya

Qamra (Arabic) Of the moon
Qamrah, Qamar, Qamara, Qamrra, Qamaria, Qamrea, Qamria

Qimat (Indian) A valuable woman
Qimate, Qimatte, Qimata, Qimatta

Qitarah (Arabic) Having a nice fragrance
Qitara, Qytarah, Qytara, Qitaria, Qitarra, Qitarria, Qytarra, Qytarria

Qoqa (Chechen) Resembling a dove

Quana (Native American) One who is aromatic; sweet-smelling
Quanah, Quanna, Quannah, Quania, Quaniya, Quanniya, Quannia, Quanea

Querida (Spanish) One who is dearly loved; beloved
Queridah, Queryda, Querydah, Querrida, Queridda, Querridda, Quereeda, Quereada

Queta (Spanish) Head of the household
Quetah, Quetta, Quettah

Quiana (American) Living with grace; heavenly
Quianah, Quianna, Quiane, Quian, Quianne, Quianda, Quiani, Quianita

Quincy (English) The fifth-born child
Quincey, Quinci, Quincie, Quincee, Quincia, Quinncy, Quinnci, Quyncy

Quintana (Latin / English) The fifth girl / queen's lawn
Quintanah, Quinella, Quinta, Quintina, Quintanna, Quintann, Quintara, Quintona

Quintessa (Latin) Of the essence
Quintessah, Quintesa, Quintesha, Quintisha, Quintessia, Quyntessa, Quintosha, Quinticia

Quinyette (American) The fifth-born child
Quinyett, Quinyet, Quinyeta, Quinyette, Quinyete

Quirina (Latin) One who is contentious
Quirinah, Quiryna, Quirynah, Quireena, Quireenah, Quireina, Quireinah, Quiriena

Quiritis (Latin) In mythology, goddess of motherhood
Quiritiss, Quiritisse, Quirytis, Quirytys, Quiritys, Quirityss

Quiterie (French) One who is peaceful; tranquil
Quiteri, Quitery, Quiterey, Quiteree, Quiterye, Quyterie, Quyteri, Quyteree

r

Rabiah (Egyptian / Arabic) Born in the springtime / of the gentle wind
Rabia, Raabia, Rabi'ah, Rabi

Rachana (Hindi) Born of the creation
Rachanna, Rashana, Rashanda, Rachna

•Rachel (Hebrew) The innocent lamb; in the Bible, Jacob's wife
Rachael, Racheal, Rachelanne, Rachelce, Rachele, Racheli, Rachell, Rachelle, Raquel

Radcliffe (English) Of the red cliffs
Radcleff, Radclef, Radclif, Radclife, Radclyffe, Radclyf, Radcliphe, Radclyphe

Radella (English) An elfin counselor
Radell, Radel, Radele, Radella, Radela, Raedself, Radself, Raidself

Radmilla (Slavic) Hardworking for the people
Radilla, Radinka, Radmila, Redmilla, Radilu

Rafi'a (Arabic) An exalted woman
Rafia, Rafi'ah, Rafee'a, Rafeea, Rafeeah, Rafiya, Rafiyah

Ragnara (Swedish) Feminine form of Ragnar; one who provides counsel to the army
Ragnarah, Ragnarra, Ragnaria, Ragnarea, Ragnari, Ragnarie, Ragnary, Ragnarey

Rahi (Arabic) Born during the springtime
Rahii, Rahy, Rahey, Rahee, Rahea, Rahie

Rahimah (Arabic) A compassionate woman; one who is merciful
Rahima, Raheema, Raheemah, Raheima, Rahiema, Rahyma, Rahymah, Raheama

Raina (Polish) Form of Regina, meaning "a queenly woman"
Raenah, Raene, Rainah, Raine, Rainee, Rainey, Rainelle, Rainy

Raja (Arabic) One who is filled with hope
Rajah

Raleigh (English) From the clearing of roe deer
Raileigh, Railey, Raley, Rawleigh, Rawley, Raly, Rali, Ralie

Ramona (Spanish) Feminine form of Ramon; a wise protector
Ramee, Ramie, Ramoena, Ramohna, Ramonda, Ramonde, Ramonita, Ramonna

Randi (English) Feminine form of Randall; shielded by wolves; form of Miranda, meaning "worthy of admiration"
Randa, Randee, Randelle, Randene, Randie, Randy, Randey, Randilyn

Raquel (Spanish) Form of Rachel, meaning "the innocent lamb"
Racquel, Racquell, Raquela, Raquelle, Roquel, Roquela, Rakel, Rakell

Rasha (Arabic) Resembling a young gazelle
Rashah, Raisha, Raysha, Rashia, Raesha

Ratana (Thai) Resembling a crystal
Ratanah, Ratanna, Ratannah, Rathana, Rathanna

Rati (Hindi) In Hinduism, goddess of passion and lust
Ratie, Ratea, Ratee, Raty, Ratey

Ratri (Indian) Born in the evening
Ratrie, Ratry, Ratrey, Ratree, Ratrea

Rawiyah (Arabic) One who recites ancient poetry
Rawiya, Rawiyya, Rawiyyah

Rawnie (English) An elegant lady
Rawni, Rawny, Rawney, Rawnee, Rawnea

Raya (Israeli) A beloved friend
Rayah

Raymonde (German) Feminine form of Raymond; one who offers wise protection
Raymondi, Raymondie, Raymondee, Raymondea, Raymonda, Raymunde, Raymunda

Rayna (Hebrew / Scandinavian) One who is pure / one who provides wise counsel
Raynah, Raynee, Rayni, Rayne, Raynea, Raynie

Reba (Hebrew) Form of Rebecca, meaning "one who is bound to God"
Rebah, Reeba, Rheba, Rebba, Ree, Reyba, Reaba

•**Rebecca** (Hebrew) One who is bound to God; in the Bible, the wife of Isaac
Rebakah, Rebbeca, Rebbecca, Rebbecka, Rebeca, Rebeccah, Rebeccea, Becky, Reba

Reese (American) Form of Rhys, meaning having great enthusiasm for life
Rhyss, Rhysse, Reece, Reice, Reise, Reace, Rease, Riece

Regan (Gaelic) Born into royalty; the little ruler
Raegan, Ragan, Raygan, Reganne, Regann, Regane, Reghan, Reagan

Regina (Latin) A queenly woman
Regeena, Regena, Reggi, Reggie, Régine, Regine, Reginette, Reginia, Raina

Rehan (Armenian) Resembling a flower
Rehane, Rehann, Rehanne, Rehana, Rehanna, Rehanan, Rehannan, Rehania

Rehoboth (Hebrew) From the city by the river
Rehobothe, Rehobotha, Rehobothia

Rekha (Indian) One who walks a straight line
Rekhah, Reka, Rekah

Remy (French) Woman from the town of Rheims
Remi, Remie, Remmy, Remmi, Remmie, Remy, Remmey, Remey

Ren (Japanese) Resembling a water lily

Renée (French) One who has been reborn
Ranae, Ranay, Ranée, Renae, Renata, Renay, Renaye, René

Reseda (Latin) Resembling the mignonette flower
Resedah, Reselda, Resedia, Reseldia

Resen (Hebrew) From the head of the stream; refers to a bridle

Reshma (Arabic) Having silky skin
Reshmah, Reshman, Reshmane, Reshmann, Reshmanne, Reshmana, Reshmanna, Reshmaan

Reya (Spanish) A queenly woman
Reyah, Reyeh, Reye, Reyia, Reyiah, Reyea, Reyeah

Reza (Hungarian) Form of Theresa, meaning "a harvester"
Rezah, Rezia, Reziah, Rezi, Rezie, Rezy, Rezee, Resi

Rezeph (Hebrew) As solid
as a stone
*Rezepha, Rezephe, Rezephia,
Rezephah, Rezephiah*

Rhea (Greek) Of the flowing stream; in mythology,
the wife of Cronus and
mother of gods and god-
desses
*Rea, Rhae, Rhaya, Rhia,
Rhiah, Rhiya, Rheya*

Rheda (Anglo-Saxon) A
divine woman; a goddess
Rhedah

Rhiannon (Welsh) The
great and sacred queen
*Rheanna, Rheanne,
Rhiana, Rhiann, Rhianna,
Rhiannan, Rhianon, Rhyan*

Rhonda (Welsh) Wielding
a good spear
*Rhondelle, Rhondene,
Rhondiesha, Rhonette,
Rhonnda, Ronda, Rondel,
Rondelle*

Rhys (Welsh) Having great
enthusiasm for life
*Rhyss, Rhysse, Reece, Reese,
Reice, Reise, Reace, Rease*

Ria (Spanish) From the
river's mouth
Riah

Riane (Gaelic) Feminine
form of Ryan; little ruler
*Riana, Rianna, Rianne,
Ryann, Ryanne, Ryana,
Ryanna, Riann*

Rica (English) Form of
Frederica, meaning "peaceful ruler"; form of Erica,
meaning "ever the ruler /
resembling heather"
*Rhica, Ricca, Ricah, Rieca,
Riecka, Rieka, Riqua, Ryca*

Riddhi (Indian) A prosper-
ous woman
*Riddhie, Riddhy, Riddhey,
Riddhee, Riddhea*

^**Rihanna** (Arabic)
Resembling sweet basil
Rihana

***Riley** (Gaelic) From the
rye clearing; a courageous
woman
*Reilley, Reilly, Rilee,
Rileigh, Ryley, Rylee,
Ryleigh, Rylie*

Rini (Japanese) Resembling
a young rabbit
*Rinie, Rinee, Rinea, Riny,
Riney*

Rio (Spanish) Woman of
the river
Rhio

Risa (Latin) One who
laughs often
*Risah, Reesa, Riesa, Rise,
Rysa, Rysah, Riseh, Risako*

Rita (Greek) Precious pearl
*Ritta, Reeta, Reita, Rheeta,
Riet, Rieta, Ritah, Reta*

Roberta (English)
Feminine form of Robert;
one who is bright with
fame
Robertah, Robbie, Robin

Rochelle (French) From
the little rock
*Rochel, Rochele, Rochell,
Rochella, Rochette, Roschella,
Roschelle, Roshelle*

Roja (Spanish) A red-
haired lady
Rojah

Rolanda (German)
Feminine form of Roland;
well-known throughout
the land
*Rolandah, Rolandia,
Roldandea, Rolande,
Rolando, Rollanda,
Rollande*

Romhilda (German) A glo-
rious battle maiden
*Romhilde, Romhild,
Romeld, Romelde, Romelda,
Romilda, Romild, Romilde*

Ronli (Hebrew) My joy is
the Lord
*Ronlie, Ronlee, Ronleigh,
Ronly, Ronley, Ronlea,
Ronia, Roniya*

Ronni (English) Form of
Veronica, meaning "dis-
playing her true image"
*Ronnie, Ronae, Ronay,
Ronee, Ronelle, Ronette,
Roni, Ronica, Ronika*

Rosalind (German /
English) Resembling a
gentle horse / form of
Rose, meaning "resem-
bling the beautiful and
meaningful flower
*Ros, Rosaleen, Rosalen,
Rosalin, Rosalina, Rosalinda,
Rosalinde, Rosaline, Chalina*

Rose (Latin) Resembling
the beautiful and mean-
ingful flower
Rosa, Rosie, Rosalind

Roseanne (English)
Resembling the graceful
rose
*Ranna, Rosana, Rosanagh,
Rosanna, Rosannah,
Rosanne, Roseann, Roseanna*

Rosemary (Latin /
English) The dew of the
sea / resembling a bitter
rose
*Rosemaree, Rosemarey,
Rosemaria, Rosemarie,
Rosmarie, Rozmary,
Rosamaria, Rosamarie*

Rowan (Gaelic) Of the red-
berry tree
*Rowann, Rowane, Rowanne,
Rowana, Rowanna*

Rowena (Welsh / German)
One who is fair and slen-
der / having much fame
and happiness
*Rhowena, Roweena,
Roweina, Rowenna,
Rowina, Rowinna,
Rhonwen, Rhonwyn*

Ruana (Indian) One who is musically inclined
Ruanah, Ruanna, Ruannah, Ruane, Ruann, Ruanne

Ruby (English) As precious as the red gemstone
Rubee, Rubi, Rubie, Rubyna, Rubea

Rudella (German) A well-known woman
Rudela, Rudelah, Rudell, Rudelle, Rudel, Rudele, Rudy, Rudie

Rue (English, German) A medicinal herb
Ru, Larue

Rufina (Latin) A red-haired woman
Rufeena, Rufeine, Ruffina, Rufine, Ruffine, Rufyna, Ruffyna, Rufyne

Ruhi (Arabic) A spiritual woman
Roohee, Ruhee, Ruhie, Ruhy, Ruhey, Roohi, Roohie, Ruhea

Rukmini (Hindi) Adorned with gold; in Hinduism, the first wife of Krishna
Rukminie, Rukminy, Rukminey, Rukminee, Rukminea, Rukminni, Rukminii

Rumah (Hebrew) One who has been exalted
Ruma, Rumia, Rumea, Rumiah, Rumeah, Rumma, Rummah

Rumina (Latin) In mythology, a protector goddess of mothers and babies
Ruminah, Rumeena, Rumeenah, Rumeina, Rumiena, Rumyna, Rumeinah, Rumienah

Rupali (Indian) A beautiful woman
Rupalli, Rupalie, Rupalee, Rupallee, Rupal, Rupa, Rupaly, Rupaley

Ruqayyah (Arabic) A gentle woman; a daughter of Muhammad
Ruqayya, Ruqayah, Ruqaya

Ruth (Hebrew) A beloved companion
Ruthe, Ruthelle, Ruthellen, Ruthetta, Ruthi, Ruthie, Ruthina, Ruthine

Ryba (Slavic) Resembling a fish
Rybah, Rybba, Rybbah

Ryder (American) An accomplished horsewoman
Rider

Rylee (American) Form of Riley, meaning from the rye clearing / a courageous woman

S

Saba (Greek / Arabic)
Woman from Sheba /
born in the morning
*Sabah, Sabaa, Sabba,
Sabbah, Sabaah*

Sabana (Spanish) From the
open plain
*Sabanah, Sabanna, Sabann,
Sabanne, Sabane, Saban*

Sabi (Arabic) A lovely
young lady
*Sabie, Saby, Sabey, Sabee,
Sabbi, Sabbee, Sabea*

Sabirah (Arabic) Having
great patience
*Sabira, Saabira, Sabeera,
Sabiera, Sabeira, Sabyra,
Sabirra, Sabyrra*

Sabra (Hebrew) Resembling
the cactus fruit; to rest
*Sabrah, Sebra, Sebrah,
Sabrette, Sabbra, Sabraa,
Sabarah, Sabarra*

Sabrina (English) A leg-
endary princess
*Sabrinah, Sabrinna,
Sabreena, Sabriena, Sabreina,
Sabryna, Sabrine, Sabryne,
Cabrina, Zabrina*

Sachet (Hindi) Having
consciousness
Sachett, Sachette

Sada (Japanese) The pure
one
*Sadda, Sadaa, Sadako,
Saddaa*

Sadella (American) A beau-
tiful fairylike princess
*Sadel, Sadela, Sadelah,
Sadele, Sadell, Sadellah,
Sadelle, Sydel*

Sadhana (Hindi) A devot-
ed woman
*Sadhanah, Sadhanna,
Sadhannah, Sadhane,
Sadhanne, Sadhann,
Sadhan*

Sadhbba (Irish) A wise
woman
Sadhbh, Sadhba

Sadie (English) Form of
Sarah, meaning "a prin-
cess; lady"
*Sadi, Sady, Sadey, Sadee,
Saddi, Saddee, Sadiey, Sadye*

Sadiya (Arabic) One who
is fortunate; lucky
*Sadiyah, Sadiyyah, Sadya,
Sadyah*

Sadzi (American) Having a
sunny disposition
*Sadzee, Sadzey, Sadzia,
Sadziah, Sadzie, Sadzya,
Sadzyah, Sadzy*

Safa (Arabic) One who is
innocent and pure
*Safah, Saffa, Sapha,
Saffah, Saphah*

Saffron (English)
Resembling the yellow
flower
*Saffrone, Saffronn,
Saffronne, Safron, Safronn,
Safronne, Saffronah, Safrona*

Saheli (Indian) A beloved
friend
*Sahelie, Sahely, Saheley,
Sahelee, Saheleigh, Sahyli,
Sahelea*

Sahila (Indian) One who
provides guidance
*Sahilah, Saheela, Sahyla,
Sahiela, Saheila, Sahela,
Sahilla, Sahylla*

Sahkyo (Native American)
Resembling the mink
Sakyo

Saida (Arabic) Fortunate
one; one who is happy
*Saidah, Sa'ida, Sayida,
Saeida, Saedah, Said,
Sayide, Sayidea*

Saihah (Arabic) One who
is useful; good
Saiha, Sayiha

Sailor (American) One
who sails the seas
*Sailer, Sailar, Saylor,
Sayler, Saylar, Saelor,
Saeler, Saelar*

Saima (Arabic) A fasting
woman
Saimah, Saimma, Sayima

Sajni (Indian) One who is
dearly loved
*Sajnie, Sajny, Sujney,
Sajnee, Sajnea*

Sakae (Japanese) One who
is prosperous
*Sakai, Sakaie, Sakay,
Sakaye*

Sakari (Native American)
A sweet girl
*Sakarie, Sakary, Sakarri,
Sakarey, Sakaree, Sakarree,
Sakarah, Sakarrie*

Sakina (Indian / Arabic)
A beloved friend / hav-
ing God-inspired peace of
mind
*Sakinah, Sakeena, Sakiena,
Sukeina, Sakyna, Sakeyna,
Sakinna, Sakeana*

Sakti (Hindi) In Hinduism,
the divine energy
*Saktie, Sakty, Sakkti,
Sackti, Saktee, Saktey,
Saktia, Saktiah*

Saku (Japanese)
Remembrance of the Lord
Sakuko

Sakura (Japanese)
Resembling a cherry blos-
som
Sakurah, Sakurako, Sakurra

Sala (Hindi) From the
sacred sala tree
Salah, Salla, Sallah

Salal (English) An evergreen shrub with flowers and berries
Sallal, Salall, Sallall, Salalle, Salale, Sallale

Salamasina (Samoan) A princess; born to royalty
Salamaseena, Salamasyna, Salamaseana, Salamaseina, Salamasiena

Salina (French) One of a solemn, dignified character
Salin, Salinah, Salinda, Salinee, Sallin, Sallina, Sallinah, Salline

Saloma (Hebrew) One who offers peace and tranquility
Salomah, Salome, Salomia, Salomiah, Schlomit, Shulamit, Salomeaexl, Salomma

Salus (Latin) In mythology, goddess of health and prosperity; salvation
Saluus, Salusse, Saluss

Salwa (Arabic) One who provides comfort; solace
Salwah

Samah (Arabic) A generous, forgiving woman
Sama, Samma, Sammah

•Samantha (Aramaic) One who listens well
Samanthah, Samanthia, Samanthea, Samantheya, Samanath, Samanatha, Samana, Samanitha

Sameh (Arabic) One who forgives
Sammeh, Samaya, Samaiya

Samina (Arabic) A healthy woman
Saminah, Samine, Sameena, Samyna, Sameana, Sameina, Samynah

Samone (Hebrew) Form of Simone, meaning "one who listens well"
Samoan, Samoane, Samon, Samona, Samonia

Samuela (Hebrew) Feminine form of Samuel; asked of God
Samuelah, Samuella, Samuell, Samuelle, Sammila, Sammile, Samella, Samielle

Sana (Persian / Arabic) One who emanates light / brilliance; splendor
Sanah, Sanna, Sanako, Sanaah, Sane, Saneh

Sanaa (Swahili) Beautiful work of art
Sanae, Sannaa

Sandeep (Punjabi) One who is enlightened
Sandeepe, Sandip, Sandipp, Sandippe, Sandeyp, Sandeype

Sandhya (Hindi) Born at twilight; name of the daughter of the god Brahma
Sandhiya, Sandhyah, Sandya, Sandyah

Sandra (Greek) Form of
Alexandra, meaning "a
helper and defender of
mankind"
*Sandrah, Sandrine, Sandy,
Sandi, Sandie, Sandey,
Sandee, Sanda, Sandrica*

Sandrica (Greek) Form of
Sandra, meaning "a helper
and defender of mankind"
*Sandricca, Sandricah,
Sandricka, Sandrickah,
Sandrika, Sandrikah,
Sandryca, Sandrycah*

Sandrine (Greek) Form
of Alexandra, meaning
"a helper and defender of
mankind"
*Sandrin, Sandreana,
Sandreanah, Sandreune,
Sandreen, Sandreena,
Sandreenah, Sandreene*

Sangita (Indian) One who
is musical
*Sangitah, Sangeeta,
Sangeita, Sangyta,
Sangieta, Sangeata*

Saniya (Indian) A moment
in time preserved
Saniyah, Sanya, Sanea, Sania

Sanjna (Indian) A con-
scientous woman

Santana (Spanish) A saint-
ly woman
*Santa, Santah, Santania,
Santaniah, Santaniata,
Santena, Santenah,
Santenna*

Saoirse (Gaelic) An independent woman; having
freedom
Saoyrse

Sapna (Hindi) A dream
come true
*Sapnah, Sapnia, Sapniah,
Sapnea, Sapneah, Sapniya,
Sapniyah*

ᴿᵀSarah (Hebrew) A prin-
cess; lady; in the Bible,
wife of Abraham
*Sara, Sari, Sariah, Sarika,
Saaraa, Sarita, Sarina,
Sarra, Kala, Sadie*

Saraid (Irish) One who is
excellent; superior
*Saraide, Saraed, Saraede,
Sarayd, Sarayde*

Sarama (African / Hindi)
A kind woman / in
Hinduism, Indra's dog
*Saramah, Saramma,
Sarrama, Sarramma*

Saran (African) One who
brings joy to others
*Sarane, Sarran, Saranne,
Saranna, Sarana, Sarann*

Sarasvati (Hindi) In
Hinduism, goddess of
learning and the arts
*Sarasvatti, Sarasvatie,
Sarasvaty, Sarasvatey,
Sarasvatee, Sarasvatea*

Saraswati (Hindi) Owning water; in Hinduism, a river goddess
Saraswatti, Saraswatie, Saraswaty, Saraswatey, Saraswatee, Saraswatea

Sardinia (Italian) Woman from a mountainous island
Sardiniah, Sardinea, Sardineah, Sardynia, Sardyniah, Sardynea, Sardyneah

Sasa (Japanese) One who is helpful; gives aid
Sasah

Sasha (Russian) Form of Alexandra, meaning "a helper and defender of mankind"
Sascha, Sashenka, Saskia

Sauda (Swahili) A dark beauty
Saudaa, Sawda, Saudda

•Savannah (English) From the open grassy plain
Savanna, Savana, Savanne, Savann, Savane, Savanneh

Savarna (Hindi) Daughter of the ocean
Savarnia, Savarnea, Savarniya, Savarneia

Savitri (Hindi) In Hinduism, the daughter of the god of the sun
Savitari, Savitrie, Savitry, Savitarri, Savitarie, Savitree, Savitrea, Savitrey

Savvy (American) Smart and perceptive woman
Savy, Savvi, Savvie, Savvey, Savee, Savvee, Savvea, Savea

Sayyida (Arabic) A mistress
Sayyidah, Sayida, Sayyda, Seyyada, Seyyida, Seyada, Seyida

Scarlett (English) Vibrant red color; a vivacious woman
Scarlet, Scarlette, Skarlet

Scota (Irish) Woman of Scotland
Scotta, Scotah, Skota, Skotta, Skotah

Sea'iqa (Arabic) Thunder and lightning
Seaqa, Seaqua

Season (Latin) A fertile woman; one who embraces change
Seazon, Seeson, Seezon, Seizon, Seasen, Seasan, Seizen, Seizan

Sebille (English) In Arthurian legend, a fairy
Sebylle, Sebill, Sebile, Sebyle, Sebyl

Secunda (Latin) The second-born child
Secundah, Secuba, Secundus, Segunda, Sekunda

Seda (Armenian) Voices of
the forest
Sedda, Sedah, Seddah

Sedona (American)
Woman from a city in
Arizona
*Sedonah, Sedonnu,
Sedonnah, Sedonia,
Sedonea*

Seema (Greek) A symbol;
a sign
*Seyma, Syma, Seama,
Seima, Siema*

Sefarina (Greek) Of a
gentle wind
*Sefarinah, Sefareena,
Sefareenah, Sefaryna,
Sefarynah, Sefareana,
Sefareanah*

Seiko (Japanese) The force
of truth

Selene (Greek) Of the moon
*Sela, Selena, Selina, Celina,
Zalina*

Sema (Arabic) A divine
omen; a known symbol
Semah

Senalda (Spanish) A sign;
a symbol
*Senaldah, Senaldia, Senaldiya,
Senaldea, Senaldya*

September (American)
Born in the month of
September
*Septimber, Septymber,
Septemberia, Septemberea*

Sequoia (Native American)
Of the giant redwood tree
Sekwoya, Lequoia

Serafina (Latin) A seraph;
a heavenly winged angel
*Serafinah, Serafine,
Seraphina, Serefina,
Seraphine, Sera*

Serena (Latin) Having a
peaceful disposition
*Serenah, Serene, Sereena,
Seryna, Serenity, Serenitie,
Serenitee, Serepta, Cerina,
Xerena*

Serendipity (American)
A fateful meeting; having
good fortune
*Serendipitey, Serendipitee,
Serendipiti, Serendipitie,
Serendypyty*

Serenity (Latin) peaceful

Sevati (Indian)
Resembling the white rose
*Sevatie, Sevatti, Sevate,
Sevatee, Sevatea, Sevaty,
Sevatey, Sevti*

Shabana (Arabic) A maid-
en belonging to the night
*Shabanah, Shabanna,
Shabaana, Shabanne,
Shabane*

Shabnan (Persian) A fall-
ing raindrop
*Shabnane, Shabnann,
Shabnanne*

Shadha (Arabic) An aromatic fragrance
Shadhah

Shafiqa (Arabic) A compassionate woman
Shafiqah, Shafiqua, Shafeeqa, Shafeequa

Shai (Gaelic) A gift of God
Shay, Shae, Shayla, Shea, Shaye

Sha'ista (Arabic) One who is polite and well-behaved
Shaistah, Shaista, Shaa'ista, Shayista, Shaysta

Shakila (Arabic) Feminine form of Shakil; beautiful one
Shakilah, Shakela, Shakeela, Shakeyla, Shakyla, Shakeila, Shakiela, Shakina

Shakira (Arabic) Feminine form of Shakir; grateful; thankful
Shakirah, Shakiera, Shaakira, Shakeira, Shakyra, Shakeyra, Shakura, Shakirra

Shakti (Indian) A divine woman; having power
Shaktie, Shakty, Shaktey, Shaktee, Shaktye, Shaktea

Shaliqa (Arabic) One who is sisterly
Shaliqah, Shaliqua, Shaleeqa, Shaleequa, Shalyqa, Shalyqua

Shamima (Arabic) A woman full of flavor
Shamimah, Shameema, Shamiema, Shameima, Shamyma, Shameama

Shandy (English) One who is rambunctious; boisterous
Shandey, Shandee, Shandi, Shandie, Shandye, Shandea

Shani (African) A marvelous woman
Shanie, Shany, Shaney, Shanee, Shanni, Shanea, Shannie, Shanny

Shanley (Gaelic) Small and ancient woman
Shanleigh, Shanlee, Shanly, Shanli, Shanlie, Shanlea

Shannon (Gaelic) Having ancient wisdom; river name
Shanon, Shannen, Shannan, Shannin, Shanna, Shannae, Shannun, Shannyn

Shaquana (American) Truth in life
Shaqana, Shaquanah, Shaquanna, Shaqanna, Shaqania

Sharifah (Arabic) Feminine form of Sharif; noble; respected; virtuous
Sharifa, Shareefa, Sharufa, Sharufah, Sharyfa, Sharefa, Shareafa, Shariefa

Sharik (African) One who is a child of God
Shareek, Shareake, Sharicke, Sharick, Sharike, Shareak, Sharique, Sharyk

Sharikah (Arabic) One who is a good companion
Sharika, Shareeka, Sharyka, Shareka, Shariqua, Shareaka

Sharlene (French) Feminine form of Charles; petite and womanly
Sharleene, Sharleen, Sharla, Sharlyne, Sharline, Sharlyn, Sharlean, Sharleane

Sharon (Hebrew) From the plains; a flowering shrub
Sharron, Sharone, Sharona, Shari, Sharis, Sharne, Sherine, Sharun

Shasta (Native American) From the triple-peaked mountain
Shastah, Shastia, Shastiya, Shastea, Shasteya

Shawnee (Native American) A tribal name
Shawni, Shawnie, Shawnea, Shawny, Shawney, Shawnea

Shayla (Irish) Of the fairy palace; form of Shai, meaning "a gift of God"
Shaylah, Shaylagh, Shaylain, Shaylan, Shaylea, Shayleah, Shaylla, Sheyla

Shaylee (Gaelic) From the fairy palace; a fairy princess
Shalee, Shayleigh, Shailee, Shaileigh, Shaelee, Shaeleigh, Shayli, Shaylie

Sheehan (Celtic) Little peaceful one; peacemaker
Shehan, Sheyhan, Shihan, Shiehan, Shyhan, Sheahan

Sheela (Indian) One of cool conduct and character
Sheelah, Sheetal

Sheena (Gaelic) God's gracious gift
Sheenah, Shena, Shiena, Sheyna, Shyna, Sheana, Sheina

Sheherezade (Arabic) One who is a city dweller

Sheila (Irish) Form of Cecilia, meaning "one who is blind"
Sheilah, Sheelagh, Shelagh, Shiela, Shyla, Selia, Sighle, Sheiletta

Shelby (English) From the willow farm
Shelbi, Shelbey, Shelbie, Shelbee, Shelbye, Shelbea

Sheridan (Gaelic) One who is wild and untamed; a searcher
Sheridann, Sheridanne, Sherydan, Sherridan, Sheriden, Sheridon, Sherrerd, Sherida

Sheshebens (Native American) Resembling a small duck

Shifra (Hebrew) A beautiful midwife
Shifrah, Shiphrah, Shiphra, Shifria, Shifriya, Shifrea

Shikha (Indian) Flame burning brightly
Shikhah, Shikkha, Shekha, Shykha

Shima (Native American) Little mother
Shimah, Shimma, Shyma, Shymah

Shina (Japanese) A virtuous woman; having goodness
Shinah, Shinna, Shyna, Shynna

Shobha (Indian) An attractive woman
Shobhah, Shobbha, Shoba, Shobhan, Shobhane

Shoshana (Arabic) Form of Susannah, meaning "white lily"
Shosha, Shoshan, Shoshanah, Shoshane, Shoshanha, Shoshann, Shoshanna, Shoshannah

Shradhdha (Indian) One who is faithful; trusting
Shraddha, Shradha, Shradhan, Shradhane

Shruti (Indian) Having good hearing
Shrutie, Shruty, Shrutey, Shrutee, Shrutye, Shrutea

Shunnareh (Arabic) Pleasing in manner and behavior
Shunnaraya, Shunareh, Shunarreh

Shyann (English) Form of Cheyenne, meaning "unintelligible speaker"
Shyanne, Shyane, Sheyann, Sheyanne, Sheyenne, Sheyene

Shysie (Native American) A quiet child
Shysi, Shysy, Shysey, Shysee, Shycie, Shyci, Shysea, Shycy

Sibyl (English) A prophetess; a seer
Sybil, Sibyla, Sybella, Sibil, Sibella, Sibilla, Sibley, Sibylla

Siddhi (Hindi) Having spiritual power
Sidhi, Syddhi, Sydhi

Sidero (Greek) In mythology, stepmother of Pelias and Neleus
Siderro, Sydero, Sideriyo

Sieglinde (German) Winning a gentle victory

Sienna (Italian) Woman with reddish-brown hair
Siena, Siennya, Sienya, Syennu, Syinna

Sierra (Spanish) From the jagged mountain range
Siera, Syerra, Syera, Seyera, Seeara

Sigfreda (German) A woman who is victorious
Sigfreeda, Sigfrida, Sigfryda, Sigfreyda, Sigfrieda, Sigfriede, Sigfrede

Sigismonda (Teutonic) A victorious defender
Sigismunda

Signia (Latin) A distinguishing sign
Signiya, Signea, Signeia, Signeya, Signa

Sigyn (Norse) In mythology, the wife of Loki

Sihu (Native American) As delicate as a flower

Silka (Latin) Form of Cecelia, meaning "one who is blind"
Silke, Silkia, Silkea, Silkie, Silky, Silkee, Sylka, Sylke

Sima (Arabic) One who is treasured; a prize
Simma, Syma, Simah, Simia, Simiya

Simone (French) One who listens well
Sim, Simonie, Symone, Samone

Sine (Scottish) Form of Jane, meaning "God is gracious"
Sinead, Sineidin, Sioned, Sionet, Sion, Siubhan, Siwan, Sineh

Sinobia (Greek) Form of Zenobia, meaning "child of Zeus"
Sinobiah, Sinobya, Sinobe, Sinobie, Sinovia, Senobia, Senobya, Senobe

Sinopa (Native American) Resembling a fox

Sinope (Greek) In mythology, one of the daughters of Asopus

Siran (Armenian) An alluring and lovely woman

Siren (Greek) In mythology, a sea nymph whose beautiful singing lured sailors to their deaths; refers to a seductive and beautiful woman
Sirene, Sirena, Siryne, Siryn, Syren, Syrena, Sirine, Sirina

Siria (Spanish / Persian) Bright like the sun / a glowing woman
Siriah, Sirea, Sireah, Siriya, Siriyah, Sirya, Siryah

Siroun (Armenian) A lovely woman
Sirune

Sirpuhi (Armenian) One who is holy; pious
Sirpuhie, Sirpuhy, Sirpuhey, Sirpuhea, Sirpuhee

Sissy (English) Form of Cecilia, meaning "one who is blind"
Sissey, Sissie, Sisley, Sisli, Sislee, Sissel, Sissle, Syssy

Sita (Hindi) In Hinduism, goddess of the harvest and wife of Rama

Sive (Irish) A good and sweet girl
Sivney, Sivny, Sivni, Sivnie, Sivnee, Sivnea

Skylar (English) One who is learned, a scholar
Skylare, Skylarr, Skyler, Skylor, Skylir

Sloane (Irish) A strong protector; a woman warrior
Sloan, Slone

Smita (Indian) One who smiles a lot

Snow (American) Frozen rain
Snowy, Snowie, Snowi, Snowey, Snowee, Snowea, Sno

Snowdrop (English) Resembling a small white flower

Solana (Latin / Spanish) Wind from the east / of the sunshine
Solanah, Solanna, Solann, Solanne

Solange (French) One who is religious and dignified

Solaris (Greek) Of the sun
Solarise, Solariss, Solarisse, Solarys, Solaryss, Solarysse, Sol, Soleil

Solita (Latin) One who is solitary
Solitah, Solida, Soledad, Soledada, Soledade

Somatra (Indian) Of the excellent moon

Sona (Arabic) The golden one
Sonika, Sonna

Sonora (Spanish) A pleasant-sounding woman
Sonorah, Sonoria, Sonorya, Sonoriya

Soo (Korean) Having an excellent long life

****Sophia** (Greek) Form of Sophie, meaning great wisdom and foresight
Sofia, Sofiya

*ᵀ**Sophie** (Greek) Wisdom
*Sophia, Sofiya, Sofie, Sofia,
Sofi, Sofiyko, Sofronia,
Sophronia, Zofia*

Sorina (Romanian)
Feminine form of Sorin;
of the sun
*Sorinah, Sorinna, Sorinia,
Soriniya, Sorinya, Soryna,
Sorynia, Sorine*

Sorrel (French) From the
surele plant
*Sorrell, Sorrelle, Sorrele,
Sorrela, Sorrella*

Sparrow (English)
Resembling a small song-
bird
*Sparro, Sparroe, Sparo,
Sparow, Sparowe, Sparoe*

Sslama (Egyptian) One
who is peaceful

Stacey (English) Form of
Anastasia, meaning "one
who shall rise again"
*Stacy, Staci, Stacie, Stacee,
Stacia, Stasia, Stasy, Stasey*

^**Stella** (English) Star of
the sea
*Stela, Stelle, Stele, Stellah,
Stelah*

Stephanie (Greek)
Feminine form of Stephen;
crowned in victory
*Stephani, Stephany,
Stephaney, Stephanee,
Stephene, Stephana,
Stefanie, Stefani*

Stevonna (Greek) A
crowned lady
*Stevonnah, Stevona,
Stevonah, Stevonia,
Stevonea, Stevoniya*

Styx (Greek) In mythology,
the river of the underworld
Stixx, Styxx, Stix

Suave (American) A
smooth and courteous
woman
Swave

Subhadra (Hindi) In
Hinduism, the sister of
Krishna

Subhaga (Indian) A fortunate person

Subhuja (Hindi) An auspicious celestial damsel

Subira (African) One who
is patient
*Subirah, Subirra, Subyra,
Subyrra, Subeera, Subeara,
Subeira, Subiera*

Suhaila (Arabic) Feminine
form of Suhail; the second
brightest star
*Suhayla, Suhaela, Suhala,
Suhailah, Suhaylah,
Suhaelah, Suhalah*

Sulwyn (Welsh) One who
shines as bright as the
sun
*Sulwynne, Sulwynn,
Sulwinne, Sulwin, Sulwen,
Sulwenn, Sulwenne*

Sumana (Indian) A good-natured woman
Sumanah, Sumanna, Sumane, Sumanne, Sumann

Sumi (Japanese) One who is elegant and refined
Sumie

Sumitra (Indian) A beloved friend
Sumitrah, Sumita, Sumytra, Sumyta, Sumeetra, Sumeitra, Sumietra, Sumeatra

Summer (American) Refers to the season; born in summer
Sommer, Sumer, Somer, Somers

Suna (Turkish) A swan-like woman

Sunanda (Indian) Having a sweet character
Sunandah, Sunandia, Sunandiya, Sunandea, Sunandya

Sunila (Indian) Feminine form of Sunil; very blue
Sunilah, Sunilla, Sunilya, Suniliya

Sunniva (English) Gift of the sun
Synnove, Synne, Synnove, Sunn

Surabhi (Indian) Having a lovely fragrance
Surbhii, Surabhie, Surabhy, Surabhey, Surabhee, Surabhea

Susannah (Hebrew) White lily
Susanna, Susanne, Susana, Susane, Susan, Suzanna, Suzannah, Suzanne, Shoshana, Huhana

Sushanti (Indian) A peaceful woman; tranquil
Sushantie, Sushanty, Sushantey, Sushantee, Sushantea

Suzu (Japanese) One who is long-lived
Suzue, Suzuko

Swanhilda (Norse) A woman warrior; in mythology, the daughter of Sigurd
Swanhild, Swanhilde, Svanhilde, Svanhild, Svenhilde, Svenhilda

Swarupa (Indian) One who is devoted to the truth

Sydney (English) Of the wide meadow
Sydny, Sydni, Sydnie, Sydnea, Sydnee, Sidney, Sidne, Sidnee

t

Taariq (Swahili) Resembling the morning star
Tariq, Taarique, Tarique

Tabia (African / Egyptian) One who makes incantations / a talented woman
Tabiah, Tabya, Tabea, Tabeah, Tabiya

Tabita (African) A graceful woman
Tabitah, Tabyta, Tabytah, Tabeeta, Tabeata, Tabieta, Tabeita

Tabitha (Greek) Resembling a gazelle; known for beauty and grace
Tabithah, Tabbitha, Tabetha, Tabbetha, Tabatha, Tabbatha, Tabotha, Tabbotha

Tabora (Spanish) One who plays a small drum
Taborah, Taborra, Taboria, Taborya

Tacincala (Native American) Resembling a deer
Tacincalah, Tacyncala, Tacyncalah, Tacincalla, Tacyncalla

Tahsin (Arabic) Beautification; one who is praised
Tahseen, Tahsene, Tahsyne, Tasine, Tahseene, Tahsean, Tahseane

Tahzib (Arabic) One who is educated and cultured
Tahzeeb, Tahzebe, Tahzybe, Tazib, Tazyb, Tazeeb, Tahzeab, Tazeab

Taithleach (Gaelic) A quiet and calm young lady

Takako (Japanese) A lofty child

Takoda (Native American) Friend to everyone
Takodah, Takodia, Takodya, Takota

Tala (Native American) A stalking wolf
Talah, Talla

Talia (Hebrew / Greek) Morning dew from heaven / blooming
Taliah, Talea, Taleah, Taleya, Tallia, Talieya, Taleea, Taleia

Talihah (Arabic) One who seeks knowledge
Taliha, Talibah, Taliba, Talyha, Taleehah, Taleahah

Taline (Armenian) Of the monestary
Talene, Taleen, Taleene, Talyne, Talinia, Talinya, Taliniya

Talisa (American)
Consecrated to God
*Talisah, Talysa, Taleesa,
Talissa, Talise, Taleese,
Talisia, Talisya*

Talisha (American) A
damsel; an innocent
*Talesha, Taleisha, Talysha,
Taleesha, Tylesha, Taleysha,
Taleshia, Talishia*

Talitha (Arabic) A maiden;
young girl
*Talithah, Taletha, Taleetha,
Talytha, Talithia, Talethia,
Tiletha, Talith*

Tamanna (Indian) One
who is desired
*Tamannah, Tamana,
Tamanah, Tammana,
Tammanna*

Tamasha (African)
Pageant winner
*Tamasha, Tomosha,
Tomasha, Tamashia,
Tamashya*

Tamesis (Celtic) In
mythology, the goddess of
water; source of the name
for the river Thames
Tamesiss, Tamesys, Tamesyss

Tangia (American) The
angel
*Tangiah, Tangya, Tangiya,
Tangeah*

Tani (Japanese /
Melanesian / Tonkinese)
From the valley / a sweet-
heart / a young woman
*Tanie, Tany, Taney, Tanee,
Tanni, Tanye, Tannie,
Tanny*

Tania (Russian) Queen of
the fairies
*Tanya, Tannie, Tanny,
Tanika*

Tanner (English) One who
tans hides
*Taner, Tannar, Tannor,
Tannis*

Tansy (English / Greek) An
aromatic yellow flower /
having immortality
*Tansey, Tansi, Tansie,
Tansee, Tansye, Tansea,
Tancy, Tanzy*

Tanushri (Indian) One
who is beautiful; attractive
*Tanushrie, Tanushry,
Tanushrey, Tanushree,
Tanushrea*

Tanvi (Indian) Slender and
beautiful woman
*Tanvie, Tanvy, Tanvey,
Tanvee, Tanvye, Tannvi,
Tanvea*

Tapati (Indian) In mythology, the daughter of the
sun god
*Tapatie, Tapaty, Tapatey,
Tapatee, Tapatye, Tapatea*

Taphath (Hebrew) In the Bible, Solomon's daughter
Tafath, Taphathe, Tafathe

Tara (Gaelic / Indian) Of the tower; rocky hill / star; in mythology, an astral goddess
Tarah, Tarra, Tayra, Taraea, Tarai, Taralee, Tarali, Taraya

Tarachand (Indian) Silver star
Tarachande, Tarachanda, Tarachandia, Tarachandea, Tarachandiya, Tarachandya

Taree (Japanese) A bending branch
Tarea, Tareya

Taregan (Native American) Resembling a crane
Tareganne, Taregann

Tareva-chine(shanay) (Native American) One with beautiful eyes

Tariana (American) From the holy hillside
Tariana, Tarianna, Taryana, Taryanna

Tarika (Indian) A starlet
Tarikah, Taryka, Tarykah, Taricka, Tarickah

Tarisai (African) One to behold; to look at
Tarysai

Tasanee (Thai) A beautiful view
Tasane, Tasani, Tasanie, Tasany, Tasaney, Tasanye, Tasanea

Taskin (Arabic) One who provides peace; satisfaction
Taskine, Taskeen, Taskeene, Taskyne, Takseen, Taksin, Taksyn

Tasnim (Arabic) From the fountain of paradise
Tasnime, Tasneem, Tasneeme, Tasnyme, Tasnym, Tasneam, Tasneame

Tatum (English) Bringer of joy; spirited
Tatom, Tatim, Tatem, Tatam, Tatym

Tavi (Aramaic) One who is well-behaved
Tavie, Tavee, Tavy, Tavey, Tavea

Taylor (English) Cutter of cloth; one who alters garments
Tailor, Taylore, Taylar, Tayler, Talour, Taylre, Tailore, Tailar

Teagan (Gaelic) One who is attractive
Teegan

Tehya (Native American) One who is precious
Tehyah, Tehiya, Tehiyah

Teigra (Greek) Resembling a tiger
Teigre

Telephassa (Latin) In mythology, the queen of Tyre
Telephasa, Telefassa, Telefasa

Temperance (English) Having self-restraint
Temperence, Temperince, Temperancia, Temperanse, Temperense, Temperinse

Tendai (African) Thankful to God
Tenday, Tendae, Tendaa, Tendaye

Tender (American) One who is sensitive; young and vulnerable
Tendere, Tendera, Tenderia, Tenderre, Tenderiya

Teranika (Gaelic) Victory of the earth
Teranikah, Teranieka, Teraneika, Teraneeka, Teranica, Teranicka, Teranicca, Teraneaka

Teresa (Greek) A harvester
Theresa, Theresah, Theresia, Therese, Thera, Tresa, Tressa, Tressam, Reese, Reza

Terpsichore (Greek) In mythology, the muse of dancing and singing
Terpsichora, Terpsichoria, Terpsichoriya

Terra (Latin) From the earth; in mythology, an earth goddess
Terrah, Terah, Teralyn, Terran, Terena, Terenah, Terenna, Terrena

Terrian (Greek) One who is innocent
Terriane, Terrianne, Terriana, Terianna, Terian, Terianne

Tessa (Greek) Form of Teresa, meaning "a harvester"

Tetsu (Japanese) A strong woman
Tetsue

Tetty (English) Form of Elizabeth, meaning "my God is bountiful; God's promise"
Tettey, Tetti, Tettie, Tettee, Tettea

Tevy (Cambodian) An angel
Tevey, Tevi, Tevie, Tevee, Tevea

Thandiwe (African) The loving one
Thandywe, Thandiewe, Thandeewe, Thandie, Thandi, Thandee, Thandy, Thandey

Thara (Arabic) One who is
wealthy; prosperous
*Tharah, Tharra, Tharrah,
Tharwat*

Thelma (Greek) One who
is ambitious and willful
*Thelmah, Telma, Thelmai,
Thelmia, Thelmalina*

Thelred (English) One
who is well-advised
*Thelrede, Thelread,
Thelredia, Thelredina,
Thelreid, Thelreed, Thelryd*

Thema (African) A queen
*Themah, Theema, Thyma,
Theyma, Theama*

Theora (Greek) A watcher
*Theorra, Theoria, Theoriya,
Theorya*

Theta (Greek) Eighth letter
of the Greek alphabet
Thetta

Thistle (English)
Resembling the prickly,
flowered plant
Thistel, Thissle, Thissel

Thomasina (Hebrew)
Feminine form of
Thomas; a twin
*Thomasine, Thomsina,
Thomasin, Tomasina,
Tomasine, Thomasa,
Thomaseena, Thomaseana*

Thoosa (Greek) In mythol-
ogy, a sea nymph
*Thoosah, Thoosia,
Thoosiah, Thusa, Thusah,
Thusia, Thusiah, Thousa*

Thorberta (Norse)
Brilliance of Thor
Thorbiartr, Thorbertha

Thordia (Norse) Spirit of
Thor
*Thordiah, Thordis, Tordis,
Thordissa, Tordissa,
Thoridyss*

Thuy (Vietnamese) One
who is gentle and pure
Thuye, Thuyy, Thuyye

Thy (Vietnamese / Greek)
A poet / one who is
untamed
Thye

Tia (Spanish / Greek) An
aunt / daughter born to
royalty
*Tiah, Tea, Teah, Tiana,
Teea, Tya, Teeya, Tiia*

Tiberia (Italian) Of the
Tiber river
*Tiberiah, Tiberiya, Tiberya,
Tiberia, Tibearia, Tibieria,
Tibeiria*

Tiegan (Aztec) A little
princess in a big valley
Tiegann, Tieganne

Tierney (Gaelic) One who is regal; lordly
Tiernie, Tierni, Tiernee, Tierny, Tiernea

Tiffany (Greek) Lasting love
Tiffaney, Tiffani, Tiffanie, Tiffanee, Tifany, Tifaney, Tifanee, Tifani

Timothea (English) Feminine form of Timothy; honoring God
Timotheah, Timothia, Timothya, Timothiya

Tina (English) From the river; also shortened form of names ending in -tina
Tinah, Teena, Tena, Teyna, Tyna, Tinna, Teana

Ting (Chinese) Graceful and slim woman

Tirza (Hebrew) One who is pleasant; a delight
Tirzah

Tisa (African) The ninth-born child
Tisah, Tiza

Tita (Latin) Holding a title of honor
Titah, Teeta, Tyta, Teata

Tivona (Hebrew) Lover of nature
Tivonna, Tivone, Tivonia, Tivoniya

Toan (Vietnamese) Form of An-toan, meaning "safe and secure"
Toane, Toanne

Toinette (French) Form of Antoinette, meaning "praiseworthy"
Toinett, Toinete, Toinet, Toineta, Toinetta, Tola

Toki (Japanese / Korean) One who grasps opportunity; hopeful / resembling a rabbit
Tokie, Toky, Tokey, Tokye, Tokiko, Tokee, Tokea

Tola (Polish / Cambodian) Form of Toinette, meaning "praiseworthy" / born during October
Tolah, Tolla, Tollah

Topanga (Native American) From above or a high place
Topangah

Topaz (Latin) Resembling a yellow gemstone
Topazz, Topaza, Topazia, Topaziya, Topazya, Topazea

Tordis (Norse) A goddess
Tordiss, Tordisse, Tordys, Tordyss, Tordysse

Torny (Norse) New; just discovered
Torney, Tornie, Torni, Torne, Torn, Tornee, Tornea

Torunn (Norse) Thor's
love
Torun, Torrun, Torrunn

Tory (American) Form of
Victoria, meaning "victorious
woman; winner; conquerer"
*Torry, Torey, Tori, Torie,
Torree, Tauri, Torye, Toya*

Tosca (Latin) From the
Tuscany region
*Toscah, Toscka, Toska,
Tosckah, Toskah*

Tosha (English) Form of
Natasha, meaning "born
on Christmas"
*Toshah, Toshiana, Tasha,
Tashia, Tashi, Tassa*

Tourmaline (Singhalese)
A stone of mixed colors
*Tourmalyne, Tourmalina,
Tourmalinia*

Tova (Hebrew) One who is
well-behaved
*Tovah, Tove, Tovi, Toba,
Toibe, Tovva*

Treasa (Irish) Having
great strength
*Treasah, Treesa, Treisa,
Triesa, Treise, Treese,
Toirease*

·Trinity (Latin) The holy
three
*Trinitey, Triniti, Trinitie,
Trinitee, Trynity, Trynitey,
Tryniti, Trynitie*

Trisha (Latin) Form of
Patricia, meaning "of
noble descent"
*Trishah, Trishia, Tricia,
Trish, Trissa, Trisa*

Trishna (Polish) In
mythology, the goddess of
the deceased, protector of
graves
*Trishnah, Trishnia,
Trishniah, Trishnea,
Trishneah, Trishniya,
Trishniyah, Trishnyu*

Trisna (Indian) The one
desired
*Trisnah, Trisnia, Trisniah,
Trisnea, Trisneah, Trisniya,
Trisniyah, Trisnya*

Trudy (German) Form
of Gertrude, meaning
"adored warrior"
*Trudey, Trudi, Trudie,
Trude, Trudye, Trudee,
Truda, Trudia*

Trupti (Indian) State of
being satisfied
*Truptie, Trupty, Truptey,
Truptee, Trupte, Truptea*

Tryamon (English) In
Arthurian legend, a fairy
princess
*Tryamonn, Tryamonne,
Tryamona, Tryamonna*

Tryna (Greek) The third-
born child
Trynah

Tsifira (Hebrew) One who is crowned
Tsifirah, Tsifyra, Tsiphyra, Tsiphira, Tsipheera, Tsifeera

Tuccia (Latin) A vestal virgin

Tula (Hindi) Balance; a sign of the zodiac
Tulah, Tulla, Tullah

Tullia (Irish) One who is peaceful
Tulliah, Tullea, Tulleah, Tullya, Tulia, Tulea, Tuleah, Tulya

Tusti (Hindi) One who brings happiness and peace
Tustie, Tusty, Tustey, Tustee, Tuste, Tustea

Tutilina (Latin) In mythology, the protector goddess of stored grain
Tutilinah, Tutileena, Tutileana, Tutilyna, Tutileina, Tutiliena, Tutilena, Tutylina

Tuuli (Finnish) Of the wind
Tuulie, Tuulee, Tuula, Tuuly, Tuuley, Tuulea

Tuyet (Vietnamese) Snow white woman
Tuyett, Tuyete, Tuyette, Tuyeta, Tuyetta

Tyler (English) Tiler of roofs

Tyme (English) The aromatic herb thyme
Time, Thyme, Thime

Tyne (English) Of the river
Tyna

Tyro (Greek) In mythology, a woman who bore twin sons to Poseidon

Tzidkiya (Hebrew) Righteousness of the Lord
Tzidkiyah, Tzidkiyahu

Tzigane (Hungarian) A gypsy
Tzigan, Tzigain, Tzigaine, Tzigayne

U

Uadjit (Egyptian) In mythology, a snake goddess
Ujadet, Uajit, Udjit, Ujadit

Ualani (Hawaiian) Of the heavenly rain
Ualanie, Ualany, Ualaney, Ualanee, Ualanea, Ualania, Ualana

Udavine (American) A thriving woman
Udavyne, Udavina, Udavyna, Udevine, Udevyne, Udevina, Udevyna

Udele (English) One who is wealthy; prosperous
Udelle, Udela, Udella, Udelah, Udellah, Uda, Udah

Uela (American) One who is devoted to God
Uelah, Uella, Uellah

Uganda (African) From the country in Africa
Ugandah, Ugaunda, Ugaundah, Ugawnda, Ugawndah, Ugonda, Ugondah

Ugolina (German) Having a bright spirit; bright mind
Ugolinah, Ugoleena, Ugoliana, Ugolyna, Ugoline, Ugolyn, Ugolyne

Ulalia (Greek) Form of Eulalia, meaning "well-spoken"
Ulaliah, Ulalya, Ulalyah

Ulan (African) Firstborn of twins
Ulann, Ulanne

Ulima (Arabic) One who is wise and astute
Ulimah, Ullima, Ulimma, Uleema, Uleama, Ulyma, Uleima, Uliema

Ulla (German) A willful woman
Ullah, Ullaa, Ullai, Ullae

Uma (Hindi) Mother; in mythology, the goddess of beauty and sunlight
Umah, Umma

Umberla (French) Feminine form of Umber; providing shade; of an earth color
Umberlah, Umberly, Umberley, Umberlee, Umberleigh, Umberli, Umberlea, Umberlie

Ummi (African) Born of my mother
Ummie, Ummy, Ummey, Ummee, Umi

Unity (American) Woman who upholds oneness; togetherness
Unitey, Unitie, Uniti, Unitee, Unitea, Unyty, Unytey, Unytie

Ura (Indian) Loved from the heart
Urah, Urra

Ural (Slavic) From the mountains
Urall, Urale, Uralle

Urbai (American) One who is gentle
Urbae, Urbay, Urbaye

Urbana (Latin) From the city; city dweller
Urbanah, Urbanna, Urbane, Urbania, Urbanya, Urbanne

Uriela (Hebrew) The angel of light
Uriella, Urielle, Uriel, Uriele, Uriell

Urta (Latin) Resembling the spiny plant
Urtah

Utah (Native American) People of the mountains; from the state of Utah

Uzoma (African) One who takes the right path
Uzomah, Uzomma, Uzommah

Uzzi (Hebrew / Arabic) God is my strength / a strong woman
Uzzie, Uzzy, Uzzey, Uzzee, Uzi, Uzie, Uzy, Uzey

V

Vala (German) The chosen one; singled out
Valah, Valla

Valda (Teutonic / German) Spirited in battle / famous ruler
Valdah, Valida, Velda, Vada, Vaida, Vayda, Vaeda

Valdis (Norse) In mythology, the goddess of the dead
Valdiss, Valdys, Valdyss

Valencia (Spanish) One who is powerful; strong; from the city of Valencia
Valenciah, Valyncia, Valencya, Valenzia, Valancia, Valenica, Valanca, Valecia

^**Valentina** (Latin) One who is vigorous and healthy
Valentinah, Valentine, Valenteena, Valenteana, Valentena, Valentyna, Valantina, Valentyne

*†**Valeria** (Latin) Form of Valerie, meaning strong and valiant
Valara, Valera, Valaria, Valeriana, Veleria, Valora

***Valerie** (Latin) Feminine form of Valerius; strong and valiant
Valeri, Valeree, Valerey, Valery, Valarie, Valari, Valeria, Vallery

Vandani (Hindi) One who is honorable and worthy
Vandany, Vandaney, Vandanie, Vandanee, Vandania, Vandanya

*†**Vanessa** (Greek) Resembling a butterfly
Vanessah, Vanesa, Vannesa, Vannessa, Vanassa, Vanasa, Vanessia, Vanysa, Yanessa

Vanity (English) Having
excessive pride
*Vanitey, Vanitee, Vaniti,
Vanitie, Vanitty, Vanyti,
Vanyty, Vanytie*

Vanmra (Russian) A
stranger; from a foreign
place
Vanmrah

Varda (Hebrew)
Resembling a rose
*Vardah, Vardia, Vardina,
Vardissa, Vardita, Vardysa,
Vardyta, Vardit*

Varuna (Hindi) Wife of
the sea
*Varunah, Varuna, Varun,
Varunani, Varuni*

Vashti (Persian) A lovely
woman
*Vashtie, Vashty, Vashtey,
Vashtee*

Vasta (Persian) One who
is pretty
Vastah

Vasteen (American) A
capable woman
*Vasteene, Vastiene, Vastien,
Vastein, Vasteine, Vastean,
Vasteane*

Vasuda (Hindi) Of the
earth
*Vasudah, Vasudhara,
Vasundhara, Vasudhra,
Vasundhra*

Vayu (Hindi) A vital life
force; the air
Vuyyu

Vedette (French) From the
guard tower
*Vedete, Vedett, Vedet,
Vedetta, Vedeta*

Vedi (Sanskrit) Filled with
wisdom
*Vedie, Vedy, Vedey, Vedee,
Vedea, Vedeah*

Vega (Latin) A falling star
Vegah

Vellamo (Finnish) In
mythology, the goddess of
the sea
Velamo, Vellammo

Ventana (Spanish) As
transparent as a window
*Ventanah, Ventanna,
Ventane, Ventanne*

Venus (Greek) In mythology, the goddess of love
and beauty
*Venis, Venys, Vynys,
Venusa, Venusina, Venusia*

Veradis (Latin) One who is
genuine; truthful
*Veradise, Veradys, Veradisa,
Verdissa, Veradysa,
Veradyssa, Veradisia,
Veraditia*

Verda (Latin) Springlike; one who is young and fresh
Verdah, Verdea, Virida, Verdy, Verdey, Verde, Verdi, Verdie

Verenase (Swedish) One who is flourishing
Verenese, Verennase, Vyrenase, Vyrennase, Vyrenese, Verenace, Vyrenace

Veronica (Latin) Displaying her true image
Veronicah, Veronic, Veronicca, Veronicka, Veronika, Veronicha, Veronique, Veranique, Ronni

Vesna (Slavic) Messenger; in mythology, the goddess of spring
Vesnah, Vezna, Vesnia, Vesnaa

Vespera (Latin) Evening star; born in the evening
Vesperah, Vespira, Vespeera, Vesperia, Vesper

Vevila (Gaelic) Woman with a melodious voice
Vevilah, Veveela, Vevyla, Vevilla, Vevylla, Vevylle, Vevyle, Vevillia

Vibeke (Danish) A small woman
Vibekeh, Vibeek, Vibeeke, Vybeke, Viheke

Vibhuti (Hindi) Of the sacred ash; a symbol
Vibuti, Vibhutie, Vibhutee

•Victoria (Latin) Victorious woman; winner; conqueror
Victoriah, Victorea, Victoreah, Victorya, Victorria, Victoriya, Vyctoria, Victorine, Tory

Vidya (Indian) Having great wisdom
Vidyah

Viet (Vietnamese) A woman from Vietnam
Vyet, Viett, Vyett, Viette, Vyette

Vigilia (Latin) Wakefulness; watchfulness
Vigiliah, Vygilia, Vygylia, Vijilia, Vyjilia

Vignette (French) From the little vine
Vignete, Vignet, Vignetta, Vignett, Vigneta, Vygnette, Vygnete, Vygnet

Vilina (Hindi) One who is dedicated
Vilinah, Vileena, Vileana, Vylina, Vyleena, Vyleana, Vylyna, Vilinia

Villette (French) From the small village
Vilette, Villete, Vilete, Vilet, Vilett, Villet, Villett, Vylet

Vimala (Indian) Feminine form of Vamal; clean and pure
Vimalah, Vimalia, Vimalla

Vincentia (Latin) Feminine form of Vincent; conqueror; triumphant
Vincentiah, Vincenta, Vincensia, Vincenzia, Vyncentia, Vyncyntia, Vyncenzia, Vycenzya

Violet (French) Resembling the purplish-blue flower
Violett, Violette, Violete, Vyolet, Vyolett, Vyolette, Vyolete, Violeta

Virginia (Latin) One who is chaste; virginal; from the state of Virginia
Virginiah, Virginnia, Virgenya, Virgenia, Virgeenia, Virgeena, Virgena, Ginny

Virtue (Latin) Having moral excellence, chastity, and goodness
Virtu, Vyrtue, Vyrtu, Vertue, Vertu

Viveka (German) Little woman of the strong fortress
Vivekah, Vivecka, Vyveka, Viveca, Vyveca, Vivecca, Vivika, Vivieka

Vivian (Latin) Lively woman
Viv, Vivi, Vivienne, Bibiana

Vixen (American) A flirtatious woman
Vixin, Vixi, Vixie, Vixee, Vixea, Vixeah, Vixy, Vixey

Vlasta (Slavic) A friendly and likeable woman
Vlastah, Vlastia, Vlasteu, Vlastiah, Vlasteah

Voleta (Greek) The veiled one
Voletah, Voletta, Volita, Volitta, Volyta, Volytta, Volet, Volett

Volva (Scandinavian) In mythology, a female shaman
Volvah, Volvya, Volvaa, Volvae, Volvai, Volvay, Volvia

Vondila (African) Woman who lost a child
Vondilah, Vondilla, Vondilya, Vondilia, Vondyla, Vondylya

Vonna (French) Form of Yvonne, meaning "young archer"
Vonnah, Vona, Vonah, Vonnia, Vonnya, Vonia, Vonya, Vonny

Vonshae (American) One who is confident
Vonshay, Vonshaye, Vonshai

Vor (Norse) In mythology, an omniscient goddess
Vore, Vorr, Vorre

Vulpine (English) A cunning woman; like a fox
Vulpyne, Vulpina, Vulpyna

Vyomini (Indian) A gift of the divine
Vyominie, Vyominy, Vyominey, Vyominee, Vyomyni, Vyomyny, Viomini, Viomyni

W

Wafa (Arabic) One who is faithful; devoted
Wafah, Wafaa, Waffa, Wapha, Waffah, Waphah

Wagaye (African) My sense of value; my price
Wagay, Wagai, Wagae

Wainani (Hawaiian) Of the beautiful waters
Wainanie, Wainany, Wainaney, Wainanee, Wainanea, Wainaneah

Wajihah (Arabic) One who is distinguished; eminent
Wajiha, Wajeeha, Wajyha, Wajeehah, Wajyhah, Wajieha, Wajiehah, Wajeiha

Wakanda (Native American) One who possesses magical powers
Wakandah, Wakenda, Wakinda, Wakynda

Wakeishah (American) Filled with happiness
Wakeisha, Wakieshah, Wakiesha, Wakesha

Walda (German) One who has fame and power
Waldah, Wallda, Walida, Waldine, Waldina, Waldyne, Waldyna, Welda

Walker (English) Walker of the forests
Wallker, Walkher

Walta (African) One who acts as a shield
Waltah

Wanetta (English) A pale-skinned woman
Wanettah, Wanette, Wannette, Wannetta, Wonetta, Wonette, Wonitta, Wonitte

Wangari (African) Resembling the leopard
Wangarie, Wangarri, Wangary, Wangarey, Wangaria, Wangaree

Wanyika (African) Of the bush
Wanyikka, Wanyicka, Wanyicca, Wanyica

Waqi (Arabic) Falling; swooping
Waqqi

Warma (American) A caring woman
Warm, Warme, Warmia, Warmiah, Warmea, Warmeah

Warna (German) One who defends her loved ones
Warnah

Washi (Japanese) Resembling an eagle
Washie, Washy, Washey, Washee, Washea, Washeah

Waynette (English) One who makes wagons
Waynett, Waynet, Waynete, Wayneta, Waynetta

Wednesday (American) Born on a Wednesday
Wensday, Winsday, Windnesday, Wednesdae, Wensdae, Winsdae, Windnesdae, Wednesdai

Welcome (English) A welcome guest
Welcom, Welcomme

Wendy (Welsh) Form of Gwendolyn, meaning "one who is fair; of the white ring"
Wendi, Wendie, Wendee, Wendey, Wenda, Wendia, Wendea, Wendya

Wesley (English) From the western meadow
Wesly, Weslie, Wesli, Weslee, Weslia, Wesleigh, Weslea, Weslei

Whisper (English) One who is soft-spoken
Whysper, Wisper, Wysper

Whitley (English) From the white meadow
Whitly, Whitlie, Whitli, Whitlee, Whitleigh, Whitlea, Whitlia, Whitlya

Whitney (English) From the white island
Whitny, Whitnie, Whitni, Whitnee, Whittney, Whitneigh, Whytny, Whytney

Wicapi Wakan (Native American) A holy star

Wijida (Arabic) An excited seeker
Wijidah, Weejida, Weejidah, Wijeeda, Wijeedah, Wijyda, Wijydah, Wijieda

Wileen (Teutonic) A firm defender
Wiline, Wilean, Wileane, Wilyn, Wileene, Wilene, Wyleen, Wyline

Wilhelmina (German)
Feminine form of
Wilhelm; determined
protector
*Wilhelminah, Wylhelmina,
Wylhelmyna, Willemina,
Wilhelmine, Wilhemina,
Wilhemine, Helma, Ilma*

Winetta (American) One
who is peaceful
*Wineta, Wynetta, Wyneta,
Winet, Winett, Winette,
Wynet, Wynett*

Wing (Chinese) Woman
of glory
Winge, Wyng

Winnielle (African) A vic-
torious woman
*Winniell, Winniele,
Winniel, Winniella*

Winola (German) Gracious
and charming friend
*Winolah, Wynola, Winolla,
Wynolla, Wynolah,
Winollah, Wynollah*

Winta (African) One who
is desired
*Wintah, Whinta, Wynta,
Whynta, Whintah,
Wyntah, Whyntah*

Wisconsin (French)
Gathering of waters; from
the state of Wisconsin
Wisconsyn, Wisconsen

Woody (American) A
woman of the forest
*Woodey, Woodi, Woodie,
Woodee, Woodea, Woodeah,
Woods*

Wren (English) Resembling
a small songbird
*Wrenn, Wrene, Wrena,
Wrenie, Wrenee, Wreney,
Wrenny, Wrenna*

Wynda (Scottish) From the
narrow passage
Wyndah, Winda, Windah

X

Xalvadora (Spanish) A
savior
*Xalvadorah, Xalbadora,
Xalbadorah, Xalvadoria,
Xalbadoria*

Xanadu (African) From
the exotic paradise

Xantara (American)
Protector of the Earth
*Xantarah, Xanterra,
Xantera, Xantarra,
Xantarrah, Xanterah,
Xanterrah*

Xaquelina (Galician) Form of Jacqueline, meaning "the supplanter"
Xaqueline, Xaqueleena, Xaquelyna, Xaquelayna, Xaqueleana

Xerena (Latin) Form of Serena, meaning "having a peaceful disposition"
Xerenah, Xerene, Xeren, Xereena, Xeryna, Xereene, Xerenna

Xhosa (African) Leader of a nation
Xosa, Xhose, Xhosia, Xhosah, Xosah

Xiang (Chinese) Having a nice fragrance
Xyang, Xeang, Xhiang, Xhyang, Xheang

Xiao Hong (Chinese) Of the morning rainbow

Xin Qian (Chinese) Happy and beautiful woman

Xinavane (African) A mother; to propagate
Xinavana, Xinavania, Xinavain, Xinavaine, Xinavaen, Xinavaene

Xirena (Greek) Form of Sirena, meaning "enchantress"
Xirenah, Xireena, Xirina, Xirene, Xyrena, Xyreena, Xyrina, Xyryna

Xi-Wang (Chinese) One with hope

Xochiquetzal (Aztec) Resembling a flowery feather; in mythology, the goddess of love, flowers, and the earth

Xola (African) Stay in peace
Xolah, Xolia, Xolla, Xollah

Xue (Chinese) Woman of snow

y

Yachne (Hebrew) One who is gracious and hospitable
Yachnee, Yachney, Yachnie, Yachni, Yachnea, Yachneah

Yadra (Spanish) Form of Madre, meaning "mother"
Yadre, Yadrah

Yaffa (Hebrew) A beautiful woman
Yaffah, Yaffit, Yafit, Yafeal

Yakini (African) An honest woman
Yakinie, Yakiney, Yakiny, Yackini, Yackinie, Yackiney, Yackiny, Yakinee

Yalena (Greek) Form of Helen, meaning "the shining light"
Yalenah, Yalina, Yaleena, Yalyna, Yalana, Yaleana, Yalane, Yaleene

Yama (Japanese) From the mountain
Yamma, Yamah, Yammah

Yamin (Hebrew) Right hand
Yamine, Yamyn, Yamyne, Yameen, Yameene, Yamein, Yameine, Yamien

Yana (Hebrew) He answers
Yanna, Yaan, Yanah, Yannah

Yanessa (American) Form of Vanessa, meaning "resembling a butterfly"
Yanessah, Yanesa, Yannesa, Yannessa, Yanassa, Yanasa, Yanessia, Yanysa

Yanka (Slavic) God is good
Yancka, Yancca, Yankka

Yara (Brazilian) In mythology, the goddess of the river; a mermaid
Yarah, Yarrah, Yarra

Yareli (American) The Lord is my light
Yarelie, Yareley, Yarelee, Yarely, Yaresly, Yarelea, Yareleah

Yaser (Arabic) One who is wealthy and prosperous
Yasera, Yaseria

Yashira (Japanese) Blessed with God's grace
Yashirah, Yasheera, Yashyra, Yashara, Yashiera, Yashierah, Yasheira, Yasheirah

Yashona (Hindi) A wealthy woman
Yashonah, Yashawna, Yashauna, Yaseana, Yashawnah, Yashaunah, Yaseanah

Yasmine (Persian) Resembling the jasmine flower
Yasmin, Yasmene, Yasmeen, Yasmeene, Yasmen, Yasemin, Yasemeen, Yasmyn

Yatima (African) An orphan
Yatimah, Yateema, Yatyma, Yateemah, Yatymah, Yatiema, Yatiemah, Yateima

Yedidah (Hebrew) A beloved friend
Yedida, Yedyda, Yedydah, Yedeeda, Yedeedah

Yeira (Hebrew) One who is illuminated
Yeirah, Yaira, Yeyra, Yairah, Yeyrah

Yenge (African) A hardworking woman
Yenga, Yengeh, Yengah

Yeshi (African) For a thousand
Yeshie, Yeshey, Yeshy, Yeshee, Yeshea, Yesheah

Yessica (Hebrew) Form of Jessica, meaning "the Lord sees all"
Yesica, Yessika, Yesika, Yesicka, Yessicka, Yesyka, Yesiko

Yetta (English) Form of Henrietta, meaning "ruler of the house"
Yettah, Yeta, Yette, Yitta, Yettie, Yetty

Yi Min (Chinese) An intelligent woman

Yi Ze (Chinese) Happy and shiny as a pearl

Yihana (African) One deserving congratulations
Yihanah, Yhana, Yihanna, Yihannah, Yhanah, Yhanna, Yhannah

Yinah (Spanish) A victorious woman
Yina, Yinna, Yinnah

Yitta (Hebrew) One who emanates light
Yittah, Yita, Yitah

Ynes (French) Form of Agnes, meaning "pure; chaste"
Ynez, Ynesita

Yogi (Hindi) One who practices yoga
Yogini, Yoginie, Yogie, Yogy, Yogey, Yogee, Yogea, Yogeah

Yohance (African) A gift from God
Yohanse

Yoki (Native American) Of the rain
Yokie, Yokee, Yoky, Yokey, Yokea, Yokeah

Yolanda (Greek) Resembling the violet flower
Yola, Yolana, Yolandah, Colanda

Yomaris (Spanish) I am the sun
Yomariss, Yomarise, Yomarris

Yon (Korean) Resembling a lotus blossom

Yoruba (African) Woman from Nigeria
Yorubah, Yorubba, Yorubbah

Yoshi (Japanese) One who is respectful and good
Yoshie, Yoshy, Yoshey, Yoshee, Yoshiyo, Yoshiko, Yoshino, Yoshea

Ysabel (Spanish) Form of Isabel, meaning "my God is bountiful; God's promise"
Ysabelle, Ysabela, Ysabele, Ysabell, Ysabella, Ysbel, Ysibel, Ysibela

Ysbail (Welsh) A spoiled girl
Ysbale, Ysbayle, Ysbaile, Ysbayl, Ysbael, Ysbaele

Yue (Chinese) Of the moonlight

Yuette (American) A capable woman
Yuett, Yuete, Yuet, Yueta, Yuetta

Yulan (Spanish) A splendid woman
Yulann

Yuna (African) A gorgeous woman
Yunah, Yunna, Yunnah

Yuta (Hebrew / Japanese) One who is awarded praise / one who is superior
Yutah, Yoota, Yootah

Yvonne (French) Young archer
Yvone, Vonne, Vonna

Z

Zabrina (American) Form of Sabrina, meaning "a legendary princess"
Zabreena, Zabrinah, Zabrinna, Zabryna, Zabryne, Zabrynya, Zabreana, Zabreane

Zachah (Hebrew) Feminine form of Zachary; God is remembered
Zacha, Zachie, Zachi, Zachee, Zachea, Zacheah

Zafara (Hebrew) One who sings
Zaphara, Zafarra, Zapharra, Zafarah, Zafarrah, Zapharah, Zapharrah

Zagir (Armenian) Resembling a flower
Zagiri, Zagirie, Zagiree, Zagirea, Zagireah, Zagiry, Zagirey, Zagira

Zahiya (Arabic) A brilliant woman; radiant
Zahiyah, Zehiya, Zehiyah, Zeheeya, Zaheeya, Zeheeyah, Zaheeyah, Zaheiya

Zahra (Arabic / Swahili)
White-skinned / flowerlike
*Zahrah, Zahraa, Zahre,
Zahreh, Zahara, Zaharra,
Zahera, Zahira*

Zainab (Arabic) A fragrant
flowering plant
Zaynab, Zaenab

Zainabu (Swahili) One
who is known for her
beauty
Zaynabu, Zaenabu

Zalina (French) Form of
Selene, meaning "of the
moon"; in mythology
Selene was the Greek god-
dess of the moon
*Zalinah, Zaleana, Zaleena,
Zalena, Zalyna, Zaleen,
Zaleene, Zalene*

Zama (Latin) One from
the town of Zama
Zamah, Zamma, Zammah

Zambda (Hebrew) One
who meditates
Zambdah

Zamella (Zulu) One who
strives to succeed
*Zamellah, Zamy, Zamie,
Zami, Zamey, Zamee,
Zamea, Zameah*

Zamilla (Greek) Having
the strength of the sea
*Zamillah, Zamila,
Zamilah, Zamylla,
Zamyllah, Zamyla,
Zamylah*

Zamora (Spanish) From
the city of Zamora
*Zamorah, Zamorrah,
Zamorra*

Zana (Romanian / Hebrew)
In mythology, the three
graces / shortened form of
Susanna, meaning "lily"
Zanna, Zanah, Zannah

Zane (Scandinavian) One
who is bold
*Zain, Zaine, Zayn, Zayne,
Zaen, Zaene*

Zanta (Swahili) A beautiful young woman
Zantah

Zarahlinda (Hebrew) Of
the beautiful dawn
*Zaralinda, Zaralynda,
Zarahlindah, Zaralyndah,
Zarahlynda, Zarahlyndah,
Zaralenda, Zarahlenda*

Zarifa (Arabic) One who
is successful; moves with
grace
*Zarifah, Zaryfa, Zaryfah,
Zareefa, Zareefah, Zariefa,
Zariefah, Zareifa*

Zarna (Hindi) Resembling
a spring of water
Zarnah, Zarnia, Zarniah

Zarqa (Arabic) Having
bluish-green eyes; from
the city of Zarqa
Zarqaa

Zaylee (English) A heavenly woman
Zayleigh, Zayli, Zaylie, Zaylea, Zayleah, Zayley, Zayly, Zalee

Zaypana (Tibetan) A beautiful woman
Zaypanah, Zaypo, Zaypanna, Zaypannah

Zaza (Hebrew / Arabic) Belonging to all / one who is flowery
Zazah, Zazu, Zazza, Zazzah, Zazzu

Zdenka (Slovene) Feminine form of Zdenek, meaning "from Sidon"
Zdena, Zdenuska, Zdenicka, Zdenika, Zdenyka, Zdeninka, Zdenynka

Zebba (Persian) A known beauty
Zebbah, Zebara, Zebarah, Zebarra, Zebarrah

Zelia (Greek / Spanish) Having great zeal / of the sunshine
Zeliah, Zelya, Zelie, Zele, Zelina, Zelinia

Zenaida (Greek) White-winged dove; in mythology, a daughter of Zeus
Zenaidah, Zenayda, Zenaide, Zenayde, Zinaida, Zenina, Zenna, Zenaydah

Zenechka (Russian) Form of Eugenia, meaning "a well-born woman"

Zenobia (Greek) Child of Zeus
Sinobia

Zephyr (Greek) Of the west wind
Zephyra, Zephira, Zephria, Zephra, Zephyer, Zefiryn, Zefiryna, Zefyrin

Zera (Hebrew) A sower of seeds
Zerah, Zeria, Zeriah, Zera'im, Zerra, Zerrah

Zeraldina (Polish) One who rules with the spear
Zeraldinah, Zeraldeena, Zeraldeenah, Zeraldiena, Zeraldienah, Zeraldeina, Zeraldeinah, Zeraldyna

Zerdali (Turkish) Resembling the wild apricot
Zerdalie, Zerdaly, Zerdaley, Zerdalya, Zerdalia, Zerdalee, Zerdalea, Zerdalea

Zesta (American) One with energy and gusto
Zestah, Zestie, Zestee, Zesti, Zesty, Zestey, Zestea, Zesteah

Zetta (Portuguese) Resembling the rose
Zettah

Zhen (Chinese) One who is precious and chaste
Zen, Zhena, Zenn, Zhenni

Zhi (Chinese) A woman of high moral character

Zhong (Chinese) An honorable woman

Zi (Chinese) A flourishing young woman

Zia (Arabic) One who emanates light; splendor
Ziah, Zea, Zeah, Zya, Zyah

Zilias (Hebrew) A shady woman; a shadow
Zilyas, Zylias, Zylyas

Zillah (Hebrew) The shadowed one
Zilla, Zila, Zyla, Zylla, Zilah, Zylah, Zyllah

Zilpah (Hebrew) One who is frail but dignified; in the Bible, a concubine of Jacob
Zilpa, Zylpa, Zilpha, Zylpha, Zylpah, Zilphah, Zylphah

Zimbab (African) Woman from Zimbabwe
Zymbab, Zimbob, Zymbob

Zinat (Arabic) A decoration; graceful beauty
Zeenat, Zynat, Zienat, Zeinat, Zeanat

Zinchita (Incan) One who is dearly loved
Zinchitah, Zinchyta, Zinchytah, Zincheeta, Zincheetah, Zinchieta, Zinchietah, Zincheita

Zintkala Kinyan (Native American) Resembling a flying bird
Zintkalah Kinyan

Ziona (Hebrew) One who symbolizes goodness
Zionah, Zyona, Zyonah

Zipporah (Hebrew) A beauty; little bird; in the Bible, the wife of Moses
Zippora, Ziporah, Zipora, Zypora, Zyppora, Ziproh, Zipporia

Zira (African) The pathway
Zirah, Zirra, Zirrah, Zyra, Zyrah, Zyrra, Zyrrah

Zisel (Hebrew) One who is sweet
Zissel, Zisal, Zysel, Zysal, Zyssel, Zissal, Zyssal

Zita (Latin / Spanish) Patron of housewives and servants / little rose
Zitah, Zeeta, Zyta, Zeetah

Ziwa (Swahili) Woman of the lake
Ziwah, Zywa, Zywah

Zizi (Hungarian)
Dedicated to God
*Zeezee, Zyzy, Ziezie,
Zeazea, Zeyzey*

Zoa (Greek) One who is
full of life; vibrant

•Zoe (Greek) A life-giving
woman; alive
*Zoee, Zowey, Zowie, Zowe,
Zoelie, Zoeline, Zoelle, Zoey*

Zofia (Slavic) Form of
Sophia, meaning "wis-
dom"
*Zofiah, Zophia, Zophiah,
Zophya, Zofie, Zofee, Zofey*

Zora (Slavic) Born at
dawn; aurora
*Zorah, Zorna, Zorra,
Zorya, Zorane, Zory,
Zorrah, Zorey*

Zoria (Basque) One who
is lucky
Zoriah

Zoriona (Basque) One who
is happy

Zubeda (Swahili) The best
one
Zubedah

Zudora (Arabic) A laborer;
hardworking woman
Zudorah, Zudorra

Zula (African) One who is
brilliant; from the town
of Zula
*Zul, Zulay, Zulae, Zulai,
Zulah, Zulla, Zullah*

Zuni (Native American)
One who is creative
*Zunie, Zuny, Zuney,
Zunee, Zunea, Zuneah*

Zurafa (Arabic) A lovely
woman
*Zurafah, Zirafa, Zirafah,
Ziraf, Zurufa, Zurufah*

Zuri (Swahili / French) A
beauty / lovely and white
*Zurie, Zurey, Zuria,
Zuriaa, Zury, Zuree,
Zurya, Zurisha*

Zuwena (African) One
who is pleasant and good
*Zuwenah, Zwena, Zwenah,
Zuwenna, Zuwennah,
Zuwyna, Zuwynah*

Zuyana (Sioux) One who
has a brave heart
Zuyanah, Zuyanna

Zuzena (Basque) One who
is correct
Zuzenah, Zuzenna

Zwi (Scandinavian)
Resembling a gazelle
Zui, Zwie, Zwee, Zwey